Recent Advances in Computed Tomography

Recent Advances in Computed Tomography

Editor: Robert Meyer

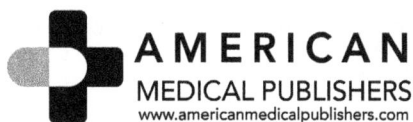

AMERICAN
MEDICAL PUBLISHERS
www.americanmedicalpublishers.com

AMERICAN
MEDICAL PUBLISHERS
www.americanmedicalpublishers.com

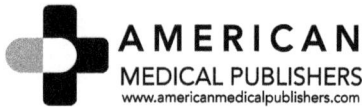

Cataloging-in-Publication Data

Recent advances in computed tomography / edited by Robert Meyer.
   p. cm.
Includes bibliographical references and index.
ISBN 978-1-63927-081-1
1. Tomography. 2. Tomography--Technological innovations. 3. Radiography, Medical.
4. Imaging systems in medicine. 5. Diagnostic imaging. I. Meyer, Robert.
RC78.7.T6 R43 2022
616.075 7--dc23

American Medical Publishers,
41 Flatbush Avenue,
1st Floor, New York,
NY 11217, USA

ISBN 978-1-63927-081-1 (Hardback)

Contents

Preface

An imaging procedure that involves the use of computer-processed combinations of many X-ray measurements is known as computed tomography or X-Ray CT. These X-ray measurements are taken from different angles in order to create cross-sectional images. The measurement focuses on specific areas of the scanned object. This technique is beneficial as it helps users to see inside the object without cutting. The most common application of X-ray computed tomography is medical imaging. Cross section images of this procedure are utilized for diagnostic and therapeutic purposes in various medical disciplines. Apart from X-ray CT, there are some other types of computed tomography such as positron emission tomography and single photon emission computed tomography. CT is also used in various other fields, such as nondestructive materials testing. It also has archaeological uses such as imaging the contents of sarcophagi and ceramics. This book contains some path-breaking studies in the field of computed tomography. It strives to provide a fair idea about this discipline and to help develop a better understanding of the latest advances within this field. The book is appropriate for students seeking detailed information in this area as well as for experts.

The researches compiled throughout the book are authentic and of high quality, combining several disciplines and from very diverse regions from around the world. Drawing on the contributions of many researchers from diverse countries, the book's objective is to provide the readers with the latest achievements in the area of research. This book will surely be a source of knowledge to all interested and researching the field.

In the end, I would like to express my deep sense of gratitude to all the authors for meeting the set deadlines in completing and submitting their research chapters. I would also like to thank the publisher for the support offered to us throughout the course of the book. Finally, I extend my sincere thanks to my family for being a constant source of inspiration and encouragement.

Editor

Computed tomography measurements of different dimensions of maxillary and frontal sinuses

Pernilla Sahlstrand-Johnson[1*†], Magnus Jannert[1†], Anita Strömbeck[2†] and Kasim Abul-Kasim[2†]

Abstract

Background: We have previously proposed the use of Doppler ultrasound to non-invasively stage sinus infection, as we showed that acoustic streaming could be generated in nonpurulent sinus secretions and helped to distinguish it from mucopurulent sinus secretions. In order to continue this development of a clinically applicable Doppler equipment, we need to determine different dimensions of the paranasal sinuses, especially the thickness of the anterior wall of the maxillary sinus (at the canine fossa). To the best of our knowledge, this is the first report on the thickness of the canine fossa. This study aimed to (a) estimate different dimensions of the maxillary and frontal sinuses measured on computed tomography (CT) of the head, (b) define cut-off values for the normal upper and lower limits of the different measured structures, (c) determine differences in age, side and gender, (d) compare manually and automatically estimated maxillary sinuses volumes, and (e) present incidental findings in the paranasal sinuses among the study patients.

Methods: Dimensions of 120 maxillary and frontal sinuses from head CTs were measured independently by two radiologists.

Results: The mean value of the maxillary sinus volume was 15.7 ± 5.3 cm^3 and significantly larger in males than in females (P = 0.004). There was no statistically significant correlation between the volume of maxillary sinuses with age or side. The mean value of the bone thickness at the canine fossa was 1.1 ± 0.4 mm. The automatically estimated volume of the maxillary sinuses was 14-17% higher than the calculated volume. There was high interobserver agreement with regard to the different measurements performed in this study. Different types of incidental findings of the paranasal sinuses were found in 35% of the patients.

Conclusion: We presented different dimensions of the maxillary and frontal sinuses on CTs. We believe that our data are necessary for further development of a clinically applicable Doppler equipment for staging rhinosinusitis.

Background

The paranasal sinuses are complex anatomical structures with a significant inter-individual variation. The use of computed tomography (CT) instead of plain radiography in the work-up of paranasal sinus pathology was recommended in the beginning of the 1990's [1]. Since then CT has become mandatory in the preoperative work-up of sinus surgery. In addition, CT has become an essential aid in navigation during the functional endoscopic sinus surgery (FESS).

The different anatomical dimensions of the paranasal sinuses can also be obtained from CT images. Kawarai's report on volume quantification of the paranasal sinuses on three-dimensional CT scans [2] was followed by different studies as this technique has been continuously developed and improved [3-5]. Although there are published studies on the anatomy of the paranasal sinuses, there are still dimensions of the maxillary sinus and the surrounding structures that need to be investigated.

We have previously demonstrated the potential for a new application of the Doppler ultrasound technique that makes it possible to determine the properties of

---
* Correspondence: pernilla.sahlstrand_johnson@med.lu.se
† Contributed equally
[1]Department of Oto-Rhino-Laryngology, Faculty of Medicine, Lund University, Skåne University Hospital, Malmö, Sweden
Full list of author information is available at the end of the article

paranasal sinus fluids safely and non-invasively [6,7]. Our findings have supported the hypothesis that non-purulent sinus secretions (which have a low viscosity) can be distinguished from mucopurulent sinus secretions (which have a high viscosity) with Doppler ultrasound, since acoustic streaming can be generated and detected in serous sinus fluid but not in mucopurulent sinus secretions [6]. Consequently, this method has the potential to improve the diagnosis of rhinosinusitis and potentially imply a decrease of the prescription of antibiotics. In order to continue the development of this new Doppler application, we needed to estimate the anatomical dimensions of the maxillary and frontal sinuses. The delivery of acoustic intensity into the sinus cavity is highly dependant on the thickness of the anterior bony wall of the sinuses. In addition, we have established that the choice of radius of the ultrasound beam is dependant on the radius of the sinus cavity [7].

Upon performing Doppler ultrasound, the probe is usually placed on the patient's cheek at the level of the nostril at the canine fossa, which is a rounded depression below the infraorbital foramen where levator anguli oris muscle originate. Bovine bone samples with a thickness of 1.08 ± 0.7 mm were used in our experimental studies to mimic the anterior wall of the maxillary sinus [7]. However, the choice of bone thickness in those experiments was based on surgical experience, as we were not able to find any published data on the thickness of the bone in this area in human series. Subsequently, clinically relevant dimensions of the paranasal sinuses and the adjacent soft tissue are still lacking. As the maxillary sinuses are situated just below the orbit, separated only by a thin bony wall, the knowledge of the anatomical dimensions is also of importance when considering safety aspects of the usage of Doppler ultrasound in this area. To the best of our knowledge, this is the first report in literature on the thickness of the bony and the soft tissue structures at the canine fossa. Moreover, there is no comparison in the literature between manually and automatically estimated sinus volumes. As manual estimation of sinus volume is easier to perform and less time consuming, finding a quotient to manually measure the maxillary sinus volume would be advantageous.

The aims of this study were to estimate different dimensions of the maxillary and frontal sinuses measured on head CTs, define a cut-off values for the normal upper and lower limits of the different measured structures, and to find out if age, side or gender of the individuals had any correlation with the different measured structures. Furthermore, we compared manually and automatically estimated sinus volume of the maxillary sinuses, and we aimed to define a quotient that helps a manual estimation of the maxillary sinus

volume. Finally, we present the incidental findings in the paranasal sinuses among the study patients.

Methods

Head CTs of 60 consecutive patients (32 females and 28 males) with mean age of 40 ± 14 years (median 41 and range 18-65 years) were included in this retrospective analysis. The Local Ethics Committee of Lund approved the study protocol. The patient's age was equally distributed with 20 patients in each age group: 18-32, 33-49, and 50-65 years. All patients were examined on a multi-slice CT scanner (SOMATOM Sensation 16, Siemens AG, Forchheim, Germany). The indications for Head CTs were: trauma (n = 16), headache (n = 16), neurological deficit and stroke (n = 13), epilepsy (n = 5), vertigo (n = 5), others (N = 5: visual disturbance, facial pain, tinnitus, anosmia, nausea). Patients with midfacial injuries were excluded. No patients with tumor, mucocele or evidence of previous sinus surgery were found among the patients included in the analyses of this study. Images were obtained with slice collimation of 0.75 mm. Axial and coronal images with slice thickness of 4.5 and 3 mm, respectively using skeletal algorithm and skeletal window (window center 700 and window width 2600) were used for analysis in the Picture Archive and Communication System (PACS, SECTRA). The following measurements were performed independently by two neuroradiologists:

(1) Maxillary sinuses: (a) maximal craniocaudal diameter, (b) maximal depth (anteroposterior diameter), (c) maximal width, (d) the width at the middle of the maxillary sinus on the axial slices, and (e) the thickness of the bony anterior wall (canine fossa). The latter was measured 1.5 cm below margo infraorbitalis (the proposed positions of the canine fossa). Measurement (a) was performed on coronal images whereas the remaining measurements were performed on axial images.

(2) The thickness of soft tissue between the anterior wall of maxillary sinus at the canine fossa and the skin surface was measured on the axial images at the same level as (1e).

(3) Frontal sinuses: (a) maximal depth (anteroposterior diameter), and (b) the thickness of anterior wall were measured on the axial images at the level of the orbital roof.

(4) Thickness of the orbital floor was measured on the coronal images. Figure 1 shows the way of performing the above mentioned measurements.

The given value for every measurement was the mean value of the measurements obtained by the two readers. Furthermore, the volume of the maxillary sinuses was estimated at the Leonardo work station (Siemens AG, Medical Solutions, Erlangen, Germany) using the volume application (figure 1). The estimation of the

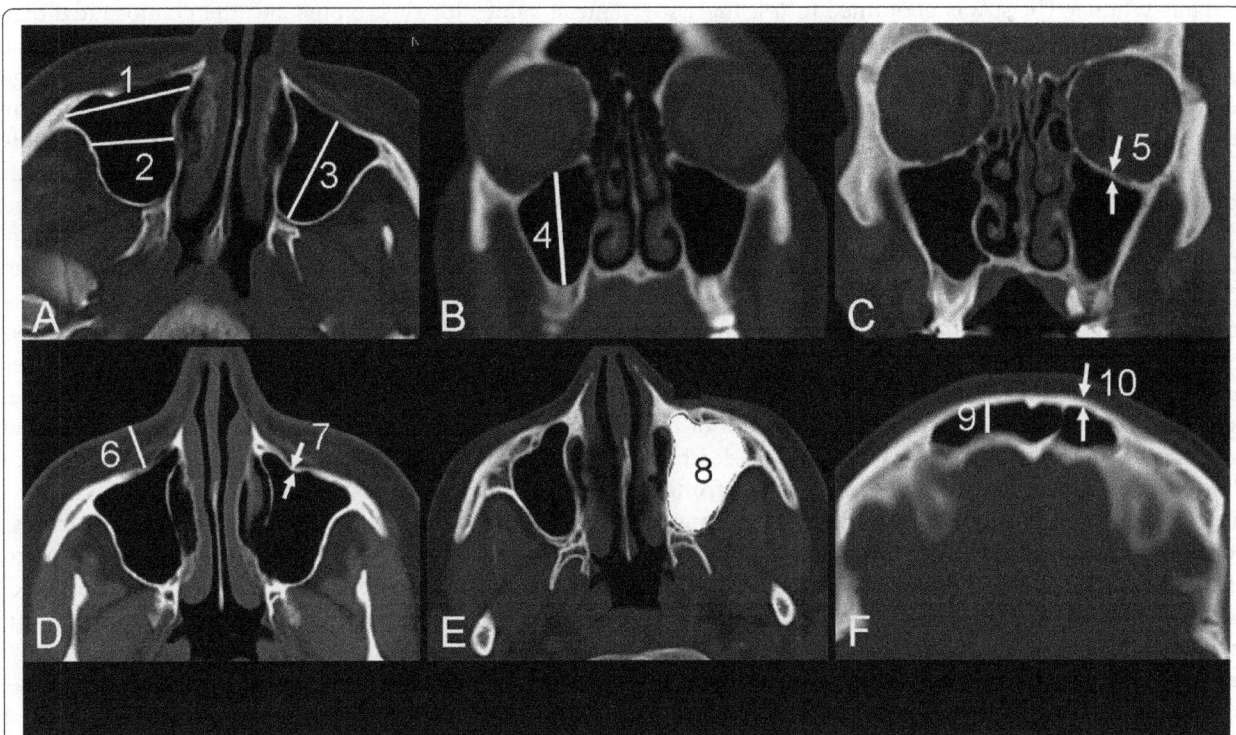

Figure 1 (A, D-F) axial CT images and (B-C) coronal CT image showing the way of the measurement of different dimensions: (1) maximal width of the maxillary sinus, (2) the width at the middle of the maxillary sinus, (3) maximal depth (anteroposterior diameter) of the maxillary sinus, (4) maximal height of the maxillary sinus, (5) thickness of the orbital floor, (6) the thickness of soft tissue between the anterior wall of maxillary sinus at the canine fossa and the skin surface, (7) the thickness of anterior wall of the maxillary sinus (canine fossa), and (8) the automatically measured volume. (9) The depth of the frontal sinus, and (10) the thickness of the anterior wall of the frontal sinus were measured at the level of the orbital roof, 1 cm lateral to the midline. All measurements were made on images with skeletal settings.

attenuation of the gas in the maxillary sinus enabled an automatic estimation of the volume of each maxillary sinus for every individual patient included in the study. Maxillary sinuses with mucous membrane swelling, cysts and/or fluid was subjected to 2-step estimation of their total volume by estimation of the volume of the gas containing portion followed by estimation of the volume of the consolidated portion of the sinus. The latter was estimated after measuring the attenuation of the structures filling the sinus. The range of the attenuation of the gas in the maxillary sinuses was set to -200 to -1200 HU. The mean value for the attenuation of the gas of the maxillary sinuses was -892 ± 226 HU (range -701 to -914 HU).

As all three dimensions of the maxillary sinus were measured, the volume of each maxillary sinus was also calculated using the following equation: (Width × anteroposterior × craniocaudal diameter × 0.5). The width used for this calculation was the mean value for the maximal width and the width at the middle of the maxillary sinus on the axial slices (measurements marked 1 and 2 in figure 1a).

Statistical analysis

Statistical analysis was performed with SPSS 17 (originally; Statistical Package for the Social Sciences). Data is presented as proportions (%) or as mean with 95% confidence interval (95% CI) or with standard deviations (SD). Reliability analysis of the interobserver agreement with regard to the different performed measurements was done by: (1) calculating a two-way mixed model of intraclass correlation coefficient (ICC), and (2) performing a paired sample t-test to calculate the random errors for the differences. The random error was the SD of the interobserver differences of each measurement. The interpretations of the ICC were done according to the one proposed by Landis and Koch [8,9] A kappa of 1 indicates total agreement whereas a kappa of zero means poor agreement and indicates that any observed agreement is attributed to chance. A kappa of 0.81-1.00 indicates almost perfect agreement, 0.61-0.80 indicates substantial agreement, 0.41-0.60 indicates moderate agreement, 0.21-0.40 indicates fair agreement, 0-0.20 indicates slight agreement, and a kappa of <0 indicates poor agreement.

Mann-Whitney U test was performed to test the association between the different measurements of the maxillary and frontal sinuses on one hand and the different categorical variables. Spearman's correlation was used to test the correlation of the same measurements with continuous variables. Differences with a *P* value ≤ 0.05 were considered statistically significant.

Results

The results of the reliability analysis of CT as a method for the measurement of different dimensions of maxillary and frontal sinuses and other nearly related structures are shown in Table 1. The intraobserver agreement was almost perfect in the estimation of the craniocaudal diameter of maxillary sinuses, the depth of the frontal sinuses, and the anterior wall of frontal sinuses, and substantial in the estimation of the anteroposterior diameter of maxillary sinuses and the thickness of the canine fossa. The interobserver agreement in the estimation of the anterior wall of maxillary sinuses and the orbital floor was moderate with interobserver random error for differences in the measurement of these structures varying between 0.3 and 0.5 millimeter (Table 1).

The mean values of the different measured dimensions were not correlated to the patient's age (correlation coefficient 0.126, P = 0.172). The median value for the estimated volumes of the maxillary sinuses in patients of different age groups were 14.4 cm^3 for patients aged 18-33 years, 16.6 cm^3 for patients aged 34-49 years and 15.2 cm^3 for patients aged 50-65 years (P = 0.299). The

mean values for the volume and the craniocaudal diameter of maxillary sinuses as well as the anteroposterior diameter of the frontal sinus of male patients were significantly greater than the corresponding values for female patients (Table 2). The mean value, SD and median value of the volume of the maxillary sinuses of both sides were 15.7, 5.3, and 15.2 cm^3, respectively. The volume of the maxillary sinuses of both sides was significantly greater in male patients than in female patients (median 18 vs. 14.1 cm^3, P = 0.004). There was no statistically significant difference between the estimated volume of the right and the left sided maxillary sinuses (median 15.3 vs. 15.5 cm^3, P = 0.727). The mean value, SD and median value of the bony anterior wall of the maxillary sinus at the canine fossa of both sides were 1.1, 0.4, and 1 mm, respectively. There was no significant difference in anterior wall thickness of the frontal sinuses between the sexes (Table 2). Additionally, there was neither any gender difference in soft tissue thickness between anterior wall of maxillary sinus and the skin surface, nor in thickness of the orbital floor.

The degree of agreement between the automated measurement of the volume of maxillary sinuses and the volume calculated according to the equation width × anteroposterior × craniocaudal diameter × 0.5, was almost perfect (ICC 0.90-0.93 and random error of 1.9-2.4 cm^3). In 52 patients the automatically estimated volume was in average 14-17% greater than the calculated volume in the right sided maxillary sinuses (Figure 2).

In five out of 60 patients (8.3%) the frontal sinuses were not pneumatisized. Seventeen out of 120 maxillary sinuses (14%) subjected for automatic volume measurements, exhibited a volume < 10 cm^3. Maxillary sinuses with volume < 10 cm^3 was found in 11 out of 60 patients (18%) (bilateral in six patients and unilateral in the remaining five). Only one maxillary sinus exhibited a volume < 5 cm^3.

Twenty-one patients (35%) showed different types of incidental findings of paranasal sinuses. These are summarized in Table 3.

Discussion

This study has shown that CT is a robust method in the estimation of different dimensions of the maxillary sinuses, frontal sinuses and the adjacent structures as the interobserver agreement ranges from substantial to almost perfect dependent on the measurement in question (Table 1). Despite the moderate interobserver agreement with regard to the measurements of the canine fossa and the orbital floor (ICC ranging between 0.50 and 0.60), the random error was only 0.3-0.4 mm. This depends partly on the fact that these structures are very thin and partly on the limitation of measurements

Table 1 Reliability analysis showing interobserver agreement in the measurements of different anatomical structures expressed as intraclass correlation coefficient (ICC)

	ICC (95% CI)		Random error, mm	
	Right	Left	Right	Left
Maxillary sinus:				
Craniocaudal diameter	0.88 (0.80-0.92)	0.87 (0.80-0.92)	2.4	2.5
A-P diameter	0.79 (0.68-0.87)	0.79 (0.67-0.87)	2.7	2.8
Anterior wall thickness	0.58 (0.38-0.73)	0.59 (0.39-0.73)	0.4	0.4
Frontal sinus:				
A-P diameter	0.80 (0.68-0.88)	0.86 (0.77-0.91)	2.1	1.8
Anterior wall thickness	0.84 (0.74-0.90)	0.87 (0.79-0.92)	0.5	0.4
Canine fossa:				
AP-diameter	0.73 (0.58-0.83)	0.75 (0.62-0.85)	2.6	2.7
Orbital floor:				
Thickness	0.50 (0.29-0.67)	0.57 (0.37-0.72)	0.3	0.3

The table shows the random error of interobserver differences, expressed in millimeter.

95% CI indicates 95% confidence interval.

A-P diameter indicates anteroposterior diameter (depth).

Table 2 shows female:male distribution of the mean value, SD, median value, range and normal cut-off values of the measurements of different anatomical structures

	study cohort	Female			Male			P-value
	Mean ± SD	Mean ± SD (median)	Range	Normal values	Mean ± SD (median)	Range	Normal values	
Maxillary sinus:								
Volume (right)	15.4 ± 5	14 ± 3 (14)	5-19	8-20	18 ± 6 (18)	9-32	6-30	**0.002**
Volume (left)	16 ± 6	15 ± 4 (15)	7-21	7-23	18 ± 7 (18)	7-34	4-32	**0.016**
Craniocaudal diameter (right)	31.3 ± 5	30 ± 3 (31)	20-35	24-36	34 ± 5 (33)	27-43	24-44	**0.004**
Craniocaudal diameter (left)	31.3 ± 5	30 ± 3 (30)	24-34	24-36	33 ± 5 (34)	21-43	23-43	**0.020**
A-P diameter (right)	35 ± 4	35 ± 3 (35)	27-41	29-41	36 ± 3 (36)	31-46	30-42	0.056
A-P diameter (left)	35.6 ± 4	34 ± 4 (34)	27-40	26-42	35 ± 4 (36)	26-43	27-43	0.058
Width (right)	23.4 ± 4	23 ± 3 (22)	12-28	17-29	25 ± 4 (25)	18-34	17-33	**0.018**
Width (left)	23.7 ± 4	23 ± 3 (24)	16-30	17-29	25 ± 5 (25)	14-33	15-35	0.125
Anterior wall thickness at canine fossa (right)	1.1 ± 0.4	1 ± 0.4 (1)	0.6-2.3	0.2-1.8	1.1 ± 0.3 (1.2)	0.6-2.1	0.5-1.7	0.266
Anterior wall thickness at canine fossa (left)	1.1 ± 0.4	1.1 ± 0.4 (1)	0.6-2.5	0.3-1.9	1 ± 0.3 (1)	0.5-1.8	0.4-1.6	0.504
Frontal sinus:								
A-P diameter (right)	9.6 ± 3	9 ± 4 (9)	4-20	1-17	10 ± 3 (10)	6-16	4-16	**0.034**
A-P diameter (left)	10.2 ± 3.3	9 ± 3 (9)	5-20	3-15	11 ± 3 (11)	6-18	5-17	**0.046**
Anterior wall thickness (right)	2.1 ± 0.8	2 ± 0.6 (1.9)	1.2-3.5	0.8-3.2	2.1 ± 1 (1.9)	0.9-5.2	0.1-4.1	0.824
Anterior wall thickness (left)	2.1 ± 0.8	2.1 ± 0.7 (1.9)	0.8-4.1	0.7-3.5	1.9 ± 0.7 (1.7)	0.9-3.7	0.5-3.5	0.450
Soft tissue thickness between anterior wall of maxillary sinus and the skin surface								
AP-diameter (right)	11.6 ± 3	11 ± 3 (11)	5-15	5-17	12 ± 4 (11)	6-20	4-20	0.300
AP-diameter (left)	12.1 ± 4	11 ± 4 (11)	5-18	3-19	13 ± 4 (12)	5-21	5-21	0.227
Orbital floor								
Thickness (right)	0.9 ± 0.2	0.8 ± 0.2 (0.8)	0.5-1.4	0.4-1.2	0.9 ± 0.3 (0.8)	0.4-1.4	0.3-1.5	0.440
Thickness (left)	0.9 ± 0.2	0.9 ± 0.3 (0.9)	0.5-2	0.3-1.5	0.9 ± 0.3 (0.8)	0.5-1.4	0.3-1.5	0.853

SD indicates standard deviation.
The volume is given in cm^3 whereas other values are given in millimeter.
P-values of statistically significant female:male differences are written in bold style.
Normal values: The lower limit equals mean -2SD whereas the upper limit equals mean +2SD.
A-P diameter indicates anteroposterior diameter (depth).

of tiny structures in PACS. The results in the present study are of importance when setting the adjustments of a clinical applicable Doppler ultrasound equipment for the diagnose of rhinosinusitis.

Previous studies have shown that dimensions of maxillary sinuses from measurements on human skulls were similar to those obtained by CT scans [10] and the consistency of measurements of the paranasal sinuses using CT images have been evaluated in the last decade [2,5,10]. Some authors have measured the volume by directly injecting different materials into the paranasal

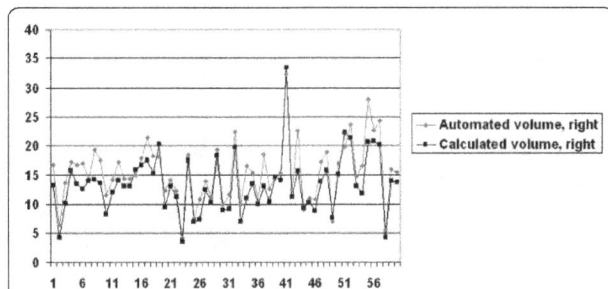

Figure 2 Diagram showing the automated and the calculated volume of the right maxillary sinus. Note that the automated volume exceeded the calculated volume in 52 out of 60 cases. The volume is presented in cm^3 on the y-axis and the patient's number is presented on the x-axis.

Table 3 summarizes the incidental findings of the paranasal sinuses among the study patients

	Right (No.)	Left (No.)	Bilateral (No.)	Total (No.)
Maxillary sinuses:				
-Non-specific MMS	5	2	1	8
-Fluid	2			2
-Retention cysts		1	2	3
Frontal sinuses: MMS			1	1
Sphenoidal sinuses: MMS		1	1	2
Ethmoidal sinuses: MMS		1	4	5
Total				21

MMS indicates mucous membrane swelling.

sinuses [11,12]. However, this procedure cannot be used in living subjects. Furthermore, using such methods in the estimation of the sinus volume usually result in underestimation of the volume in the presence of mucosal thickening and other sinus pathologies [5,11,12]. Our analysis was performed on head CT in patients subjected to trauma, and patients with headache, neurological deficit and stroke, epilepsy, and vertigo. Thus, our material represents individuals with no history of sinus pathology and can in practice be considered as "normal population".

The results of the maxillary sinuses measurements were consistent with previous reports [2,5]. The mean values of the maxillary sinus volume have been reported to range from 11.1 ± 4.5 cm^3 to 23.0 ± 6.7 cm^3 in previous studies [5].

We found that there was a significant difference of the maxillary sinus volume between males and females, mainly due to the fact that male exhibit higher and wider maxillary sinuses than females. Similarly, the anteroposterior diameter of the frontal sinus was larger in men. Some authors have reported difference of the volume of the maxillary sinuses between males and females [2,4,13] whereas others have showed no such difference [5]. Ariji et al have described the correlation between the craniocaudal diameter of the maxillary sinus and body height, body weight and age [10]. As men are generally larger than women, this could explain our observed difference in gender for maxillary sinus volume.

In our work we only included adults (age 18-65 years) and we found neither significant age difference nor significant difference between the left and right maxillary sinus volume. Previous reports suggested that the maxillary sinus volume increase with both age [14] and loss of teeth [15]. On the other hand Ariji found no significant difference between dentate and edentulous patients [10].

To our knowledge this is the first report on the thickness of the canine fossa. The bone thickness was 1.1 mm (mean value for study cohort), which correlates well with our surgical experience or when inspecting dried skulls. The thickness of the soft tissue in front of the bone of the canine fossa varied from 5 to 20 mm. These results are of special importance in our future work with the evaluation of Doppler ultrasound as a diagnostic tool for staging rhinosinusitis, as bone attenuates ultrasound waves considerably, and soft tissue does not. The volume and anteroposterior diameter of the sinuses are also relevant for the development of this new Doppler application, as we previously showed that the radius of the ultrasound transducer should correspond to half the radius of the sinus cavity [7]. This novel application of the Doppler ultrasound technique makes it possible to determine the properties of paranasal sinus fluids safely and non-invasively. It has previously been proved that the Doppler ultrasound technique can be used to identify mucopurulent rhinosinusitis [6]. This method could improve the diagnosis of rhinosinusitis, reduce the suffering of patients with rhinosinusitis and potentially decrease the prescription of antibiotics. This in turn would lead to a decrease in antibiotic resistance and a significant cost reduction for the health care services as a whole.

In our study we measured the anteroposterior diameter and the anterior wall thickness of the frontal sinuses at the level of the orbital roof (Figure 1F). We chose this reference point since one upon performing an ultrasound examination of the frontal sinuses usually hold the ultrasound probe against this area and it is consequently the dimensions of this area that affect the ultrasound wave of the prospective Doppler equipment. The thickness of the bone of the anterior wall of the frontal sinuses is approximately twice as thick as the anterior bony wall of the maxillary sinus in our material, which implies that the attenuation of the ultrasound waves would be much higher when examining the frontal sinuses. Subsequently, it would be hard to induce acoustic streaming in secretions in the frontal sinuses. The anteroposterior diameter of the frontal sinus at this reference point may not be the deepest of the frontal sinuses and consequently our data are difficult to compare to results of other authors.

This study showed a good concordance between the manual and automatically calculated volume of the maxillary sinus with ICC ranging between 0.90 and 0.93. The results from the automatically computed data were 14-17% higher than the manually calculated volumes, which enable a rough estimation of the maxillary sinus volume by measuring the sinus diameter in three planes. Although such estimation is not suitable for research purposes, we believe that this tool might be beneficial in clinical practice for approximate estimation of the maxillary sinus volume, where volume measurement applications are not available.

In our study, there were incidental findings of the paranasal sinuses in 35% of the patients which correlates well to previous reports, where mucosal changes in the paranasal sinuses have been detected in 17-42.5% of CT scans for non-rhinological disease [16-18]. Non-specific mucosal swelling was the commonest finding (27% of the patients) in our material, whereas the incidence of maxillary mucosal cysts was less frequent than previously reported (12.4 to 22%) [19,20].

The measurements of this study were done by two radiologists. One of the drawbacks of this study was that some selection bias might have occurred by the subjective selection of the slice by each reader. However, the reader's choice of the slice should have been almost identical to give such a good agreement in most of the measurements that is shown in Table 1. Other drawbacks are the retrospective nature of the study and inclusion of patients rather than healthy individuals. However, the radiation doses of head CT amounts to 2-2.5 mSv, which make the exposure of healthy individuals to such high radiation doses ethically unacceptable.

Conclusions

This study showed that CT is a reliable method for the measurement of different dimensions of the maxillary and frontal sinus. We presented data on the thickness of canine fossa, which is not previously studied or reported to our knowledge. We believe that these data are necessary for further development of a clinically applicable Doppler equipment for staging a sinus infection. Furthermore, we showed a good correlation between the manually and the automatically estimated maxillary sinuses volumes. Finally, we have described incidental findings in the paranasal sinuses, which is of importance when interpreting CT scans in patients with possible rhinosinusitis.

Acknowledgements
This study was performed with grants from Skane county council's research and development foundation.

Author details
[1]Department of Oto-Rhino-Laryngology, Faculty of Medicine, Lund University, Skåne University Hospital, Malmö, Sweden. [2]Division of Neuroradiology, Diagnostic Centre for Imaging and Functional Medicine, Faculty of Medicine, Lund University, Skåne University Hospital, Malmö, Sweden.

Authors' contributions
PSJ has contributed to conception and design of the study, analysis and interpretation of data, drafting the manuscript and has given her final approval of the version to be published. MJT has contributed to the revision of the manuscript critically for important intellectual content, and has given his final approval of the version to be published. ASK has contributed to analysis and interpretation of data, drafting the manuscript and has given her final approval of the version to be published. KAK has contributed to conception and design of the study, acquisition of data, analysis and interpretation of data, drafting the manuscript and has given his final approval of the version to be published. All four authors have read and approved the final manuscript.

Competing interests
The authors declare that they have no competing interests.

References
1. White PS, Robinson JM, Stewart IA, Doyle T: Computerized tomography mini-series: an alternative to standard paranasal sinus radiographs. *Aust N Z J Surg* 1990, **60(1)**:25-29.
2. Kawarai Y, Fukushima K, Ogawa T, Nishizaki K, Gunduz M, Fujimoto M, Masuda Y: Volume quantification of healthy paranasal cavity by three-dimensional CT imaging. *Acta Otolaryngol Suppl* 1999, **540**:45-49.
3. Sanchez Fernandez JM, Anta Escuredo JA, Sanchez Del Rey A, Santaolalla Montoya F: Morphometric study of the paranasal sinuses in normal and pathological conditions. *Acta Otolaryngol* 2000, **120(2)**:273-278.
4. Emirzeoglu M, Sahin B, Bilgic S, Celebi M, Uzun A: Volumetric evaluation of the paranasal sinuses in normal subjects using computer tomography images: a stereological study. *Auris Nasus Larynx* 2007, **34(2)**:191-195.
5. Pirner S, Tingelhoff K, Wagner I, Westphal R, Rilk M, Wahl FM, Bootz F, Eichhorn KW: CT-based manual segmentation and evaluation of paranasal sinuses. *Eur Arch Otorhinolaryngol* 2009, **266(4)**:507-518.
6. Sahlstrand-Johnson P, Jonsson P, Persson HW, Holmer NG, Jannert M, Jansson T: In vitro studies and safety assessment of Doppler ultrasound as a diagnostic tool in rhinosinusitis. *Ultrasound Med Biol* 2010, **36(12)**:2123-2131.
7. Jonsson P, Sahlstrand-Johnson P, Holmer NG, Persson HW, Jannert M, Jansson T: Feasibility of measuring acoustic streaming for improved diagnosis of rhinosinusitis. *Ultrasound Med Biol* 2008, **34(2)**:228-238.
8. Landis JR, Koch GG: The measurement of observer agreement for categorical data. *Biometrics* 1977, **33(1)**:159-174.
9. Reliability analysis. [http://www2.chass.ncsu.edu/garson/pa765/reliab.htm].
10. Ariji Y, Ariji E, Yoshiura K, Kanda S: Computed tomographic indices for maxillary sinus size in comparison with the sinus volume. *Dentomaxillofac Radiol* 1996, **25(1)**:19-24.
11. Schumacher GH, Heyne HJ, Fanghanel R: Anatomy of the human paranasal sinuses. 2. Volumetric measurement. *Anat Anz* 1972, **130(1)**:143-157.
12. Uchida Y, Goto M, Katsuki T, Akiyoshi T: A cadaveric study of maxillary sinus size as an aid in bone grafting of the maxillary sinus floor. *J Oral Maxillofac Surg* 1998, **56(10)**:1158-1163.
13. Barghouth G, Prior JO, Lepori D, Duvoisin B, Schnyder P, Gudinchet F: Paranasal sinuses in children: size evaluation of maxillary, sphenoid, and frontal sinuses by magnetic resonance imaging and proposal of volume index percentile curves. *Eur Radiol* 2002, **12(6)**:1451-1458.
14. Ariji Y, Kuroki T, Moriguchi S, Ariji E, Kanda S: Age changes in the volume of the human maxillary sinus: a study using computed tomography. *Dentomaxillofac Radiol* 1994, **23(3)**:163-168.
15. Uemura J: Morphological studies on the maxilla of the endentulous skulls and the skulls with teeth. 1. On the sinus of the maxilla (author's transl). *Shikwa Gakuho* 1974, **74(12)**:1860-1889.
16. Havas TE, Motbey JA, Gullane PJ: Prevalence of incidental abnormalities on computed tomographic scans of the paranasal sinuses. *Arch Otolaryngol Head Neck Surg* 1988, **114(8)**:856-859.
17. Bolger WE, Butzin CA, Parsons DS: Paranasal sinus bony anatomic variations and mucosal abnormalities: CT analysis for endoscopic sinus surgery. *Laryngoscope* 1991, **101(1 Pt 1)**:56-64.
18. Jones NS, Strobl A, Holland I: A study of the CT findings in 100 patients with rhinosinusitis and 100 controls. *Clinical Otolaryngology* 1997, **22(1)**:47-51.
19. Bhattacharyya N: Do maxillary sinus retention cysts reflect obstructive sinus phenomena? *Arch Otolaryngol Head Neck Surg* 2000, **126(11)**:1369-1371.
20. Harar RP, Chadha NK, Rogers G: Are maxillary mucosal cysts a manifestation of inflammatory sinus disease? *J Laryngol Otol* 2007, **121(8)**:751-754.

2

Low tube voltage CT for improved detection of pancreatic cancer: detection threshold for small, simulated lesions

Jon Holm[1,2*†], Louiza Loizou[2,3†], Nils Albiin[2,3], Nikolaos Kartalis[2,3], Bertil Leidner[2,3] and Anders Sundin[4,5]

Abstract

Background: Pancreatic ductal adenocarcinoma is associated with dismal prognosis. The detection of small pancreatic tumors which are still resectable is still a challenging problem.
The aim of this study was to investigate the effect of decreasing the tube voltage from 120 to 80 kV on the detection of pancreatic tumors.

Methods: Three scanning protocols was used; one using the standard tube voltage (120 kV) and current (160 mA) and two using 80 kV but with different tube currents (500 and 675 mA) to achieve equivalent dose (15 mGy) and noise (15 HU) as that of the standard protocol.
Tumors were simulated into collected CT phantom images. The attenuation in normal parenchyma at 120 kV was set at 130 HU, as measured previously in clinical examinations, and the tumor attenuation was assumed to differ 20 HU and was set at 110HU. By scanning and measuring of iodine solution with different concentrations the corresponding tumor and parenchyma attenuation at 80 kV was found to be 185 and 219 HU, respectively.
To objectively evaluate the differences between the three protocols, a multi-reader multi-case receiver operating characteristic study was conducted, using three readers and 100 cases, each containing 0–3 lesions.

Results: The highest reader averaged figure-of-merit (FOM) was achieved for 80 kV and 675 mA (FOM = 0,850), and the lowest for 120 kV (FOM = 0,709). There was a significant difference between the three protocols ($p < 0,0001$), when making an analysis of variance (ANOVA). Post-hoc analysis (students t-test) shows that there was a significant difference between 120 and 80 kV, but not between the two levels of tube currents at 80 kV.

Conclusion: We conclude that when decreasing the tube voltage there is a significant improvement in tumor conspicuity.

Keywords: Pancreatic adenocarcinoma, CT, Low tube voltage, Phantom

Background

Pancreatic ductal adenocarcinoma (PDAC) is associated with a dismal prognosis. The overall 5 year survival rate is less than 5% and even after potentially curative surgery this increases to only 20% [1]. Tumor size is an important prognostic factor and increasing size correlates with a higher rate of unresectable tumors and decreased survival [2]. For this reason it is important to detect pancreatic tumors while they are small and still resectable. Technological advances in multi-detector computed tomography (MDCT) combined with its wide availability have made it the modality of choice for diagnosing and staging pancreatic malignancies [3]. MDCT is highly sensitive in detecting large tumors: 100% sensitivity for tumors > 2 cm [4,5] but for small tumors, <2 cm, sensitivity is lower (60-77%) [4,5]. Recent studies have shown that MDCT and Magnetic Resonance Imaging (MRI) have comparable diagnostic accuracy [6,7] with MRI probably offering an advantage for liver metastases [7]. Our clinical impression, using a 64-channel MDCT and

* Correspondence: jon.holm@gmail.com
†Equal contributors
[1]Division of Medical Physics, Karolinska University Hospital, Huddinge, Stockholm 14186, Sweden
[2]Department of Clinical Science, Intervention and Technology (CLINTEC), Karolinska Institutet, 17177 Stockholm, Sweden
Full list of author information is available at the end of the article

a triple-phased protocol, is that the sensitivity to detect 1–2 cm tumors is higher than is stated in the literature but for very small tumors, <1 cm, the detection rate is very low and needs to be improved.

Imaging pancreatic cancer with MDCT needs contrast enhancement in at least two phases, the pancreatic parenchymal phase (PPP) and the portal venous phase (PVP). In the obligate PPP the normal pancreatic parenchyma enhances avidly whereas the vast majority of pancreatic adenocarcinomas (PDAC) are hypointense, due to the high fibrous tissue content of the tumor [8]. The key to the PDAC diagnosis is to achieve as high an attenuation difference as possible between the normal pancreatic parenchyma and the tumor [9]. Reducing the tube voltage can increase this contrast between tumor and normal parenchyma [10]. The main disadvantage of low tube voltage CT is the increased image noise, which until recently has been difficult to overcome because of limitations in the output of the x-ray tubes. The increased contrast is achieved by an increased photoelectric effect and a decreased Compton scattering, resulting in a higher attenuation of iodinated contrast media [10]. This principle has been used to reduce the radiation dose for CT of the thorax [11,12] and heart [13,14], in patients with low body mass index (BMI) and in children. In recent years, the technique has also been used to improve CT angiography of the pulmonary arteries [15-17] and to facilitate detection of hypervascular liver lesions [18]. In a recent dual-energy MDCT study, the low tube voltage technique improved the enhancement of the pancreas and peripancreatic vasculature in order to improve tumor conspicuity [19].

In this phantom study, the purpose was to investigate whether a decrease of the tube voltage from 120 kVp to 80 kVp could improve the detection of small, low attenuating, solid pancreatic tumors. We decided to assess this in an experimental model whereby small hypoattenuating simulated tumor lesions were mathematically created in a phantom.

Methods
Image acquisition
A phantom (Catphan® 600, The Phantom Laboratory, Salem, USA) was scanned with a 64-channel MDCT scanner (LightSpeed VCT, GE Healthcare, Milwaukee, USA), using three protocols A, B and C (Table 1). The phantom consisted of five separate modules with different properties. The CTP486 image uniformity module of the Catphan phantom was scanned to acquire uniform images. A body annulus, CTP579, was mounted onto the phantom to better simulate the size of the human trunk (Figure 1).

Protocol A utilizes a tube voltage of 120 kVp, which is the tube voltage in clinical use for pancreatic MDCT in our department. In the low voltage protocols B and C, the tube voltage was decreased to 80 kVp. The tube current in protocol B was increased from 160 mA to 500 mA to achieve the same mean radiation dose as in protocol A (15 mGy volume computed tomography dose index (CTDIvol)). In protocol C, the tube current was increased to 675 mA, resulting in a higher radiation dose of 20 mGy CTDIvol, to attain image noise comparable to that in protocol A (15 HU).

For all three protocols, the X-ray tube rotation time (0.6 seconds), detector configuration (64 x 0.625) and helical pitch factor (0.516) were kept constant. The acquired images were reconstructed using the soft reconstruction algorithm, a display field-of-view (DFOV) of 25 cm, a slice thickness of 3 mm and with an interval of 1.5 mm.

Creation of cases and lesions
One hundred cases were created and used for each protocol. Twenty-one images were acquired for each case with the method described above. In 57 of the 100 cases we inserted 1 to 3 simulated lesions in random positions.

Table 1 Scanning parameters

Protocol	Tube voltage [kVp]	Tube Current [mA]	CTDIvol [mGy]	Noise [HU]
A. 120 kVp	120	160	15	15
B. 80 kVp	80	500	15	17
C. 80 kVp	80	675	20	15

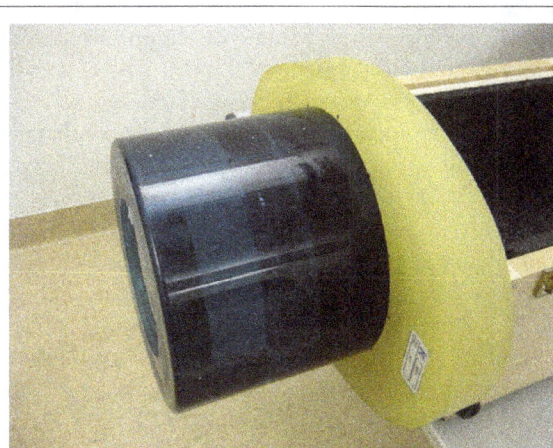

Figure 1 Image of the phantom. Image of the Catphan 600 phantom with the body anulus (CTP579) mounted on top of the image uniformity module (CTP486).

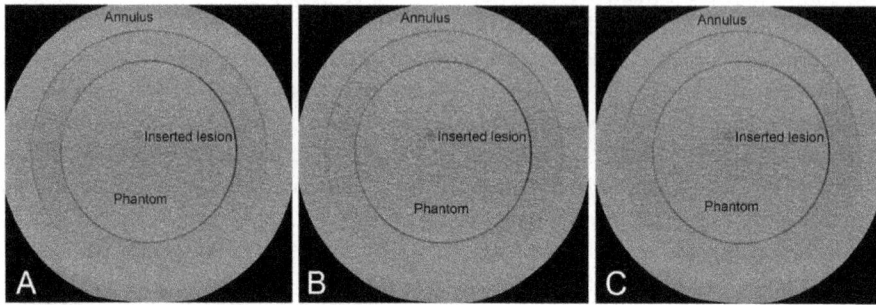

Figure 2 (A-C) Image of the phantom scanned with protocol A, B and C. The image includes an inserted lesion with 10 mm diameter and a contrast resulting from 120 kVp scanning (**A**), 80 kVp and 500 mA (**B**) and 80 kVp and 675 mA (**C**). The lesion has a random position inside the inner circle.

The lesions were created assuming a spherical shape. They were calculated by pixel-wise integration of a hemisphere, which is mathematically expressed by:

$$\iint f(x,y)dxdy = \iint \sqrt{r^2 - x^2 - y^2}dxdy \qquad (1)$$

where r is the radius of the lesion and x and y are the Cartesian coordinates in the axial plane of the CT scanner. The integration limits in the xy plane were derived from DFOV information and the size of the image matrix (512 x 512), and are in increments of 0.5 mm in both x and y directions. The integration in z direction is given from the slice thickness and its different positions. Due to the symmetry, integrations were only carried out in one of the quadrants of the hemisphere. The integrations were performed numerically using Mathematica software (Wolfram Research, Champaign, USA). Lesions with a diameter of 2, 3, 4, 5, 6, 8 and 10 mm were created (Figure 2). Because of the 3 mm slice thickness, many of the pixels in the smaller lesions did not only represent the attenuation of the lesion itself, but also the attenuation of the background phantom material, causing partial volume effect problems. Since the lesions had an attenuation close to that of the surrounding phantom material, the CT number for these pixels was computed by assuming a linear combination of the µ values according to their volumetric proportions [20].

Determination of parenchymal and lesion attenuation

After determining the proportion of lesion and surrounding phantom material in the voxels as described in the previous section, the actual attenuation of the lesion and parenchyma was measured and calculated for both tube voltages. Previous measurements from 15 clinical CT examinations of the pancreas with our standard protocol (120 kVp and 0.75 g I/kg body weight) yielded an attenuation of the normal pancreatic parenchyma of approximately 130 HU in the PPP. These measurements

had been performed in examinations reconstructed in 0.625 mm slices, to avoid the effect of partial volume averaging, and by using circular regions of interest (ROIs). The lesions that are usually missed have an attenuation very similar to that of the normal pancreas. Therefore we assumed that the simulated lesions' attenuation differs from the background by only 20 HU at 120 kVp.

Iodine contrast medium (Iomeron 400 mg I/ml) was diluted with water in six different concentrations (1.1, 2.2, 3.2, 4.3, 5.4 and 6.5 mg I/ml) in standard 10 ml plastic vials. These were inserted into the center position of a homogenous phantom (RMI Model 461A, Gammex/RMI, Middleton, USA), which was scanned at 120 kVp and 80 kVp. The attenuation values were plotted against the iodine concentration and correlated linearly (Figure 3). By using this information about attenuation at both tube voltages, all pixel values were calculated based on the assumptions detailed in the previous section.

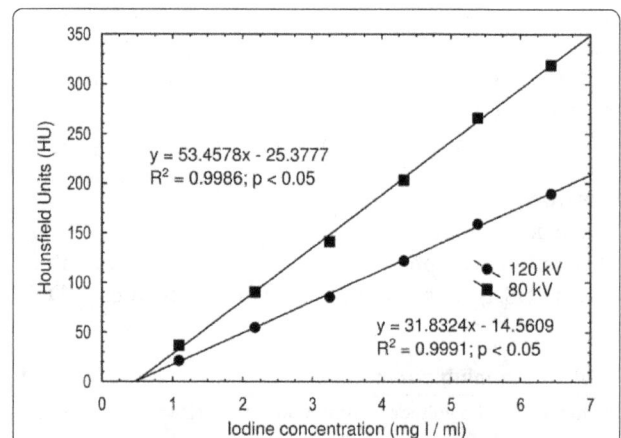

Figure 3 The mean attenuation. The mean attenuation (Hounsfield units) for the six test tubes containing different iodine concentrations, positioned in the center position of an RMI phantom and scanned at 120 kV and 80 kV.

Insertion of simulated lesions

The simulated lesions were inserted into the CT images by subtracting the lesion pixel matrix from the uniform phantom image matrix. The phantom background was also adjusted by matrix addition to achieve the same attenuation as the parenchyma. All matrix operations were carried out using Matlab (The Mathworks, Natick, USA). The lesions were randomly positioned in both xy and z planes using the random number generator in Matlab.

Radiation dose and image noise

The $CTDI_{100}$ were measured by using a pencil ionization chamber (DCT10, Wellhöfer, Germany). The measurements were performed with the chamber inside the central ($CTDI_{100,c}$) and the four peripheral holes ($CTDI_{100,p}$) of a 32 cm standard polymethylmethacrylate (PMMA) body phantom. Scans were made for both tube voltages at four different tube currents (Figure 4). Calculations for $CTDI_{vol}$ were performed by using the two well-known equations [21]:

$$CTDI_w = \frac{1}{3}CTDI_{100,c} + \frac{2}{3}CTDI_{100,p} \qquad (2)$$

$$CTDI_{vol} = \frac{CTDI_w}{pitch} \qquad (3)$$

Image noise was measured in the phantom's image uniformity module. The phantom was scanned with both tube voltages at different tube currents (Figure 5). For each scan, a circular region of interest (ROI) was used with its size adjusted to cover the whole inner part of the phantom. The standard deviation of the pixels inside each ROI was registered as the amount of the image noise.

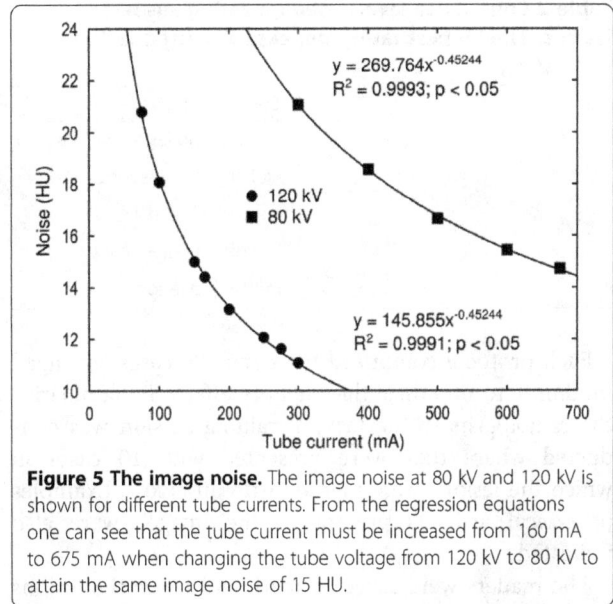

Figure 4 The radiation dose. The radiation dose measured as the CTDIvol at 80 kV and 120 kV is shown for different tube currents. From the regression equations one can see that the tube current must be increased from 160 mA to 500 mA when changing the tube voltage from 120 kV to 80 kV to attain the same CTDIvol of 15 mGy.

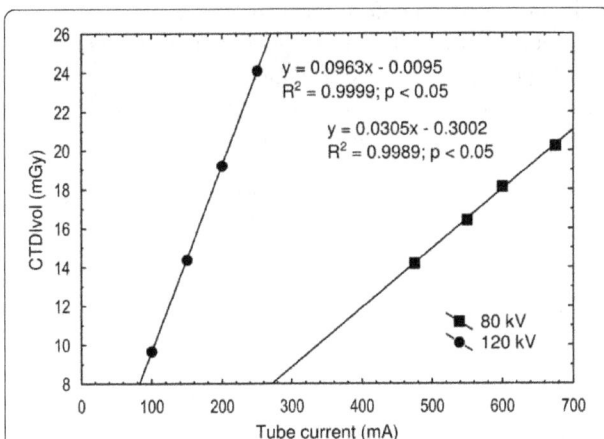

Figure 5 The image noise. The image noise at 80 kV and 120 kV is shown for different tube currents. From the regression equations one can see that the tube current must be increased from 160 mA to 675 mA when changing the tube voltage from 120 kV to 80 kV to attain the same image noise of 15 HU.

Both the radiation dose and the image noise were plotted against the tube current and correlated using appropriate functions (Figures 4 and 5). Regression equations were used to calculate the tube currents for protocols B and C.

Viewer performance

A standard Picture Archiving and Communicating System (PACS) workstation (Sectra, Linköping, Sweden) was used, with either a one mega pixel color monitor (RadiForce R12, EIZO Nanao Corporation, Ishikawa, Japan) or a three mega pixel grey scale monitor (RadiForce G31, EIZO Nanao Corporation, Ishikawa, Japan). The monitors were calibrated according to DICOM part 14 using a dedicated quality control tool (RadiCS, EIZO Nanao Corporation, Ishikawa, Japan). The images were scaled to fit the monitor, and the radiologists were not allowed to use the zoom tool. The window center was set at the attenuation of the pancreatic parenchyma, which was 130 HU for the 120 kVp images and 217 HU for the 80 kVp examinations. The window width was set to 400 HU for all protocols. Viewing time was unrestricted.

Three radiologists with 24, 21 and 7 years of experience in CT imaging participated in the study. For each scanning protocol, the radiologists were instructed to independently read the 100 cases. They were blinded to CT scanning parameters and to lesion characteristics. They were instructed to indicate suspicious lesions with an arrow marker and rate their level of confidence in the detection of each lesion according to an arbitrary scale ranging from 1 to 4, where 4 indicates the highest confidence and 1 the lowest (Table 2).

Table 2 Confidence levels used for rating suspected lesions. The highest rating per case was used as the ROC rating

Rating	Confidence level
0	Definitely no lesion (no marking)
1	Probably not a lesion
2	Possibly a lesion
3	Probably a lesion
4	Definitely a lesion

Each protocol comprised the same 100 cases, arranged randomly to minimize the memory effect. To familiarize the radiologists to the task, a training session was conducted where they were presented with 10 cases in which the lesions were marked with an arrow. Examples of typical artifacts present in the images were also indicated.

The readers were asked to mark and grade the lesions in two different reading sessions. In the first viewing session they were not allowed to adjust the window setting. In the second viewing session all readers were asked to reinterpret all images, the order of which had been rearranged to minimize the memory effect, but now the readers were instructed that they were free to adjust the window setting according to their own preferences.

Statistical analysis

The study was analyzed using the receiver operating characteristic method (ROC). The highest rated mark per case was used for the ROC evaluation and the rest of the information was used for descriptive statistics. The collected ROC data were statistically analyzed using DBM-MRMC software version 2.2 [22]. The software first calculated a figure-of-merit (FOM) for each reader and protocol. This was performed by summing the number of ratings for each level of confidence for every actually negative and actually positive case. The false positive fraction (FPF) and the true positive fraction (TPF) were calculated for all possible cut points. A cut point was defined as the point where, as above, the readers' interpretation is considered as a true positive for an actual positive (tumor case) or a false positive for an actual negative (non-tumor case) [23]. The TPF was then plotted against the FPF and the points were correlated (trapezoidally) and extrapolated to the point of (1,1). The area under the curve (AUC) was the FOM and could be interpreted as the probability that a randomly chosen, actually positive case was rated higher than a randomly chosen, actually negative case [24].

The software performed an analysis of variance (ANOVA) on the FOMs to test any difference between the various scanning protocols, as well as a following post-hoc analysis (t-test) to determine exactly where the differences were. Because we had 100 cases but only 3 readers, the analysis was performed by treating the cases as random samples and the readers as fixed samples.

Because the ROC methodology cannot handle information about the number of lesions per case and their localization, the lesion localization fraction (LLF) was calculated. A lesion localization (LL) was defined as a mark that was located not more than 1 cm from a lesion, and the LLF is the LL divided by the total number of lesions. The corresponding non-lesion localization fraction (NLF) was also calculated. A non-lesion localization (NL) was defined as a mark that was located more than 1 cm from a lesion, and the NLF is the NL divided by the total number of cases.

Results

Determination of parenchymal and lesion attenuation

The attenuation values for the lesions and the parenchyma at 120 kVp had previously been determined in clinical examinations as 110 HU and 130 HU respectively, and were therefore used for the simulated lesions and parenchyma at 120 kVp. The corresponding attenuation values for the simulated lesions and the simulated normal parenchyma scanned at 80 kVp were 183 HU and 217 HU respectively. Thus, the attenuation

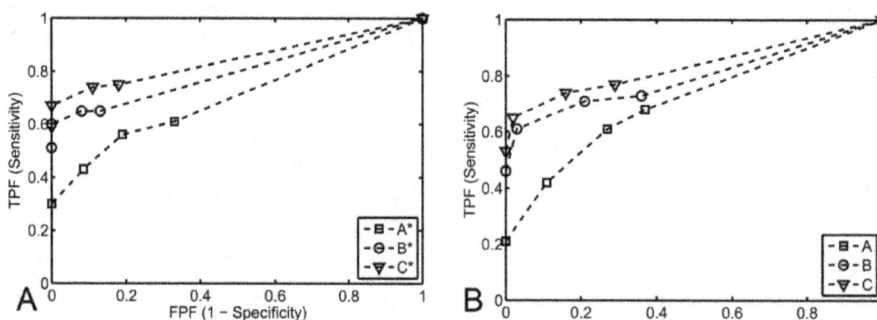

Figure 6 (A-B) ROC curves with fixed and free-choice window setting. ROC curves for each scanning protocol interpreted with the fixed window setting (**A**) and free-choice setting (**B**). The FPF is plotted against the TPF for all possible cut points and correlated trapezoidally.

difference increased from 20 HU to 34 HU at 80 kVp as compared to 120 kVp.

Radiation dose and image noise

When the tube voltage was decreased from 120 kVp to 80 kVp, the tube current had to be increased to 500 mA to achieve an equivalent absorbed radiation dose and adjusted up to 675 mA to achieve similar image noise. The CTDIvol for protocols A and B were 15 mGy and for protocol C 20 mGy.

Viewer performance

The FOMs for each reader and scanning protocol, determined from the areas under the ROC curves (Figure 6), are presented in Table 3. The highest reader-averaged FOM was acquired for protocol C using a free-choice window setting. The lowest reader-averaged FOM was acquired for protocol A, using a free-choice window setting. The reader-averaged FOM for each protocol, with range in paranthesis as a measure of the interobserver variablility, were as follows: A: 0.713 (0.679-0.741), B: 0.803 (0.785-0.829), C: 0.837 (0.834-0.840), A*: 0.709 (0.706-0.716), B*: 0.807 (0.771-0.842) and C*:0.850 (0.833-0.876). The reader-averaged FOMs differed significantly ($p < 0.0001$), which in this analysis means that at least two, but not necessarily all, protocols differ. Post-hoc analysis showed better lesion detection when the tube voltage was decreased from 120 to 80 kVp but not when the tube current was increased from 500 to 675 mA at 80 kVp (Table 4). Similar results were achieved by using the predefined fixed window setting and a free-choice window setting. The TPF and FPF for all possible cut points and protocols are presented in table 5.

When the LLF and NLF were analyzed for each lesion size (Figures 7 and 8), smaller lesions were detected with 80 kVp than with 120 kVp. A major portion of the 5 mm lesions were detected at 80 kVp while only a small fraction of these were detected at 120 kVp. Also, a major proportion of the 4 mm lesions were detected at 80 kVp and 675 mA but not at 500 mA. The detection of lesions

Table 4 Inter-protocol comparisons with the highest differences between the FOMs and the lowest p-values at the top

Protocol comparison	Δ FOM	P-value
C* - A*	0.1419	<0.0001
C* - A	0.1372	<0.0001
C - A*	0.1283	<0.0001
C - A	0.1237	<0.0001
B* - A*	0.0979	0.0003
B - A*	0.0943	0.0005
B* - A	0.0933	0.0006
B - A	0.0897	0.0010
C* - B	0.0475	0.0797
C* - B*	0.0439	0.1053
C - B	0.0340	0.2097
C - B*	0.0304	0.2621
C* - C	0.0135	0.6174
A - A*	0.0046	0.8644
B* - B	0.0036	0.8941

measuring between 2 and 3 mm was poor in all protocols.

Discussion

The Catphan phantom was utilized in this study to represent the normal pancreatic parenchyma and was scanned by using various acquisition protocols, essentially varying the tube voltage between 120 kVp and 80 kVp. Computer-simulated, low attenuating lesions of various diameters, representing hypovascularised solid pancreatic tumors, were inserted into the ensuing phantom images. The rationale for using a low kilovoltage protocol was to achieve a higher attenuation difference between the tumor and the pancreatic parenchyma, in order to improve tumor conspicuity and delineation. Generally, lesions with attenuation nearly identical to that of the normal pancreatic parenchyma are difficult to visualize. By inserting 110 HU computer-simulated lesions, 20 HU less than that of

Table 3 FOMs for each reader and scanning protocol together with a reader-averaged FOM. * Indicates a free-choice window setting

Reader	Protocol					
	Fixed window setting			Free-choice window setting		
	A. 120 kVp	B. 80 kVp	C. 80 kVp	A*. 120 kVp	B*. 80 kVp	C*. 80 kVp
1	0.720	0.785	0.840	0.706	0.771	0.833
2	0.741	0.795	0.836	0.704	0.807	0.842
3	0.679	0.829	0.834	0.716	0.842	0.876
Average	0.713	0.803	0.837	0.709	0.807	0.850

Table 5 TPF (sensitivity) and The FPF (1 – specificity) for all possible cut points and protocols

Cut point	A. 120 kVp		B. 80 kVp		C. 80 kVp	
	TPF (1-FNF)	FPF (1-TNF)	TPF (1-FNF)	FPF (1-TNF)	TPF (1-FNF)	FPF (1-TNF)
0-1	0.678	0.372	0.731	0.357	0.766	0.287
1-2	0.608	0.271	0.708	0.209	0.743	0.163
2-3	0.421	0.109	0.614	0.031	0.655	0.016
3-4	0.211	0.000	0.462	0.000	0.532	0.000

Cut point	A*. 120 kVp		B*. 80 kVp		C*. 80 kVp	
	TPF (1-FNF)	FPF (1-TNF)	TPF (1-FNF)	FPF (1-TNF)	TPF (1-FNF)	FPF (1-TNF)
0-1	0.608	0.326	0.655	0.132	0.749	0.178
1-2	0.561	0.194	0.655	0.078	0.737	0.109
2-3	0.433	0.085	0.596	0.000	0.673	0.000
3-4	0.298	0.000	0.509	0.000	0.591	0.000

the pancreatic phantom, we were able to mimic this clinical situation. When the tube voltage was decreased from 120 to 80 kVp, the mean photon energy decreased in parallel from 56.8 to 43.7 keV [18]. This lower value was closer to the K edge of iodine (33.2 keV) resulting in higher X-ray absorption and a significantly higher attenuation (67%) of the background (i.e. normal pancreatic tissue). Consequently, the attenuation difference between the digital lesions and the pancreatic background increases by 70% (from 20 HU to 34 HU).

The post-hoc analysis revealed significantly better lesion detection at 80 kVp than at 120 kVp, which means that smaller lesions and more of them are detected at 80 kVp. The main consideration for applying a lower tube voltage was the increase of image noise. In protocol C, we established the same image noise as in protocol A by using the maximum tube current possible with our 64-channel MDCT (675 mA). However, for lesions measuring ≥5 mm, the LLF at 80 kVp was not improved when the tube current was increased to 675 mA in order to establish the same image noise as in the 120 kVp protocol. In contrast, an increase of the

tube current in the 80 kVp protocol (C) to achieve similar noise as in the 120 kVp protocol (A) improved the LLF for lesions with a diameter ≤4 mm.

The receiver operating characteristic (ROC) method has long been one of the standard methods in radiology to analyze and compare diagnostic accuracy [25].

The ROC method is very powerful because it estimates and reports all combinations of sensitivity and specificity that a diagnostic test is able to provide [26] and it is therefore used in this study. In the ROC paradigm, the observer is given a number of cases in some of which some kind of abnormality is present. The observer is asked to rate every case depending on how confident he or she is about whether there is an abnormality somewhere in that case.

The resulting 2 x 2 truth-response table defines correct decisions (true positives (TP) and true negatives (TN)) and incorrect decisions (false positives (FP) and false negatives (FN)) in comparison to a gold standard.

Pancreatic cancer incidence peaks between 60 and 80 years of age [27]. The risk of developing a radiation-induced cancer is markedly age-dependent. Given an estimated less than 5% 5-year survival rate, the risk to

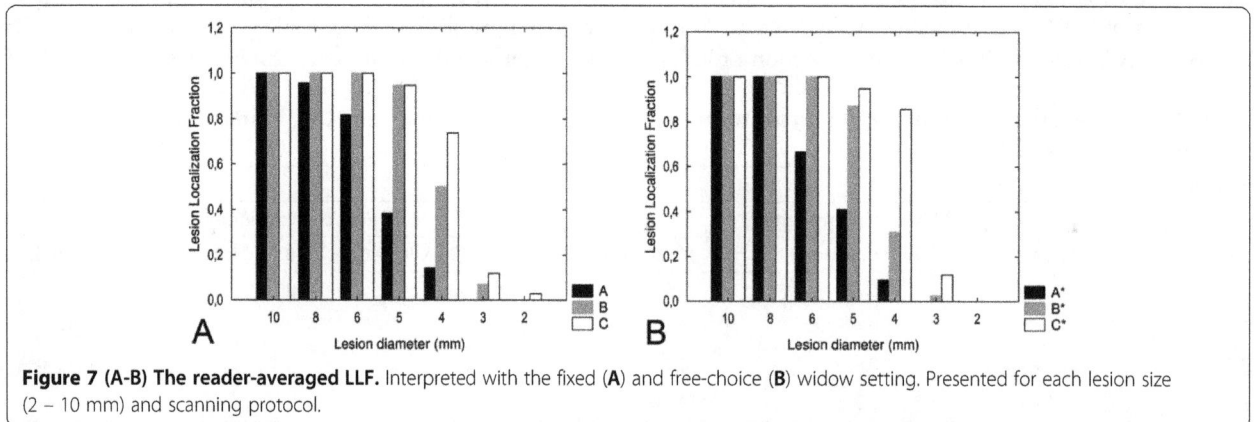

Figure 7 (A-B) The reader-averaged LLF. Interpreted with the fixed (**A**) and free-choice (**B**) widow setting. Presented for each lesion size (2 – 10 mm) and scanning protocol.

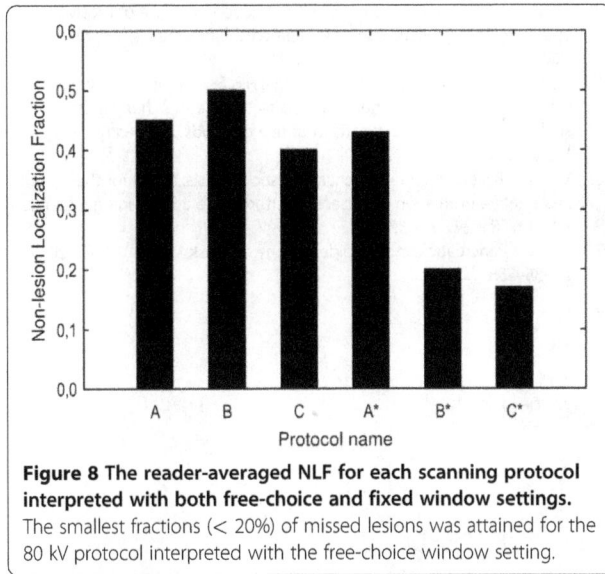

Figure 8 The reader-averaged NLF for each scanning protocol interpreted with both free-choice and fixed window settings. The smallest fractions (< 20%) of missed lesions was attained for the 80 kV protocol interpreted with the free-choice window setting.

the patient associated with an increased radiation dose in order to achieve a technically optimal MDCT is negligible. We therefore believe that for patients with a high probability of pancreatic malignancy, the examination protocol should be tailored to achieve optimal tumor conspicuity. The radiation dose must, however, be taken into account for patients with hereditary or predisposing factors for pancreatic tumors (for example familiar syndromes and chronic pancreatitis) and subjects with the multiple endocrine neoplasia syndrome Type I (MEN-I) who undergo repeated screening controls.

When designing these examination protocols, it is therefore important to remember that the radiation dose will increase when the tube voltage is decreased because at the same time the tube current needs to be adjusted to maintain similar image noise. The reason for this is that the image noise is a function of the dose to the detector and not to the patient.

This study has some limitations. In daily clinical practice we do not consider the low kilovoltage protocols suitable for large patients (> 85 kg) because of the high image noise, despite the increase in radiation dose. Real tumors are not uniformly spherical in shape and are not always located in a perfectly homogenous background. Even though the vast majority of PDACs are hypoattenuated to pancreatic parenchyma, it should be noted that 11% of solid pancreatic malignancies are isoattenuating on CT [9]. In these cases the presence of secondary signs such as pancreatic and/or biliary duct dilatation can indicate the existence of a tumor. Also, the attenuation used as reference for pancreatic parenchyma (130HU) and the pancreatic cancers (110HU) were measured in a limited number of patients (n = 15). In the experimental situation a 20 HU attenuation difference between pancreas and tumor was thus assumed

wheras in the clinical situation there is a variation in this respect. Furthermore, the simulated tumors were inserted into already reconstructed images, meaning that the lesions were not affected by the modular transfer function (MTF) of the system. In future studies, the lesions may instead be convolved with the point-spread function (PSF) before inserting them into the images in order to avoid this inconsistency.

Moreover, the study was designed as a free-response ROC (FROC), but the evaluation was performed as an ROC. Because two of the readers did not generate an appreciable amount of NLs for protocols B* and C*, the statistical analysis became less reliable. An ROC analysis was therefore performed, complemented with descriptive statistics, so that the information about the location and the number of lesions was not lost.

One of the readers did not use the same type of monitor (three mega pixel grey scale) as the other two. A one mega pixel color monitor was used instead. However, all monitors were calibrated according to DICOM part 14, and since CT images do not require high-resolution monitors, this difference was considered to be of small importance.

Conclusion

In conclusion, by using this experimental model, we have shown that the low-kilovoltage, high-current MDCT improved the depiction of small, minimally hypodense, solid pancreatic lesions. However, further studies are needed to assess what the technique yields in the clinical setting.

Competing interests
The authors declare that they have no competing interests.

Authors' contributions
JH, LL, NA, NK, BL and AS participated in planning the study, executing the experiments, collecting and analysing the data and writing the manuscript. All the authors read and approved the final manuscript.

Author details
[1]Division of Medical Physics, Karolinska University Hospital, Huddinge, Stockholm 14186, Sweden. [2]Department of Clinical Science, Intervention and Technology (CLINTEC), Karolinska Institutet, 17177 Stockholm, Sweden. [3]Department of Radiology, Karolinska University Hospital, Huddinge, 14186 Stockholm, Sweden. [4]Department of Radiology, Karolinska University Hospital, Solna, 17176 Stockholm, Sweden. [5]Department of Molecular Medicine and Surgery, Karolinska Institutet, Stockholm 17176 Sweden.

References
1. Wagner M, Redaelli C, Lietz M, Seiler CA, Friess H, Büchler HW: **Curative resection is the single most important factor determining outcome in patients with pancreatic adenocarcinoma.** *Br J Surg* 2004, **91**:586–594.
2. Garcea G, Dennison AR, Pattenden CJ, Neal CP, Sutton CD, Berry DP: **Survival following curative resection for pancreatic ductal adenocarcinoma. A systematic review of the literature.** *JOP* 2008, 9:99–132.

3. Kinney T: **Evidence-based imaging of pancreatic malignancies.** *Surg Clin North Am* 2010, **90**:235–249.

4. Pauls S, Sokiranski R, Schwarz M, Rieber A, Möller P, Brambs HJ: **Value of spiral CT and MRI (1.5 T) in preoperative diagnosis of tumo rs of the head of the pancreas.** *Rontgenpraxis* 2003, **55**:3–15.

5. Bronstein YL, Loyer EM, Kaur H, Choir H, David C, DuBrow RA, Broemeling LD, Cleary KR, Charnsangavej C: **Detection of small pancreatic tumors with multiphasic helical CT.** *AJR Am J Roentgenol* 2004, **182**:619–623.

6. Fusari M, Maurea S, Imbriaco M, Mollica C, Avitabile G, Soscia F, Camera L, Salvatore M: **Comparison between multislice CT and MR imaging in the diagnostic evaluation of patients with pancreatic masses.** *La Radiologia* 2010, **115**:453–466.

7. Tamm EP, Balachandran A, Bhosale PR, Katz MH, Fleming JB, Lee JH, Varadhachary GR: **Imaging of pancreatic adenocarcinoma: update on staging/resectability.** *Radiol Clin North Am* 2012, **50**:407–428.

8. Lu DS, Vedantham S, Krasny RM, Kadell B, Berger WL, Reber HA: **Two-phase helical CT for pancreatic tumors: pancreatic versus hepatic phase enhancement of tumor, pancreas, and vascular structures.** *Radiology* 1996, **199**:697–701.

9. Prokesch RW, Chow LC, Beaulieu CF, Bammer R, Jeffrey B: **Isoattenuating pancreatic adenocarcinoma at multi-detector row CT: secondary signs.** *Radiology* 2002, **224**:764–768.

10. Nakayama Y, Awai K, Funama Y, Hatemura M, Imuta M, Nakaura T, Ryu D, Morishita S, Sultana S, Sato N, Yamashita Y: **Abdominal CT with low tube voltage: preliminary observations about radiation dose, contrast enhancement, image quality, and noise.** *Radiology* 2005, **237**:945–951.

11. Kim JE, Newman B: **Evaluation of a radiation dose reduction strategy for pediatric chest CT.** *AJR Am J Roentgenol* 2010, **194**:1188–1193.

12. Kim MJ, Park CH, Choi SJ, Hwang KH, Kim HS: **Multidetector computed tomography chest examinations with low-kilovoltage protocols in adults: effect on image quality and radiation dose.** *J Comput Assist Tomogr* 2009, **33**:416–421.

13. Leschka S, Stolzmann P, Schmid FT, Scheffel H, Stinn B, Marincek B, Alkadhi H, Wildermuth S: **Low kilovoltage cardiac dual-source CT: attenuation, noise, and radiation dose.** *Eur Radiol* 2008, **18**:1809–1817.

14. Feuchtner GM, Jodocy D, Klauser A, Haberfellner B, Aglan I, Spoeck A, Hiehs S, Soegner P, Jaschke W: **Radiation dose reduction by using 100-kV tube voltage in cardiac 64-slice computed tomography.** *A comparative study.* 2010, **75**:51–56.

15. Szucs-Farkas Z, Kurmann L, Strautz T, Patak MA, Vock P, Schindera S: **Patient exposure and image quality of low-dose pulmonary computed tomography angiography: comparison of 100- and 80-kVp protocols.** *Invest Radiol* 2008, **43**:871–876.

16. Schueller-Weidekamm C, Schaefer-Prokop CM, Weber M, Herold CJ, Prokop M: **CT angiography of pulmonary arteries to detect pulmonary embolism: improvement of vascular enhancement with low kilovoltage settings.** *Radiology* 2006, **241**:899–907.

17. Sigal-Cinqualbre AB, Hennequin R, Abada HT, Chen X, Paul JF: **Low-kilovoltage multi-detector row chest CT in adults: feasibility and effect on image quality and iodine dose.** *Radiology* 2004, **231**:169–174.

18. Schindera ST, Nelson RC, Mukundan S Jr, Paulson EK, Jaffe TA, Miller CM, DeLong DM, Kawaji K, Yoshizumi TT, Samei E: **Hypervascular liver tumors: low tube voltage, high tube current multi-detector row CT for enhanced detection--phantom study.** *Radiology* 2008, **246**:125–132.

19. Marin D, Nelson RC, Barnhart H, Schindera ST, Ho LM, Jaffe TA, Yoshizumi TT, Youngblood R, Samei E: **Detection of pancreatic tumors, image quality, and radiation dose during the pancreatic parenchymal phase: effect of a low-tube-voltage, high-tube-current CT technique–preliminary results.** *Radiology* 2010, **256**:450–459.

20. Berthelet E, Liu M, Truong P, Czaykowski P, Kalach N, Yu C, Patterson K, Currie T, Kristensen S, Kwan W, Moravan V: **CT slice index and thickness: impact on organ contouring in radiation treatment planning for prostate cancer.** *J Appl Clin Med Phys* 2003, **4**:365–373.

21. McNitt-Gray MF: **AAPM/RSNA Physics Tutorial for Residents: Topics in CT.** *Radiation dose in CT. Radiographics* 2002, **22**:1541–1553.

22. Dorfman DD, Berbaum KS, Metz CE: **Receiver operating characteristic rating analysis. Generalization to the population of readers and patients with the jackknife method.** *Invest Radiol* 1992, **27**:723–731.

23. Obuchowski NA: **Receiver operating characteristic curves and their use in radiology.** *Radiology* 2003, **229**:3–8.

24. Lasko TA, Bhagwat JG, Zou KH, Ohno-Machado L: **The use of receiver operating characteristic curves in biomedical informatics.** *J Biomed Inform* 2005, **38**:404–415.

25. Obuchowski NA, Beiden SV, Berbaum KS, Hillis SL, Ishwaran H, Song HH, Wagner RF: **Multireader, multicase receiver operating characteristic analysis: an empirical comparison of five methods.** *Acad Radiol* 2004, **11**:980–995.

26. Metz CE: **Receiver operating characteristic analysis: a tool for the quantitative evaluation of observer performance and imaging systems.** *J Am Coll Radiol* 2006, **3**:413–422.

27. Krejs GJ: **Pancreatic cancer: epidemiology and risk factors.** *Dig Dis* 2010, **28**:355–358.

3

A pilot study using low-dose Spectral CT and ASIR (Adaptive Statistical Iterative Reconstruction) algorithm to diagnose solitary pulmonary nodules

Huijuan Xiao[1†], Yihe Liu[2†], Hongna Tan[1], Pan Liang[1], Bo Wang[1], Lei Su[1], Suya Wang[1] and Jianbo Gao[1*]

Abstract

Background: Lung cancer is the most common cancer which has the highest mortality rate. With the development of computed tomography (CT) techniques, the case detection rates of solitary pulmonary nodules (SPN) has constantly increased and the diagnosis accuracy of SPN has remained a hot topic in clinical and imaging diagnosis. The aim of this study was to evaluate the combination of low-dose spectral CT and ASIR (Adaptive Statistical Iterative Reconstruction) algorithm in the diagnosis of solitary pulmonary nodules (SPN).

Methods: 62 patients with SPN (42 cases of benign SPN and 20 cases of malignant SPN, pathology confirmed) were scanned by spectral CT with a dual-phase contrast-enhanced method. The iodine and water concentration (IC and WC) of the lesion and the artery in the image that had the same density were measured by the GSI (Gemstone Spectral Imaging) software. The normalized iodine and water concentration (NIC and NWC) of the lesion and the normalized iodine and water concentration difference (ICD and WCD) between the arterial and venous phases (AP and VP) were also calculated. The spectral HU (Hounsfield Unit) curve was divided into 3 sections based on the energy (40–70, 70–100 and 100–140 keV) and the slopes (λHU) in both phases were calculated. The IC_{AP}, IC_{VP}, WC_{AP} and WC_{VP}, NIC and NWC, and the λHU in benign and malignant SPN were compared by independent sample t-test.

Results: The iodine related parameters (IC_{AP}, IC_{VP}, NIC_{AP}, NIC_{VP}, and the ICD) of malignant SPN were significantly higher than that of benign SPN ($t = 3.310$, 1.330, 2.388, 1.669 and 3.251, respectively, $P < 0.05$). The 3 λHU values of venous phase in malignant SPN were higher than that of benign SPN ($t = 3.803$, 2.846 and 3.205, $P < 0.05$). The difference of water related parameters (WC_{AP}, WC_{VP}, NWC_{AP}, NWC_{VP} and WCD) between malignant and benign SPN were not significant ($t = 0.666$, 0.257, 0.104, 0.550 and 0.585, $P > 0.05$).

Conclusions: The iodine related parameters and the slope of spectral curve are useful markers to distinguish the benign from the malignant lung diseases, and its application is extremely feasible in clinical applications.

Keywords: Computed tomography, Spectral CT, Solitary pulmonary nodules, Adaptive statistical iterative reconstruction

* Correspondence: cjr.gaojianbo@163.vip.com
†Equal contributors
[1]The Department of Radiology, The First Affiliated Hospital of Zhengzhou University, No.1, East Jianshe Road, Zhengzhou, Henan Province 450052, China
Full list of author information is available at the end of the article

Background

Lung cancer is the most common cancer which has the highest mortality rate. In the past decades, the incidence of lung cancer has gradually increased in China [1, 2]. With the development of computed tomography (CT) techniques, the case detection rates of solitary pulmonary nodules (SPN) has constantly increased and the diagnosis accuracy of SPN has remained a hot topic in clinical and imaging diagnosis. Contrast-enhanced CT of the chest still remains the standard imaging test for the initial assessment of patients with suspected lung cancer. Using standard contrast-enhanced CT the characterization of pulmonary nodules is based on simple morphological criteria e.g., irregular or spiculated margins as a sign for malignancy or calcifications as a sign of benignity. However, in a clinical context these simple morphologic criteria are unreliable for an accurate differentiation between benign and malignant lung nodules.

X-ray computed tomography (CT) is a medical imaging modality that allows reconstruction of the internal stucture of the human body from a large number of x-ray attenuation measurements. The spectral CT in which the energy dependence of the x-ray attenuation coefficient is utilized Multiple parameters can be acquired by means of spectral CT techniques, such as monochromatic imaging, material decomposition images, spectral HU curve and effective atomic number, etc. [3, 4] ASIR (Adaptive Statistical Iterative Reconstruction) algorithm, is a compromise that relies on the accurate modeling of the noise distribution of the acquired data, rather than modeling the system optics. The result is an algorithm that is computationally fast and is effective at reducing noise, enabling radiation dose reductions that would not be possible [5–12]. The ASIR reconstruction algorithm is a promising technique for providing diagnostic quality CT images at significantly reduced radiation doses. ASIR is also helpful in improving CT image quality for obese patients.

In this study, patients with solitary pulmonary nodules (SPN) underwent dual-phase scanning by low dose spectral CT. The iodine and water concentrations were derived and the spectral HU curves were also acquired. By calculating and comparing the normalized concentration of iodine and water, the slopes of spectral curves in the benign and malignant SPN, the practical value of multiple parameters which was acquired by low dose spectral CT in SPN diagnosis are discussed. In this paper we propose an improved method to detect SPN. By analysis of different comparison parameters between benign and malignant pulmonary nodules and provide a reference for clinical diagnosis and treatment.

Methods

Design and setting

For this study, the use of medical imaging was approved by Medical Ethical Committee of The First Affiliated Hospital of Zhengzhou University. Approval was granted in accordance with Chinese legislations, and written informed consent was obtained from all participants, in accordance with the guidelines of the Chinese Ministry of Health. 64 patients with SPN received dual phase spectral CT scan between December 2013 and November 2014, but only 62 patients were included in the research. One case was excluded because the patient did not hold the breath and caused too many unacceptable motion artifacts; the other case was excluded since the solid lesion was too small to allow determination of the region of interest (ROI). The average age of 62 patients was 60 (ages from 42 to 80), including 40 males and 22 females. All the SPN cases were confirmed by surgery, trans-bronchial biopsy and pathology. Some patients with inflammatory nodules improved after anti-inflammatory therapy which was evident, clinically. There were totally 42 patients with malignant SPN (including 25 cases of adenocarcinoma; 13 cases of squamous carcinoma; 2 cases of bronchioloalveolar carcinoma; 1 case of mucoepidermoid carcinoma and 1 case of metastasis) and 20 patients with benign SPN (including 9 cases of inflammation; 7 cases of tuberculoma; 2 cases of hamartoma and 2 cases of sclerosing hemangioma). For use of these clinical materials for research purposes, prior consent from the patients and approval from the Research Ethics Committee of The First Affiliated Hospital of Zhengzhou University were obtained. All specimens were handled and made anonymous according to the ethical and legal standards.

Diagnosis method

All patients underwent a two-phase contrast-enhanced low-dose spectral CT(GE Discovery CT750HD) examination with a single tube, and fast kilovoltage switching between 80 kVp and 140 kVp in less than 0.5 ms (GSI mode). Patients were examined 30 s (artery phase) and 60 s (venous phase) after contrast medium injection respectively. The scanning parameters were: 40 % ASIR (40 % ASIR images combined with 60 % FBP reconstruction image); tube current 260 mA; helical pitch 1.375:1; rotation speed 0.8 s; slice thickness 1.25 mm; detector coverage 40 mm, field-of-view (FOV) 32 cm, and CT dose index volume (CTDIVol) of 4.17 mGy per phase. Non-ionic contrast medium Iodixanol (Visipaque® 270 mg I/ml,, GE HealthCare) with antecubital venous access through power injector (Urich REF XD 2060-Touch, Germany) at a rate of 3–4 mL/s for a total of 90–120 mL (1.5 mL/kg, 80 ~ 100 ml).

Image analysis

All the data were processed and analyzed by GSI Volume Viewer software package at AW4.6 work station (GE HealthCare, USA). The images were independently analyzed by two radiologists who had 5 and 10 years of experience, respectively. During the data analysis, the radiologists were able to adjust the window width and position based on the condition of each imaging. A circularregions of interest (ROI) was placed in the area that encompassed the entire tumor, as large as possible to reduce noise (.50 pixels), away from any peripheral fat and necrotic area. All measurements were repeated three times at the three contiguous imaging levels and average values were calculated to ensure consistency. In the iodine density image derived from the iodine/water based material decomposition image, the concentration of iodine (IC) and water (WC) in lesions (ICles and WCles) were measured in both arterial phase (AP) and venous phase (VP). In the same slice, the concentration of iodine and water in aorta descendens or subclavian artery (IC_{ao} and WC_{ao}) were also measured. The normalized iodine concentration (NIC), which is the ratio of iodine concentration in lesion and aorta descendens ($NIC = IC_{les}/IC_{ao}$) and normalized water concentration (NWC, $NWC = WC_{les}/WC_{ao}$) were calculated. The iodine concentration difference (ICD, $ICD = NIC_{VP}-NIC_{AP}$ where the NIC_{AP} and NIC_{VP} are the normalized iodine concentration in arterial phase and venous phase, respectively) was calculated, and the water concentration difference (WCD, $WCD = NWC_{VP}-NWV_{AP}$) was calculated in the same manner. The spectral HU curve was divided into 3 regions, 40–70 keV, 70–100 keV and 100–140 keV. The slope (λHU) of 40–70 keV was calculated by the equations K40-70 keV = (40 keV-70 keV) HU/70-40 which was the same with The slope (λHU) of 70–100 keV and 100–140 keV.

Statistical analysis

All data was analyzed by SPSS 17.0 software package. The measurement data was displayed as s ± d (mean ± deviation), and independent-samples t-test was used in the differential analysis ($\alpha = 0.05$). The results were considered statistically significant when $P < 0.05$.

Results

Comparison of IC, NIC and ICD in both benign and malignant SPN

In malignant SPN, the IC in both arterial and venous phase, NIC and ICD were significantly higher than benign SPN when statistically analyzed. The results are shown in Table 1.

Table 1 The comparison of IC, NIC and ICD in benign and malignant SPN

	Malignant SPN ($n = 42$)	Benign SPN ($n = 20$)	t value	P value
IC_{AP}	19.322 ± 5.554	11.711 ± 3.724	3.310	0.003
IC_{VP}	19.191 ± 6.438	15.297 ± 6.258	1.330	0.014
NIC_{AP}	0.163 ± 0.056	0.112 ± 0.028	2.388	0.027
NIC_{VP}	0.649 ± 0.888	0.286 ± 0.078	1.669	0.035
ICD	0.264 ± 0.120	0.163 ± 0.061	3.251	0.002

Comparison of WC, NWC and WCD in both benign and malignant SPN

WC in both arterial and venous phase, the NWC and WCD in malignant SPN have no statistically significant differences compared to benign SPN. The results are shown in Table 2.

Calculation and comparison of spectral curve slope (λHU) at arterial and venous phase in benign and malignant SPN

The results showed that with the increase in keV, the λHU in both benign and malignant SPN decreased, and the λHU of malignant SPN was larger than that of benign SPN, but the differences were reduced when keV increased (Fig. 1 and Fig. 2). In the arterial phase, the 3 slopes of malignant and benign SPN have no significant differences ($P > 0.05$); while in the venous phase, the 3 slopes of malignant SPN were significantly larger than that of benign SPN ($P < 0.05$).So we can use the λHU of venous phase in lower keV to identify benign with malignant nodule. The results are shown in Table 3.

Discussion

The methodology to diagnose SPN has been developing over the years from a traditional morphological examination to a dynamic functional examination. Spectral CT imaging has the potential to provide multiple techniques, such as polychromatic and monochromatic imaging, material decomposition imaging, etc. Therefore, spectral CT has been widely used in the detection of early stage cancer, qualitative diagnosis of neoplastic disease, staging diagnosis and reducing the metal artifacts and so on [13–17].

Table 2 The comparison of WC, NWC and WCD in benign and malignant SPN

	Malignant SPN ($n = 42$)	Benign SPN ($n = 20$)	t value	P value
WC_{AP}	1019.55 ± 14.407	1015.85 ± 13.438	0.666	0.511
WC_{VP}	1020.61 ± 12.598	1018.84 ± 19.568	0.257	0.801
NWC_{AP}	1.014 ± 0.021	1.015 ± 0.019	0.104	0.918
NWC_{VP}	1.005 ± 0.021	1.001 ± 0.017	0.550	0.587
WCD	0.008 ± 0.022	0.013 ± 0.021	0.585	0.563

Table 3 The slope of 3 energy decay curve sections in benign and malignant SPN

Groups	Arterial phase			Venous phase		
	40-70 keV	70-100 keV	100-140 keV	40-70 keV	70-100 keV	100-140 keV
Malignant SPN(n = 42)	3.473 ± 1.121	0.781 ± 2.975	0.359 ± 0.119	4.147 ± 1.356	1.793 ± 1.465	0.425 ± 0.141
Benign SPN(n = 20)	3.396 ± 2.578	0.835 ± 0.712	0.357 ± 0.276	2.670 ± 0.697	0.761 ± 0.351	0.289 ± 0.083
t value	0.09	0.231	0.030	3.803	2.846	3.205
P value	0.930	0.822	0.976	0.001	0.010	0.004

It was reported that tumor cells can produce angiogenic factors that stimulate and generate a large number of new blood vessels. Since the wall of these new blood vessels are immature there is a lack of hemangiopericyte and smooth muscle tissue and there is increased permeability of the blood vessels [18–20]. Lung cancer cells by themselves are highly aggressive; they can invade the corresponding artery making the terminal blood vessels get thicker and circuitous. Since there is a lack of venous and lymphatic drainage system in the cancer lesion, the

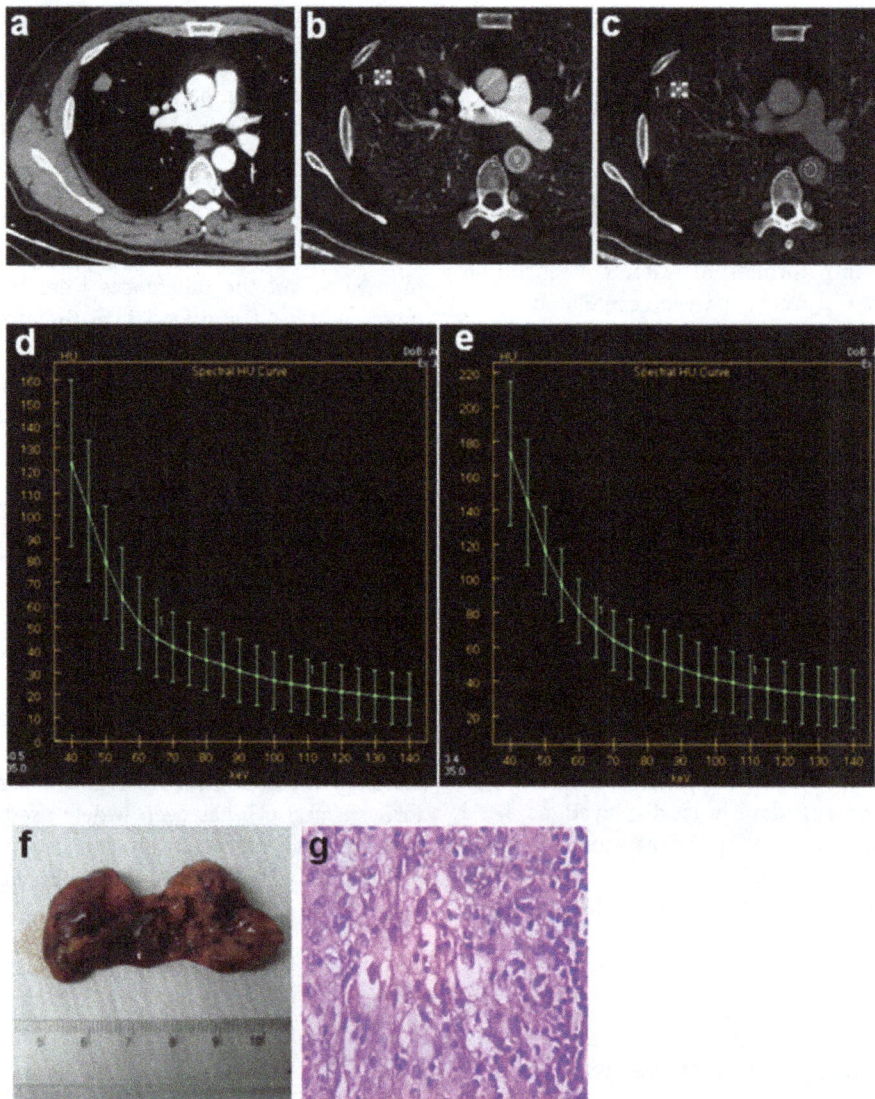

Fig. 1 Male, 47 years old. Space occupying lesion was found in the right upper lobe. Middle differentiation squamous cell carcinomas, confirmed by the postoperative pathological diagnosis. **a** monochromatic image, 70 keV, arterial and venous phase; **b** arterial phase iodine image, IC_{AP} = 13.28 mg/ml; **c** venous phase iodine image, IC_{VP} = 18.1 mg/ml; **d** arterial phase spectral energy curve; **e** venous phase spectral energy curve, the slope of 40–70, 70–100 and 100–140 keV are 3.72, 0.66, 0.36, respectively; **f** pathologic samples after surgery; **g** pathological section image (HE dye, ×400)

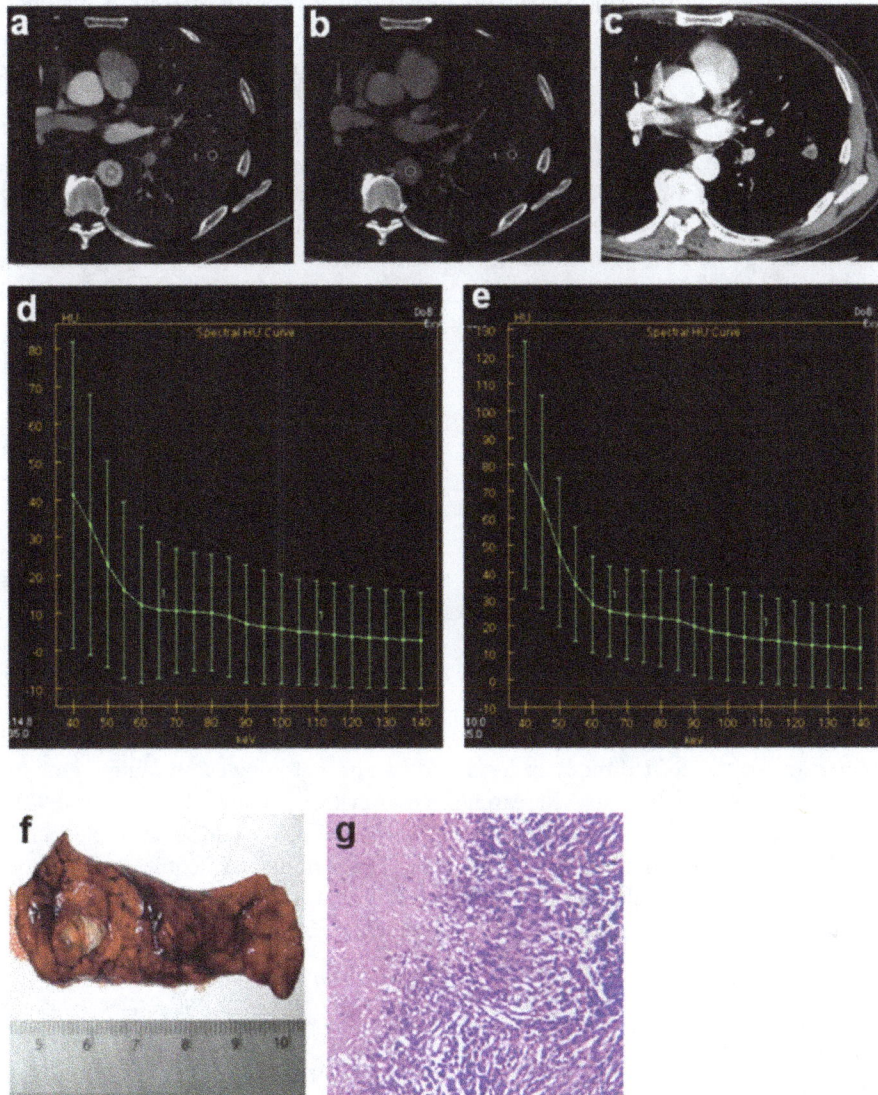

Fig. 2 Male, 57 years old. Pulmonary nodule was found in left upper lobe. Tuberculosis in lower left lobe confirmed by postoperative pathological diagnosis **a** monochromatic image, 70 *keV*, arterial and venous phase; **b** arterial phase iodine image, $IC_{AP} = 8.43$ mg/ml; **c** venous phase iodine image, $IC_{VP} = 8.55$ mg/ml; **d** arterial phase spectral energy curve; **e** venous phase spectral energy curve, the slope of 40–70, 70–100 and 100–140 *keV* are 1.84, 0.25, 0.17, respectively; **f** pathologic samples after surgery; **g** pathological section image (HE dye, ×100)

contrast agent gets diffused into the extravascular space. But in the case of benign SPN, most of them do not have abundant blood supply and the vascular basement membrane is not damaged, so the permeability of blood vessels is not increased. Tateishi et al. analyzed the correlation of tumor enhancement with MVD and VEGF expression in 130 patients with histological proven lung cancer [21]. They found a significantly higher peak enhancement of VEGF-positive tumors than in VEGF-negative tumors. In this study, the ICAP, ICVP, NIC and ICD in malignant SPN were all significantly higher than that of benign SPN. In benign SPN, the active inflammatory nodule also contains more blood vessels due to the stimulation of inflammatory substances. With the conversion of an active

nodule to a chronic inflammatory nodule, the fabric content in the lesion increases while the vascular content decreases. As a consequence, the iodine concentration in active inflammatory nodule may also be high, and comparable to a malignant nodule. In the chronic inflammatory and other benign nodule, due to the lack of blood vessel, the contrast agent diffuse slowly, therefore, in some case, the ICVP is higher than ICAP. It is similar to the study of Schmid-Bindert et al., who investigated the correlation between maximum standardized uptake value (SUV(max)) of (18) FDG PET-CT and iodine-related attenuation (IRA) of dual energy CT (DECT) of primary tumours and (18) FDG PET-CT positive thoracic lymph nodes (LN) in patients with lung cancer and a moderate correlation was found between SUV(max) and maximum IRA in all tumours [22].

In the iodine/water based material decomposition image, the water content was measured. Based on the calculation and statistical analysis, the results showed that WC, NWC and WCD in both benign and malignant SPN have no significant differences. In this study, the inflammatory nodule cases were relatively high in the benign SPN group. Since the blood flow of inflammatory nodule increases in the congestive stage, the water content in both intra- and extra-cellular is high. As for the malignant SPN, the water content in intra- and extra-cellular is also high due to the relatively higher vascular capacitance and large amount of tumor cells. The center of tuberculoma consists of caseous necrotic tissue surrounded by fibrous tissue, and the caseous necrotic tissue is a pink amorphous granular mass, which exhibits more severe necrosis: coagulative necrosis. Coagulative necrosis is enriched with lipid and less water content. In this study, the water content is high in inflammatory nodule cases, which led to the premise that water concentration related parameters (WC, NWC, WCD) are not significantly different between benign and malignant groups.

The iodine concentration in the ROI directly reflects the blood supply situation in the nodule. Research showed that the IC in malignant nodules is higher than in benign nodules [23]. Several studies have compared the CT numbers of pulmonary nodules on iodine-enhanced image with that on enhanced weighted average images The results of both the CT number on iodine-enhanced images and the degree of enhancement showed that malignant nodules showed a significantly higher enhancement than benign nodules ($P = 0.001$), and iodine-enhanced images had a higher sensitivity and accuracy than the degree of enhancement [24–28]. The spectra curve is a reflection of different lesions and different tissues or organs in the human body absorb X-rays at different rates. It shows the variation of CT values in different regions of different keV [29, 30].The difference of spectral curve needs to be correlated to the iodine concentration in the lesions when the contrast agent is applied. In this study, the slopes of spectral HU curve were decreased with the increase in keV in both benign and malignant nodules. However in all the 3 curve sections, the slopes of malignant SPN are all higher than the corresponding slopes of benign SPN.

The low dose spectral scan mode was applied in this research. The tube current was set to 260 mA, CTDIVol was 4.17 mGy per phase, which is significantly lower compared to the dose of the first generation technology. In addition, the ASIR algorithm reduced the noise and improved the imaging quality, and makes it possible to acquire good quality image in much lower dosage. The

percentage of ASIR (10–100 %) is operator selectable at the console. It reflects a linear combination of the original FBP image (0 % ASIR) and an essentially noise-free image created by full compliance with the mathematic model (100 % ASIR). A choice of 40 % ASIR implies that 40 % of the ASIR image was blended with the FBP image. A preliminary phantom analysis and clinical feasibility study of low-dose body CT using 40 % ASIR determined that it provided quantitative and qualitative image noise and quality nearly identical to those of routine-dose CT [31].

In this study, the ultralow concentration iso-osmolar contrast agent (270mgI/mL) was given to the patients; consequently, the incidence of adverse reaction was reduced, which is a better choice of contrast agent when the patients have potential renal damage or cardiac insufficiency.

Although the results in this research are concrete and convincing, this work still has several aspects that need to be explored thoroughly in further studies, such as, expanding the cases; detailed study based on different pathological types of lung cancer; distinguishing the active inflammatory nodules from malignant nodules; comparing the water content related parameters in different pathological nodules, etc. In conclusion, the combination of low dose spectral CT and ASIR algorithm can help acquire multiple parameters under the low dose mode and acquiring these parameters is highly practicable in the clinic during diagnosis of benign and malignant SPN.

Abbreviations

CT: computed tomography; ASIR: adaptive statistical iterative reconstruction; FBP: filtered back projection; SPN: solitary plmonary nodules; IC: iodine concentration; WC: water concentration; GSI: gemstone spectral imaging; NIC: normalized iodine concentration; NWC: normalized water concentration; ICD: iodine concentration difference; WCD: water concentration difference; AP: arterial phases; VP: venous phases; HU: Hounsfield Units.

Competing of interests

The authors declare no conflict of interest.

Authors' contributions

HJX carried out the Image analysis, statistical analysis, and drafted the manuscript. YHL carried out the Image analysis, statistical analysis, and drafted the manuscript. HT participated in its design and coordination .PL performed the statistical analysis. JBG participated in the design of the study, supervised the work, and corrected the final version of manuscript. LS performed the Image analysis. SW performed the statistical analysis. BW and helped to draft the manuscript. All authors read and approved the final manuscript.

Acknowledgments

We thank Dr. Dengyan Zhu and Dr. Xianzheng Gao for helpful discussion. This work was supported by Foundation for Outstanding Scholarship in Henan Province (grant number 144200510008) and Foundation for key project of Science and Technology Department in Henan Province (grant number 112102310091).

Author details

[1]The Department of Radiology, The First Affiliated Hospital of Zhengzhou University, No.1, East Jianshe Road, Zhengzhou, Henan Province 450052,

China. [2]The No.7 People's Hospital of Zhengzhou, 17 Jingnan 5th Road, Zhengzhou Economic and Technological Development Zone, Zhengzhou, Henan Province 450000, China.

References

1. She J, Yang P, Hong Q, Bai C. Lung cancer in china: challenges and interventions. Chest. 2013;143(4):1117–26.
2. Rami-Porta R, Crowley JJ, Goldstraw P. The revised TNM staging system for lung cancer. Ann Thorac Cardiovasc Surg. 2009;15(1):4–9.
3. Johnson TR, Krauss B, Sedlmair M, Grasruck M, Bruder H, Morhard D, et al. Material differentiation by dual energy CT: initial experience. Eur Radiol. 2007;17(6):1510–7.
4. Chae EJ, Song JW, Seo JB, Krauss B, Jang YM, Song KS. Clinical utility of dual-energy CT in the evaluation of solitary pulomonary nodules: initial experience. Radiology. 2008;249(2):671–81.
5. Vorona GA, Ceschin RC, Clayton BL, Sutcavage T, Tadros SS, Panigrahy A. Reducing abdominal CT radiation dose with the adaptive statistical iterative reconstruction technique in children: a feasibility study. Pediatr Radiol. 2011;41(9):1174–82.
6. Rapalino O, Kamalian S, Kamalian S, Payabvash S, Souza LC, Zhang D, et al. Cranial CT with adaptive statistical iterative reconstruction: improved image quality with concomitant radiation dose reduction. AJNR Am J Neuroradiol. 2012;33(4):609–15.
7. Leipsic J, Nguyen G, Brown J, Sin D, Mayo JR. A prospective evaluation of dose reduction and image quality in chest CT using Adaptive statistical iterative reconstruction . AJR Am J Roentgenol. 2010;195(5):1095–9.
8. Qi L-P, Li Y, Tang L, Li YL, Li XT, Cui Y, et al. Evaluation of dose reduction and image quality in chest CT using adaptive statistical iterative reconstruction with the same group of patients . Br J Radiol. 2012;85(1018):e906–11.
9. Fontarensky M, Alfidja A, Perignon R, Schoenig A, Perrier C, Mulliez A, et al. Reduced Radiation Dose with Model-based Iterative Reconstruction versus Standard Dose with Adaptive Statistical Iterative Reconstruction in Abdominal CT for Diagnosis of Acute Renal Colic. Radiology. 2015;276(1):156–66.
10. Koc G, Courtier JL, Phelps A, Marcovici PA, MacKenzie JD. Computed tomography depiction of small pediatric vessels with model-based iterative reconstruction. Pediatr Radiol. 2014;44(7):787–94.
11. Neroladaki A, Botsikas D, Boudabbous S, Becker CD, Montet X. Computed tomography of the chest with model-based iterative reconstruction using a radiation exposure similar to chest X-ray examination: preliminary observations. Eur Radiol. 2013;23(2):360–6.
12. Xu Y, He W, Chen H, Hu Z, Li J, Zhang T. Impact of the adaptive statistical iterative reconstruction technique on image quality in ultra-low-dose CT. Clin Radiol. 2013;68(9):902–8.
13. Kim YK, Park BK, Kim CK, Park SY. Adenoma characterization: adrenal protocol with dual-energy CT. Radiology. 2013;267(1):155–63.
14. Karçaaltıncaba M, Aktaş A. Dual-energy CT revisited with multidetector CT: review of principles and clinical applications. Diagn Interv Radiol. 2011;17(3):181–94.
15. Altenbernd J, Heusner TA, Ringelstein A, Ladd SC, Forsting M, Antoch G. Dual-energy-CT of hypervascular liver lesions in patients with HCC: investigation of image quality and sensitivity. Eur Radiol. 2011;21(4):738–43.
16. Graser A, Becker CR, Staehler M, Clevert DA, Macari M, Arndt N, et al. Single-phase dual-energy CT allows for characterization of renal masses as benign or malignant. Invest Radiol. 2010;45(7):399–405.
17. Apfaltrer P, Meyer M, Meier C, Henzler T, Barraza JM Jr, Dinter DJ, et al. Contrast-Enhanced Dual-Energy CT of Gastrointestinal Stromal Tumors: Is Iodine-Related Attenuation a Potential Indicator of Tumor Response? Invest Radiol. 2012;47(1):65–70.
18. Goo HW, Yang DH, Kim N, Park SI, Kim DK, Kim EA. Collateral ventilation to congenital hyperlucent lung lesions assessed on xenon-enhanced dynamic dual-energy CT: an initial experience. Korean J Radiol. 2011;12(1):25–33.
19. Hur S, Lee JM, Kim SJ, Park JH, Han JK, Choi BI. 80-kVp CT using Iterative Reconstruction in Image Space algorithm for the detection of hypervascular hepatocellular carcinoma: phantom and initial clinical experience. Korean J Radiol. 2012;13(2):152–64.
20. Ruoslahti E. Specialization of tumor vasculature. Nat Rev Cancer. 2012;2:83–90.
21. Tateishi U, Kusumoto M, Nishihara H, Nagashima K, Morikawa T, Moriyama N. Contrast-enhanced dynamic computed tomography for the evaluation of tumor angiogenesis in patients with lung carcinoma. Cancer. 2002;95(4):835–42.
22. Schmid-Bindert G, Henzler T, Chu TQ, Meyer M, Nance JW Jr, Schoepf UJ, et al. Functional imaging of lung cancer using dual energy CT: how does iodine related attenuation correlate with standardized uptake value of 18FDG-PET-CT? Eur Radiol. 2012;22(1):93–103.
23. Lee SH, Hur J, Kim YJ, Lee HJ, Hong YJ, Choi BW. Additional value of dual-energy CT to differentiate between benign and malignant mediastinal tumors: an initial experience. Eur J Radiol. 2013;82(11):2043–9.
24. Swensen SJ, Viggiano RW, Midthun DE, Müller NL, Sherrick A, Yamashita K, et al. Lung nodule enhancement at CT: multicenter study. Radiology. 2000;214(1):73–80.
25. Swensen SJ, Brown LR, Colby TV, Weaver AL. Pulmonary nodules: CT evaluation of enhancement with iodinated contrast material. Radiology. 1995;194(2):393–8.
26. Yamashita K, Matsunobe S, Tsuda T, Nemoto T, Matsumoto K, Miki H, et al. Solitary pulmonary nodule: preliminary study of evaluation with incremental dynamic CT. Radiology. 1995;194(2) :399–405.
27. Swensen SJ, Morin RL, Aughenbaugh GL, Leimer DW. CT reconstruction algorithm selection in the evaluation of solitary pulmonary nodules. J Comput Assist Tomogr. 1995;19(6):932–5.
28. Henzler T, Shi J, Jafarov H, Schoenberg SO, Manegold C, Fink C, et al. Functional CT imaging techniques for the assessment of angiogenesis in lung cancer. Transl Lung Cancer Res. 2012;1(1):78–83.
29. Musturay K, Aykut A. Dual-energy CT revisited with multidetector CT: review of Pinciples and clinical applications . Dian Interv Radiol. 2010;17(3):181–94.
30. Remy-Jardin M, Faivre JB, Pontana F, Hachulla AL, Tacelli N, Santangelo T, et al. Thoracic applications of dual energy . Radiol Clin North Am. 2010;48(1):193–205.
31. Flicek KT, Hara AK, Silva AC, Wu Q, Peter MB, Johnson CD. Reducing the radiation dose for CT colonography using adaptive statistical iterative reconstruction: a pilot study . AJR Am J Roentgenol. 2010;195(1):126–31.

4

CT of the chest with model-based, fully iterative reconstruction: comparison with adaptive statistical iterative reconstruction

Yasutaka Ichikawa, Kakuya Kitagawa[*], Naoki Nagasawa, Shuichi Murashima and Hajime Sakuma

Abstract

Background: The recently developed model-based iterative reconstruction (MBIR) enables significant reduction of image noise and artifacts, compared with adaptive statistical iterative reconstruction (ASIR) and filtered back projection (FBP). The purpose of this study was to evaluate lesion detectability of low-dose chest computed tomography (CT) with MBIR in comparison with ASIR and FBP.

Methods: Chest CT was acquired with 64-slice CT (Discovery CT750HD) with standard-dose (5.7 ± 2.3 mSv) and low-dose (1.6 ± 0.8 mSv) conditions in 55 patients (aged 72 ± 7 years) who were suspected of lung disease on chest radiograms. Low-dose CT images were reconstructed with MBIR, ASIR 50% and FBP, and standard-dose CT images were reconstructed with FBP, using a reconstructed slice thickness of 0.625 mm. Two observers evaluated the image quality of abnormal lung and mediastinal structures on a 5-point scale (Score 5 = excellent and score 1 = non-diagnostic). The objective image noise was also measured as the standard deviation of CT intensity in the descending aorta.

Results: The image quality score of enlarged mediastinal lymph nodes on low-dose MBIR CT (4.7 ± 0.5) was significantly improved in comparison with low-dose FBP and ASIR CT (3.0 ± 0.5, $p = 0.004$; 4.0 ± 0.5, $p = 0.02$, respectively), and was nearly identical to the score of standard-dose FBP image (4.8 ± 0.4, $p = 0.66$). Concerning decreased lung attenuation (bulla, emphysema, or cyst), the image quality score on low-dose MBIR CT (4.9 ± 0.2) was slightly better compared to low-dose FBP and ASIR CT (4.5 ± 0.6, $p = 0.01$; 4.6 ± 0.5, $p = 0.01$, respectively). There were no significant differences in image quality scores of visualization of consolidation or mass, ground-glass attenuation, or reticular opacity among low- and standard-dose CT series. Image noise with low-dose MBIR CT (11.6 ± 1.0 Hounsfield units (HU)) were significantly lower than with low-dose ASIR (21.1 ± 2.6 HU, $p < 0.0005$), low-dose FBP CT (30.9 ± 3.9 HU, $p < 0.0005$), and standard-dose FBP CT (16.6 ± 2.3 HU, $p < 0.0005$).

Conclusion: MBIR shows greater potential than ASIR for providing diagnostically acceptable low-dose CT without compromising image quality. With radiation dose reduction of >70%, MBIR can provide equivalent lesion detectability of standard-dose FBP CT.

Keywords: Model-based iterative reconstruction, Adaptive statistical iterative reconstruction, Filtered back projection, Low-dose computed tomography, Radiation dose reduction, Chest

* Correspondence: kakuya@clin.medic.mie-u.ac.jp
Department of Radiology, Mie University Hospital, 2-174 Edobashi, Tsu, Mie 514-8507, Japan

Background

Radiation associated with diagnostic computed tomography (CT) has recently come under scrutiny because of the known association between ionizing radiation and malignancy. The lifetime cancer risk based on current CT use has been estimated to be as high as 2.0% [1]. There is a compelling need for high quality CT images acquired with reduced radiation doses.

The filtered back projection (FBP) technique is currently the most widespread CT reconstruction algorithm. However, this reconstruction technique does have significant limitations, mainly because it relies on several assumptions. The FBP technique assumes that there is a focal point source on the anode, a pencil-shaped beam emerging from the anode, a point-like interaction of the beam with the voxel, and a point-like interaction of the beam with the detector [2]. In actuality, all these assumptions about the x-ray beam are incorrect. These assumptions lead to substantial limitations in spatial resolution and noise generation. Furthermore, there is no general statistical consideration for noise. As a result, FBP images are prone to high levels of noise, streak artifacts, and low-contrast detectability in low-dose acquisitions [2].

Recently, adaptive statistical iterative reconstruction (ASIR) was introduced as a way to reduce image noise [3-6]. With this technique, projection data are first reconstructed with a FBP, and are then compared with an ideal noise model until the algorithm converges. Previous studies have demonstrated that there is a significant reduction in image noise, and, on average, a 25-50% dose reduction can be achieved [3,6-9]. One limitation, however, is that the ASIR technique continues to assume an ideal x-ray system.

Model-based iterative reconstruction (MBIR) is the most advanced of the various iterative reconstruction schemes as it attempts to model the entire x-ray beam as it travels from the cathode to the detector [10]. This includes modeling of the shape of the focal spot on the anode, the shape of the beam as it emerges from the anode, the 3-dimensional interaction of the beam with the voxel in the patient, and the 2-dimensional interaction of the beam with the detector [2]. By modeling these optical effects, MBIR can substantially improve image quality and spatial resolution, and reduce streaking artifacts. Recent studies demonstrated that low-dose MBIR images had significantly lower image noise than low-dose ASIR images [11,12]. However, the lesion detectability of low-dose MBIR CT has not been sufficiently studied yet. The purpose of this study was to evaluate the lesion detectability of low-dose chest CT reconstructed with MBIR and ASIR in comparison with standard-dose FBP CT.

Methods

Patients

This study was approved by the local institutional review board (Mie University Medical Research Ethics Committee). Informed consent was obtained from all participating patients. The study prospectively enrolled 55 patients (mean age, 72 ± 7 years; male / female = 25 / 30) who were referred for chest CT examinations between February 2011 and June 2011 because of suspected lung disease on chest radiograms. Patients were considered ineligible if they were younger than 60 years old. The mean body mass index (BMI) was $22.1 \pm 3.4 \text{ kg/m}^2$.

CT scanning protocol

All 55 subjects underwent standard-dose and low-dose chest CT with a 64-section multi-detector row CT scanner (GE Discovery CT750 HD; GE Healthcare, Milwaukee, WI). A weight-based adjustment of a combined modulation type (Auto mA 3D) automatic exposure control technique was used for both CT scans. For standard-dose CT, a noise index of 18.33 was employed on the basis of vendor recommendation. For low-dose CT, a noise index of 36.66 was used to reduce the radiation dose by approximately 75% compared with standard-dose CT. With the exception of the noise index, all remaining scanning parameters were held identical for standard-dose and low-dose CT examinations. These parameters included helical scanning mode, 0.5 second gantry rotation time, minimum and maximum mA of 75 and 740, respectively, 120 kVp, 0.984:1 beam pitch, and a 40 mm table feed per gantry rotation. Standard-dose CT images were reconstructed with FBP using standard and bone kernels. Low-dose CT images were reconstructed with the FBP and ASIR technique using standard and bone kernels, and the MBIR algorithm. A blending factor of 50% was used for ASIR. All images are reconstructed with a 0.625 mm slice thickness which is standard for reading high resolution CT of the chest in our institute. Each image data set was coded, patient information was removed, and the sets were randomized by a study coauthor (N.N., with 12 years of experience) to enable double-blinded evaluation. All images were transferred to a commercially available workstation (Advantage Windows 4.2; GE Healthcare). A 21.2" color monitor with 1536×2048 of resolution was used for evaluation.

Assessment of lesion detectability

First, one thoracic radiologist (S.M. with 25 years of experience) evaluated the presence or absence of abnormal structures in the lung and mediastinum on standard-dose FBP CT. Abnormal lung structures were assessed in four categories: consolidation or mass, ground-glass attenuation, reticular opacity, and decreased lung attenuation (bulla, emphysema, or cyst). The abnormal mediastinal structures were assessed in one category: lymph node enlargement (>1 cm along the minor axis).

Then, two thoracic radiologists (Y.I., with 14 years of experience, and K.K., with 15 years of experience) were asked to evaluate the image quality of those abnormal structures by consensus. Each image series was displayed in the blinded and randomized manner. The observers were previously informed of the presence and location of the lesions in the lung and mediastinum for evaluation. The radiologists were not aware of the clinical information, patient data, or image reconstruction techniques. Visualization of abnormal structures was evaluated on a 5-point scale (5 = excellent image quality with demarcation of structures, 4 = slight increase in noise or artifact, 3 = moderate increase in noise or artifact, 2 = severe increase in noise or artifact, and 1 = not applicable for the evaluation). Images were displayed in the lung image setting (window level, -500 HU; window width, 1500 HU) and in the mediastinal image setting (window level, 40 HU; window width, 350 HU) for evaluation. The observers were allowed to change the window width and window level and to use the pan/zoom functions.

Image noise analysis

Objective assessment of image noise was performed by measuring the standard deviation of pixel values in homogeneous regions-of-interest (ROI) within the descending aorta at the level of the ventricular cavities on the standard kernel images. Care was taken to avoid superimposition of the ROI on the inner portion of the aortic wall.

The visual perception of noise, defined by a grainy appearance of the CT images, was evaluated by two thoracic radiologists (Y.I., with 14 years of experience, and K.K., with 15 years of experience) who were not aware of any clinical information or image reconstruction techniques. Images were displayed in the lung image setting (window level, -500 HU; window width, 1500 HU) and in the mediastinal image setting (window level, 40 HU; window width, 350 HU) for evaluation. Both readers evaluated image quality for the CT images reconstructed with the FBP, ASIR, and MBIR techniques by consensus. On each series of lung and mediastinal images, the image noise was graded on a 5-point scale (5 = minimum, 4 = less than average noise, 3 = average noise with an acceptable image, 2 = above average noise, and 1 = unacceptable image noise).

Radiation dose analysis

To assess the radiation dose associated with the chest CT examinations, the total dose-length product, which represents the total absorbed dose for all the scan series, was recorded. Estimated effective doses were calculated from the total dose-length product using a revised normalized effective dose constant of 0.014 [13].

Statistical analysis

Data were recorded on worksheets (Excel; Microsoft, Redmond, WA) and analyzed using Excel and SPSS for Windows, version 19 (SPSS, Inc, Chicago, IL). Continuous values are presented as mean ± standard deviation. Differences in objective image noise measurements, image noise scores, lesion conspicuity scores, and radiation dose were analyzed by the Wilcoxon signed-rank test. Differences by ages between male and female subjects were tested with the unpaired Student's t-test. A P value of less than 0.05 was considered to represent a statistically significant difference.

Results

There were no statistically significant differences associated with age in both male and the female patients in the present study (p = 0.05). Of the 55 patients evaluated, 45 patients (82%) had abnormal lung or mediastinal structures detected on chest CT. Abnormal structures were distributed as follows: areas of consolidation or mass in 27 patients, ground-glass attenuation in 22 patients, reticular opacity in 7 patients, areas of decreased lung attenuation (bulla, emphysema, or cyst) in 18 patients, and enlargement of mediastinal lymph nodes in 10 patients.

Lesion conspicuity

Figure 1 shows a representative case with mediastinal lymph node enlargement. In Table 1, the results of lesion conspicuity on the chest CT are summarized. Concerning visualization of mediastinal lymph node enlargement, the image quality score on low-dose MBIR CT (4.7 ± 0.5) was significantly improved in comparison with low-dose FBP and ASIR CT (3.0 ± 0.5, p = 0.004; 4.0 ± 0.5, p = 0.02, respectively), and was nearly identical to the score of standard-dose FBP image (4.8 ± 0.4, p = 0.66). Image quality score of consolidation or mass, ground-glass attenuation, or reticular opacity on low-dose MBIR CT was 4.9 ± 0.2, 4.8 ± 0.4, and 5.0 ± 0, respectively, showing no significant differences in comparison with low-dose ASIR, low- and standard-dose FBP CT. As to areas of decreased lung attenuation (bulla, emphysema, or cyst), the image quality score on low-dose MBIR CT (4.9 ± 0.2) was slightly better compared to low-dose FBP and ASIR CT (4.5 ± 0.6, p = 0.01; 4.6 ± 0.5, p = 0.01, respectively). Figure 2 shows a comparison of image quality between standard-dose FBP and low-dose MBIR CT in a patient with lung cavities and reticular opacity. Low-dose CT with MBIR offers equivalent image quality compared with standard-dose FBP CT in this patient.

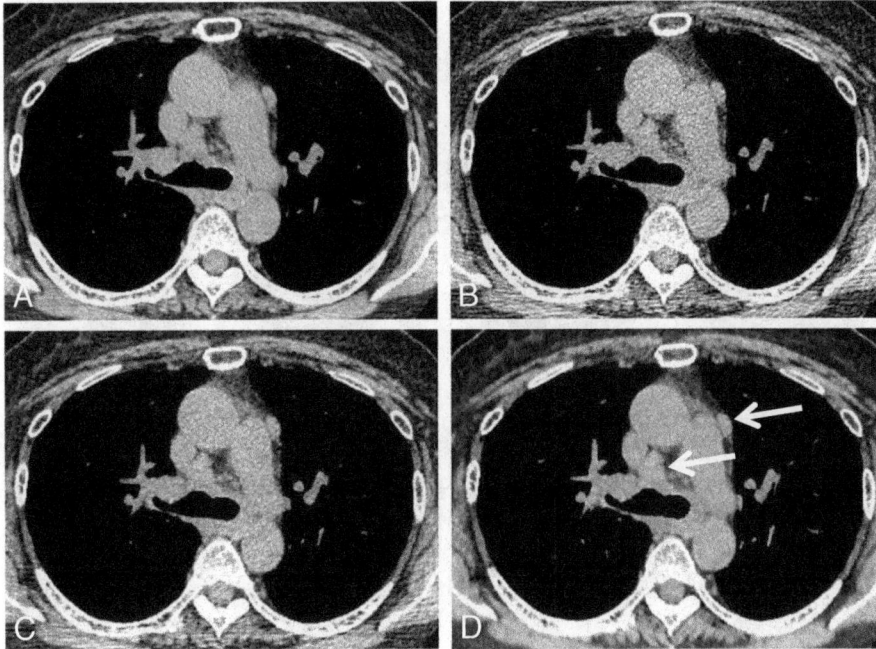

Figure 1 Transverse chest CT through the ascending aorta in a 64 year-old woman with mediastinal lymph node enlargement (arrows). Images were obtained with standard-dose FBP CT **(A)**, low-dose FBP CT **(B)**, low-dose ASIR 50% **(C)**, and low-dose MBIR method **(D)**. Note the excellent depiction of mediastinal lymph nodes on the low-dose MBIR image (lesion conspicuity score 5), compared with low-dose CT with FBP (score 3) and ASIR (score 4). Objective image noise on low-dose MBIR CT is 12.12 HU, showing higher than those on standard-dose FBP (17.72 HU), low-dose FBP (27.69 HU), and low-dose ASIR CT (20.76 HU) in this patient.

Image noise

In Figure 3, the mean values of objective noise measurements at the level of the descending aorta are summarized. Image noise on low-dose MBIR CT (11.6 ± 1.0 HU) were significantly lower than those on low-dose FBP CT (30.9 ± 3.9 HU, $p < 0.001$) and low-dose ASIR CT (21.1 ± 2.6 HU, $p < 0.001$), with mean noise reductions of $62.1 \pm 3.3\%$ and $44.5 \pm 4.9\%$, respectively. In addition, low-dose MBIR CT demonstrated significantly reduced image noise in comparison with standard-dose FBP CT (16.6 ± 2.3 HU, $p < 0.001$) with a mean noise reduction of $29.3 \pm 8.2\%$. The results of image noise scores on chest CT images are shown in Figure 4. There was a significant reduction in the level of subjective image noise on low-dose MBIR CT (4.6 ± 0.5) compared with that of low-dose FBP (2.5 ± 0.6, $p < 0.001$) and ASIR CT (3.5 ± 0.6, $p = 0.01$) on the mediastinal images. For the lung images, there was a slight but significant improvement in image noise with the MBIR technique (5.0 ± 0.2), compared with the FBP (4.6 ± 0.5, $p < 0.001$) and ASIR techniques (4.9 ± 0.4, $p = 0.01$) on low-dose CT. There were no significant differences in image noise scores on the lung images between low-dose MBIR and standard-dose FBP CT (5.0 ± 0.2 vs 4.9 ± 0.2, $p = 0.32$).

Radiation dose

The mean dose-length product and estimated effective dose of low-dose chest CT was 112.5 ± 55.6 mGy·cm

Table 1 Comparison of lesion conspicuity between filtered back projections and iterative reconstructions

	Standard-dose CT with FBP	Low-dose CT with FBP	Low-dose CT with ASIR	Low-dose CT with MBIR
Consolidation or mass	4.9 ± 0.2	4.7 ± 0.6	4.8 ± 0.4	4.9 ± 0.2
Ground-glass attenuation	5.0 ± 0.2	4.8 ± 0.4	4.8 ± 0.4	4.8 ± 0.4
Reticular opacity	5.0 ± 0	4.9 ± 0.4	5.0 ± 0	5.0 ± 0
Decreased lung attenuation (bulla, emphysema, or cyst)	4.9 ± 0.2	4.5 ± 0.6 *§	4.6 ± 0.5 *§	4.9 ± 0.2
Mediastinal lymph node enlargement	4.8 ± 0.4	3.0 ± 0.5 *§	4.0 ± 0.5 *§	4.7 ± 0.5

CT Computed tomography, *FBP* Filtered back projection, *ASIR* Adaptive statistical iterative reconstruction, *MBIR* Model-based iterative reconstruction.
The comparisons of lesion conspicuity scores were made by the Wilcoxon signed-rank test. * refers to statistically significant differences with standard-dose FBP CT (* $p < 0.05$). § refers to statistically significant differences with low-dose MBIR CT (§ $p < 0.05$).

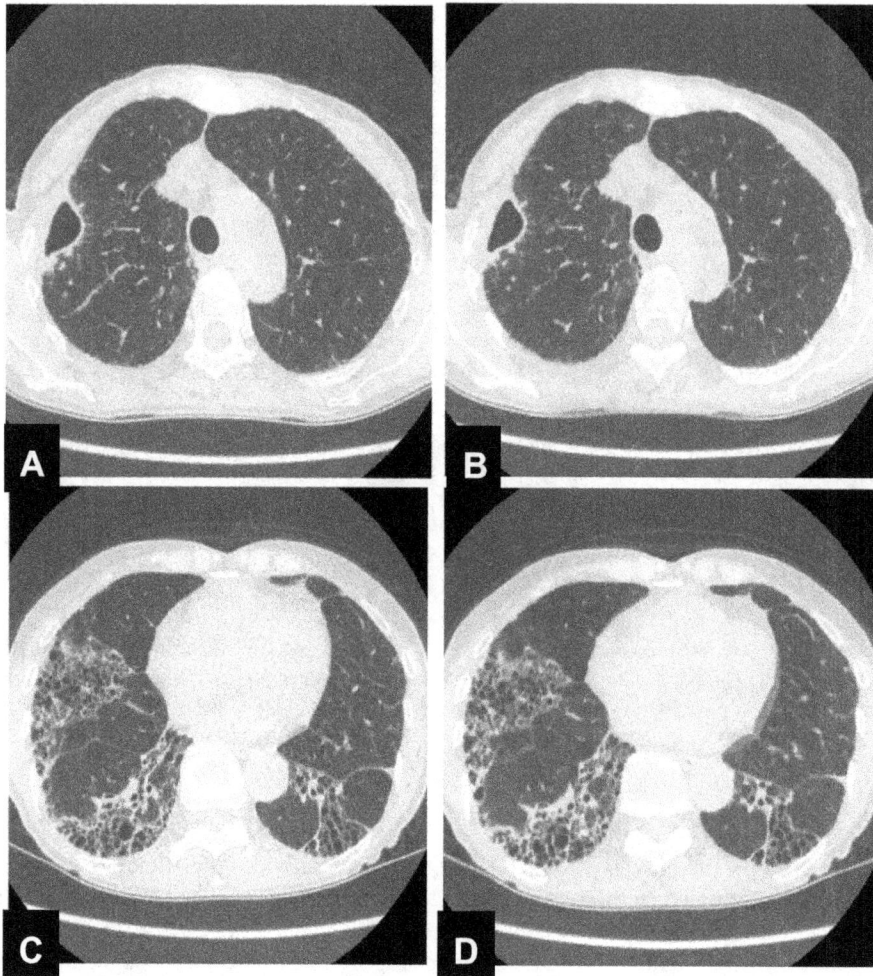

Figure 2 Standard-dose FBP CT images at the level of aortic arch (A) and at the level of lower lung lobe (C), and low-dose MBIR CT images at the corresponding level (B and D) in a 67 year-old woman with lung cavities and reticular opacity. Image quality score for those lesions on low-dose MBIR CT are both graded 5, showing equivalent on standard-dose FBP CT. Objective image noise measured is 13.04 on standard-dose FBP CT and 11.09 on low-dose MBIR CT in this patient.

and 1.6 ± 0.8 mSv, respectively. This was significantly lower than that of standard-dose chest CT (410.6 ± 165.2 mGy·cm, $p < 0.001$; 5.7 ± 2.3 mSv, $p < 0.0005$). The mean percentage of radiation dose reduction was $73.3 \pm 3.0\%$ with the low-dose CT protocol.

Discussion

The current prospective study demonstrated that MBIR techniques enabled an average of >70% radiation dose reduction compared with routine-dose FBP techniques for chest CT examinations without compromising diagnostic image quality. No significant differences were seen between low-dose MBIR and standard-dose FBP chest CT with regards to lesion detectability for lung consolidation or mass, ground-glass attenuation, or reticular opacity. On low-dose chest CT, the image quality of mediastinal lymph nodes and low attenuation

lung diseases were significantly improved by MBIR techniques in comparison with ASIR techniques. Objective image noise on low-dose MBIR CT was significantly lower than that on low-dose ASIR CT.

Over the past several years, there has been a concerted effort to reduce radiation exposure in thoracic CT with various methods including tube current modulation, BMI-based tube voltage reduction, decreased scan length, low tube current scanning, and ASIR [3,6-9,14-22]. Recently developed MBIR is a more advanced and complex iterative reconstruction technique in compared with ASIR in that the reconstruction algorithm includes modeling of the x-ray optic system. Prior phantom studies have reported the potential of MBIR in reduction of image noise and artifacts [10,23,24]. A recent *ex vivo* study [25] demonstrated that the MBIR method leads to significantly decreased image noise accompanied

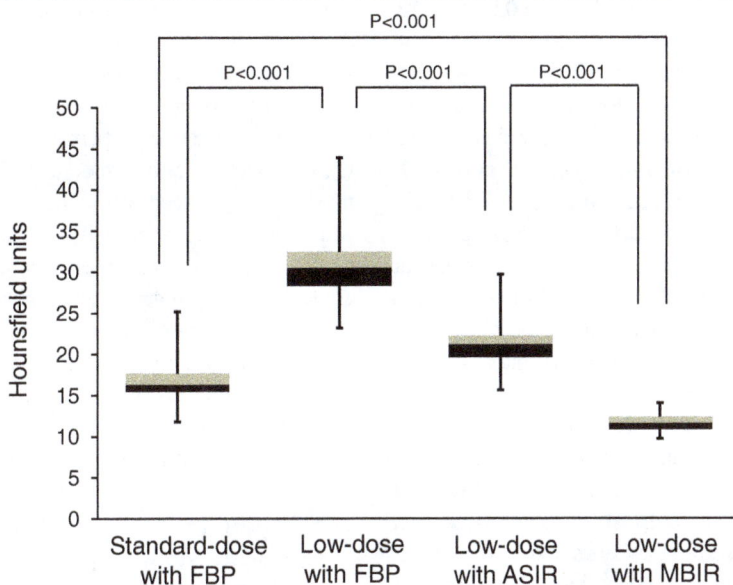

Figure 3 Comparison of objective image noise measurements. Images at the level of the descending aorta on the standard-dose CT with FBP and low-dose CT with FBP, ASIR, and MBIR. Low-dose MBIR CT demonstrated significantly reduced image noise in comparison with standard-dose FBP CT (p < 0.001) with a mean noise reduction of 29.3 ± 8.2%.

with a substantial improvement of image quality and contrast-noise-ratio compared to the FBP and ASIR techniques. Katsura M, et al. [12] showed that low-dose MBIR chest CT images had significantly lower objective image noise (16.93 ± 3.00) than low-dose ASIR (49.24 ± 9.11, p < 0.01) and standard-dose ASIR images (24.93 ± 4.65, p < 0.01). In line with these previous studies, image noise with low-dose MBIR CT (11.6 ± 1.0 HU) in our study was significantly lower than that with low-dose FBP CT (30.9 ± 3.9 HU, p < 0.001) and low-dose ASIR

CT (21.1 ± 2.6 HU, p < 0.001), with a mean noise reduction of 62.1 ± 3.3% and 44.5 ± 4.9%, respectively.

On the other hand, few data are available regarding its effect on diagnostic acceptability and lesion detectability on low-dose CT. We found that MBIR method is quite useful for improving image quality of mediastinal structures on low-dose chest CT. The present study demonstrated the lesion conspicuity score for mediastinal lymph node enlargement on low-dose MBIR CT (4.7 ± 0.5) was also significantly improved in comparison with

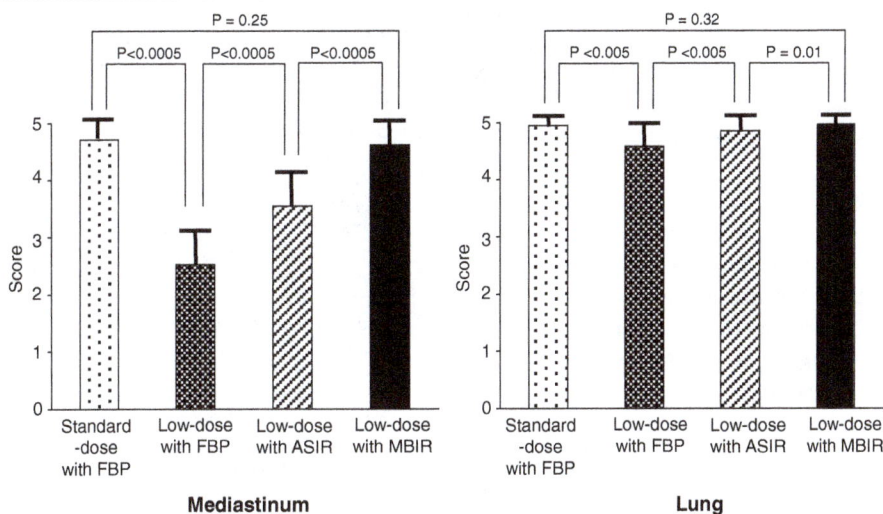

Figure 4 Subjective image noise score. Mediastinal and lung images of standard-dose CT aquired with FBP and low-dose CT with FBP, ASIR, and MBIR. The MBIR algorithm yields significantly improved image noise scores, especially of the mediastinal structures on low-dose chest CT.

low-dose FBP and ASIR CT (3.0 ± 0.5, p = 0.004; 4.0 ± 0.5, p = 0.02, respectively), and nearly identical to the conspicuity score for standard-dose FBP CT (4.8 ± 0.4, p = 0.66). The image quality score for decreased lung attenuation (bulla, emphysema, or cyst) on low-dose MBIR CT was slightly better than on low-dose FBP and ASIR CT, and similar to that on standard-dose FBP CT. Concerning visualization of consolidation or mass, ground-glass attenuation, or reticular opacity, there was no significant differences between low-dose MBIR CT and standard-dose FBP CT. Considering marked improvement of mediastinal image quality, low-dose MBIR CT can be alternative to standard-dose FBP CT. Although dose reduction is desirable for all patients, this new reconstruction algorithm may thus have significant impact in imaging young patients requiring CT, patients requiring serial CT follow-up, and the pregnant patients in whom imaging is deemed medically necessary. However, MBIR does have some drawbacks in the current setting. First, image processing is extremely slow. This is because MBIR is a complicated algorithm which uses multiple iterations and multiple models. Even with use of parallel processors, more than an hour is needed to process a typical 600-slice dataset. Because of this lengthy reconstruction time, initial application of this technique to clinical practice will mainly focus on patients with nonurgent or nonemergent conditions. Fortunately, in most practices, the majority of CT scans are performed in the outpatient setting, and immediate assessment is not mandatory. Furthermore, it is possible to have a preliminary set of ASIR images for immediate review. Second, the MBIR technique cannot be used for reconstruction of the electrocardiographic-gated CT images. It has already been reported that the ASIR technique can reduce image noise on coronary CT angiography [7]. Third, MBIR CT images have a slightly different "look and feel" compared with images reconstructed with FBP because images are reconstructed in a statistically optimal fashion. In this regard, Xu et al. recently raised a practical concern that statistical reconstruction might give an impression of somewhat reduced diagnostic value by radiologists who are used to FBP image appearance [26]. However, in the present study, standard dose FBP and low dose MBIR demonstrated equivalent diagnostic information. It is possible that interpreters can adapt themselves to the new look of MBIR in a relatively short period of time, particularly if they have preliminary experience with images from other iterative reconstruction techniques.

There were several limitations to the present study design. First, the sample size was small owing to the need for written informed consent for the additional radiation dose to participating patients. Second, image analysis was made by consensus between two readers and did not include assessment of inter- or intra-observer agreement between the two radiologists enrolled in this analysis. Because of the recent introduction of MBIR technique, this study design was considered a preliminary evaluation. Third, chest CT images with a noise index >36.33 were not assessed. It is possible that radiation doses of chest CT may be further decreased with MBIR. Fourth, for the ASIR method, a 50% blending factor was selected on the basis of vendor recommendations. It is conceivable that a higher ASIR percentage would allow even greater noise reduction and subsequent dose reduction. This idea needs to be balanced with concerns about loss of image detail with a higher degree of ASIR [6]. Fifth, the body size of the patients in this study was generally small. MBIR has not yet been assessed in extremely large or obese patients. Sixth, in this study, the observers evaluated the images in a blinded and randomized manner; however, they could recognize the reconstruction algorithms of the images to some extent because of differences in the appearances of the image data sets. This could be a potential source of observer bias.

Conclusion

In conclusion, MBIR shows greater potential than ASIR for providing diagnostically acceptable low-dose CT without compromising image quality. With radiation dose reduction of >70%, MBIR can provide equivalent lesion detectability of standard-dose FBP CT.

Abbreviations
ASIR: Adaptive statistical iterative reconstruction; CT: Computed tomography; FBP: Filtered back projection; MBIR: Model-based iterative reconstruction.

Competing interests
The authors have no competing interests to declare.

Authors' contributions
Author contributions were as following; conception and design (YI, KK, NN, SM, and HS), analysis and interpretation of data (YI and KK), drafting of the manuscript (YI), and revising it critically for important intellectual content (KK, SM, HS). All authors have read and approved the final version of the manuscript.

References
1. Brenner DJ, Hall EJ: Computed tomography: an increasing source of radiation exposure. N Engl J Med 2007, 357:2277–2284.
2. Nelson RC, Feuerlein S, Boll DT: New iterative reconstruction techniques for cardiovascular computed tomography: how do they work, and what are the advantages and disadvantages? J Cardiovac Comput Tomgr 2011, 5:286–292.
3. Prakash P, Kalra MK, Ackman JB, Digmarthy SR, Hsieh J, Do S, et al: Diffuse lung disease: CT of the chest with adaptive statistical iterative reconstruction technique. Radiology 2010, 256:261–269.
4. Marin D, Nelson RC, Schindera ST, Richard S, Youngblood RS, Yoshizumi TT, et al: Low-tube-voltage, high-tube-current multidetector abdominal CT: improved image quality and decreased radiation dose with adaptive statistical iterative reconstruction algorithm – initial clinical experience. Radiology 2010, 254:145–153.
5. Leipsic J, Nguyen G, Brown J, Sin D, Mayo JR: A prospective evaluation of dose reduction and image quality in chest CT using adaptive statistical iterative reconstruction. AJR Am J Roentgenol 2010, 195:1095–1099.
6. Singh S, Kalra MK, Gilman MD, Hseigh J, Pien HH, Digmarthy SR, et al: Adaptive statistical iterative reconstruction technique for radiation dose reduction in chest CT: a pilot study. Radiology 2011, 259:565–573.
7. Leipsic J, Labountry TM, Heilbron B, Min JK, Mancini GB, Lin FY, Taylor C, Dunning A, Earls JP: Adaptive statistical iterative reconstruction: assessment of image noise and image quality in coronary CT angiography. AJR Am J Roentgenol 2010, 195:649–654.

8. Sagara Y, Hara A, Pavlicek W, Silva AC, Paden RG, Wu Q: **Abdominal CT: comparison of low-dose CT with adaptive statistical iterative reconstruction and routine-dose CT with filtered back projection in 53 patients.** *AJR Am J Roentgenol* 2010, **195:**713–719.
9. Prakash P, Kalra MK, Kambadakone AK, Pien H, Hsieh J, Blake MA, Sahani DV: **Reducing abdominal CT radiation dose with adaptive statistical iterative reconstruction technique.** *Invest Radiol* 2010, **45:**202–210.
10. Thibault JB, Sauer KD, Bouman CA, Hsieh J: **A three-dimensional statistical approach to improved image quality for multislice helical CT.** *Med Phys* 2007, **34:**4526–4544.
11. Yamada Y, Jinzaki M, Tanami Y, *et al*: **Model-based iterative reconstruction technique for ultralow-dose computed tomography of the lung. A pilot study.** *Invest Radiol* 2012, **47:**482–489.
12. Katsura M, Matsuda I, Akahane M, *et al*: **Model-base iterative reconstruction technique for radiation dose reduction in chest CT: comparison with adaptive statistical reconstruction technique.** *Eur Radiol* 2012, **22:**1613–1623.
13. EUR 16262: *European guidelines on quality criteria for computed tomography*; 2009. http://www.drs.dk/guidelines/ct/quality.
14. Funama Y, Awai K, Miyazaki O, *et al*: **Improvement of low-contrast detectability in low-dose hepatic multidetector computed tomography using a novel adaptive filter: evaluation with a computer- simulated liver including tumors.** *Invest Radiol* 2006, **41:**1–7.
15. Funama Y, Awai K, Nakayama Y, *et al*: **Radiation dose reduction without degradation of low-contrast detectability at abdominal multisection CT with a low-tube voltage technique: phantom study.** *Radiology* 2005, **237:**905–910.
16. Kalra MK, Maher MM, Blake MA, *et al*: **Detection and characterization of lesions on low-radiation-dose abdominal CT images postprocessed with noise reduction filters.** *Radiology* 2004, **232:**791–797.
17. Kalra MK, Maher MM, Toth TL, *et al*: **Strategies for CT radiation dose optimization.** *Radiology* 2004, **230:**619–628.
18. Linton OW, Mettler FA Jr: **National conference ondose reduction in CT, with an emphasis on pediatric patients.** *AJR* 2003, **181:**321–329.
19. Nakayama Y, Awai K, Funama Y, *et al*: **Abdominal CT with low tube voltage: preliminary observations about radiation dose, contrast enhancement, image quality, and noise.** *Radiology* 2005, **237:**945–951.
20. Okumura M, Ota T, Kainuma K, Sayre JW, Mc-Nitt-Gray M, Katada K: **Effect of edge-preserving adaptive image filter on low-contrast detectability in CT systems: application of ROC analysis.** *Int J Biomed Imaging* 2008, **2008:**379486.
21. Valentin J: **International Commission on Radiation Protection. Managing patient dose in multidetector computed tomography (MDCT): ICRP publication 102.** *Ann ICRP* 2007, **37:**1–79.
22. Kalra MK, Maher MM, Sahani DV, *et al*: **Low dose CT of the abdomen: evaluation of image improvement with use of noise reduction filters pilot study.** *Radiology* 2003, **228:**251–256.
23. Ziegler A, Kohler T, Proska R: **Noise and resolution in images reconstructed with FBP and OSC algorithms for CT.** *Med Phys* 2007, **34:**585–598.
24. Yu Z, Thibault J, Bouman C, Sauer K, Hsieh J: **Fast model-base X-ray CT reconstruction using spatially non-homogeneous ICD optimization.** *IEEE Trans Image Process* 2011, **20:**161–175.
25. Scheffel H, Stolzmann P, Schlett CL, *et al*: **Coronary artery plaques: Cardiac CT with model-based and adaptive-statistical iterative reconstruction technique.** *Eur J Radiol* 2011. in press.
26. Xu J, Mahesh M, Tsui BMW: **Is iterative reconstruction ready for MDCT?** *J Am Coll Radiol* 2009, **6:**274–276.

5

Increased pelvic incidence may lead to arthritis and sagittal orientation of the facet joints at the lower lumbar spine

Thorsten Jentzsch[1*], James Geiger[1], Samy Bouaicha[1], Ksenija Slankamenac[1], Thi Dan Linh Nguyen-Kim[2] and Clément ML Werner[1]

Abstract

Background: Correct sagittal alignment with a balanced pelvis and spine is crucial in the management of spinal disorders. The pelvic incidence (PI) describes the sagittal pelvic alignment and is position-independent. It has barely been investigated on CT scans. Furthermore, no studies have focused on the association between PI and facet joint (FJ) arthritis and orientation. Therefore, our goal was to clarify the remaining issues about PI in regard to (1) physiologic values, (2) age, (3) gender, (4) lumbar lordosis (LL) and (5) FJ arthritis and orientation using CT scans.

Methods: We retrospectively analyzed CT scans of 620 individuals, with a mean age of 43 years, who presented to our traumatology department and underwent a whole body CT scan, between 2008 and 2010. The PI was determined on sagittal CT planes of the pelvis by measuring the angle between the hip axis to an orthogonal line originating at the center of the superior end plate axis of the first sacral vertebra. We also evaluated LL, FJ arthritis and orientation of the lumbar spine.

Results: 596 individuals yielded results for (1) PI with a mean of 50.8°. There was no significant difference for PI and (2) age, nor (3) gender. PI was significantly and linearly correlated with (4) LL ($p = < 0.0001$). Interestingly, PI and (5) FJ arthritis displayed a significant and linear correlation ($p = 0.0062$) with a cut-off point at 50°. An increased PI was also significantly associated with more sagitally oriented FJs at L5/S1 ($p = 0.01$).

Conclusion: PI is not correlated with age nor gender. However, this is the first report showing that PI is significantly and linearly associated with LL, FJ arthritis and more sagittal FJ orientation at the lower lumbar spine. This may be caused by a higher contact force on the lower lumbar FJs by an increased PI. Once symptomatic or in the event of spinal trauma, patients with increased PI and LL could benefit from corrective surgery and spondylodesis.

Keywords: Pelvic incidence, Age, Gender, Lumbar Lordosis, Facet joint arthritis, Orientation

Background

Pelvic rotation has emerged from the genesis of an erect position of the human spine [1]. Nowadays, a proper sagittally oriented pelvis, which acts as a basis for the building block of the entire spine, and an ideal lordotic curvature of the spine equilibrate each other in regard to overall spinal balance [2,3]. Nevertheless, aging and spinal deformities, such as spondylolisthesis may change spinal balance [4]. Thus, the establishment of a neutral upright sagittal alignment with the pelvis and spine in sync is essential in the management of spinal disorders [5,6].

Although other parameters have been suggested to be superior in the study of spinal balance, pelvic incidence (PI) remains the most studied parameter [7]. It was introduced by Duval-Beaupère et al. [8] in 1992. Describing the sagittal pelvic alignment, it constitues a true anatomic parameter, since it does not change with position, e.g. standing or supine [9]. This attributes to the fact that the sacrum does not move within the rigid pelvic ring, but rotates around the bicoxofemoral axis as a whole unit [10,11]. Measurements are carried out by putting the center of the superior end plate of the first

* Correspondence: thorsten.jentzsch@usz.ch
[1]Division of Trauma Surgery, Department of Surgery, University Hospital Zuerich, Zuerich, Switzerland
Full list of author information is available at the end of the article

sacral vertebra in relation to the bicoxofemoral axis (Figure 1). Normal values range around 57°, with a variability of up to 10°, whereby higher values indicate a more tilted pelvis [12-15]. Nonetheless, the optimal spinal balance remains poorly definced [16].

Yet, there are a handful of remaining issues about the PI. (1) It has been studied extensively on X-rays [17,18]. But overlap or magnification of structures my falsify the measured angle [7,17]. Furthermore, very few studies [4,12,13] in the English literature have investigated the PI on CT scans, which are more more precise and more commonly used nowadays. (2) PI has been reported to increase until the age of ten and than stabilize [19-21], but other reports [22-26] have shown an increase later on during life, especially with spinal deformities, such as spondylolisthesis, or sacral fractures. (3) Even though most studies [14,27-29] have not found a gender difference, another study [18] has documented significant higher values for females. (4) Interestingly, PI may increase in order to compensate for a decrease in lumbar lordosis (LL) [24,25]. A simple predictive equation has been proposed recently [30]: LL = PI +9° (+/− 9°). (5) Facet joint (FJ) arthritis may arise from several misbalanced forces, such as increased LL, which leads to higher contact forces on the FJs, compression, rotation, and shear as well as more sagittal orientation of the lower lumbar spine, which may lead to spondylolysis and spondylolisthesis [31-36]. However, this may be prevented by compensatory mechanisms of the pelvis and a previous osteologic study [37] has linked increased pelvic lordosis to FJ arthritis at L5/S1. Other previous studies [38,39] have also found an association between the pelvic geometry and lumbar degenerative processes. However, none have focused on the association between PI and FJ arthritis, let alone PI and FJ orientation. Therefore, we hypothesized that increased PI is associated with FJ arthritis and changes in FJ orientation.

Therefore, our goal was to clarify the remaining issues about PI in regard to (1) physiologic values, (2) age, (3) gender, (4) LL and, according to our main hypothesis (5) FJ arthritis and orientation using CT scans.

Methods

The study has been approved by the local research ethics review committee (Kantonale Ethikkommission Zürich (KEK-ZH)-Nr.2011-0507). We included and retrospectively analyzed CT scans of 620 individuals (2480 functional units consisting of two FJs and one intervertebral disc on each level between L2 and S1) [40], with a median age of 39 (IQR 27–54), who presented to our traumatology department and underwent a whole body CT scan, including the pelvis and lumbar spine, between 2008 and 2010. Exclusion criteria involved fractures of the lumbar spine and pelvis that may have changed the spino-pelvic alignment and CT studies that did not include sagittally reconstructed pelvic cross-sections. A dual-source computed tomography scanner (Somatom Definition, Siemens Healthcare, Forchheim, Germany) was used [41]. Our study utilized CT scans instead of plain radiographs, because there is a paucity on studies about the PI and FJs are more accurately displayed [12,13,42].

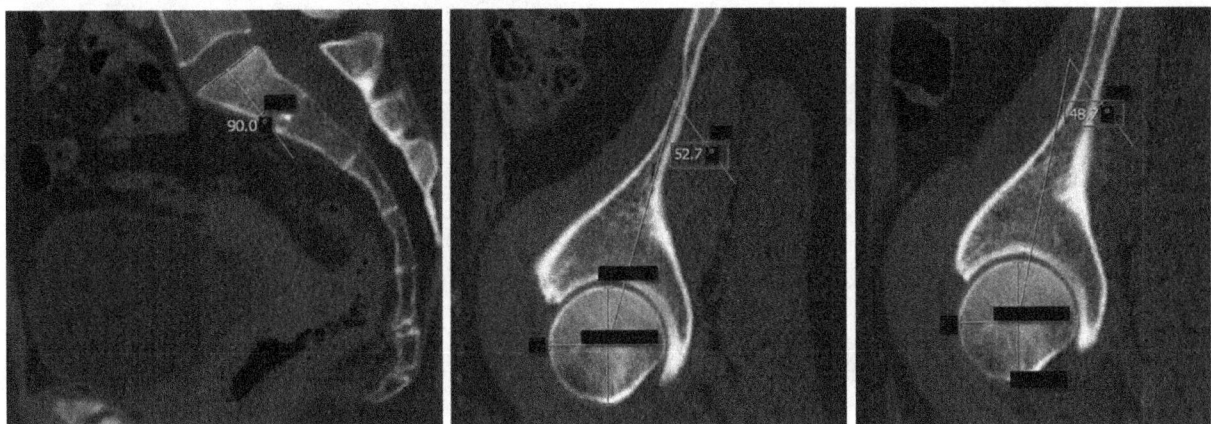

Figure 1 Pelvic Incidence (PI): The PI was determined on sagittal CT planes of the pelvis. A line was drawn along the axis of the superior end plate of S1 (left image). Then, originating at the center of this axis, an orthogonal line was drawn (left image). Secondly, the middle of the femoral head was determined by the intersecting point of a vertical and horizontal line within the femoral head (middle and right image). Finally, a line was drawn from the middle of the each femoral head to the center of the superior end plate axis and the angle was measured in regard to the orthogonal line originating at this point (middle and right image). The red box indicates the PI. The blacked out numbers were disregarded because they were created automatically by our software and contained irrelevant information. In order to acquire the superposition of the two femoral heads, left and right, the PI was measured for both sides and the mean was stated.

(1) The PI was determined on sagittal CT planes of the pelvis using the AGFA® Impax viewer by measuring the angle between the hip axis to an orthogonal line originating at the center of the superior end plate axis of the first sacral vertebra [8] (Figure 1). Precisely, this was done in the following manner: Firstly, a line was drawn along the axis of the superior end plate of S1. Then, an orthogonal line originating at the center of this axis was drawn. Secondly, the middle of the femoral head was determined by the intersecting point of a vertical and horizontal line within the femoral head. Finally, a line was drawn from the middle of the each femoral head to the center of the superior end plate axis and the angle was measured in regard to the orthogonal line originating at this point, In order to acquire the superposition of the two femoral heads, left and right, the PI was measured for both sides and the mean was stated. (2) Individuals were grouped into different age groups according to low, i.e. 40 years, and high, i.e. 70 years, cut-off points chosen by Kalichman et al. [43] as well as the assumption of different activity levels and degenerative processes in younger individuals ≤ 30 years, middle-aged individuals between 31–50 years and aging individuals between 51–70 years. The first group included individuals ≤ 40 and ≥ 41 years and the second group included individuals ≤ 30 years, 31–50 years, 51–70 years and ≥ 71 years. (3) Gender was also evaluated. (4) LL was evaluated on the middle of the sagittal planeby measuring the angle between the superior endplates of L1 and S1, based on the definition of Stokes and the Scoliosis Research Society [27,44] (Figure 2). The middle of the sagittal plane could be easily determined in Agfa® Impax viewer by a coexisting alignment line at the axial plane that can be viewed on the frame right next to the sagittal plane. (5) FJs of the lumbar spine were evaluated between the second lumbar and the first sacral level [45] (Figure 3). Axial planes with the largest intersecting set of the superior and inferior FJ process were chosen. Assessment of FJ arthritis was carried out as previously described in similar studies, where a grading scale described by Pathria was used [46,47]. Grade 0 (normal) indicates a normal facet joint, whereas grades 1 – 3 display increasing signs of FJ arthritis with each grade including signs of the lower grade. Grade 1 (mild) shows joint space narrowing, grade 2 (moderate) demonstrates sclerosis and grade 3 (severe) reveals osteophytes [48]. FJ orientation in the axial plane was evaluated by measuring the angle between the midline of the sagittal plane and the midline of the FJ as described by Schuller and Mahato [49,50]. The midline of the sagittal planes corresponds to a line drawn through the center of the vertebral body and spinous process. Therefore, each FJ was compared against this line. The overall FJ orientation was calculated by averaging the angles between the right and left side of the FJs. We

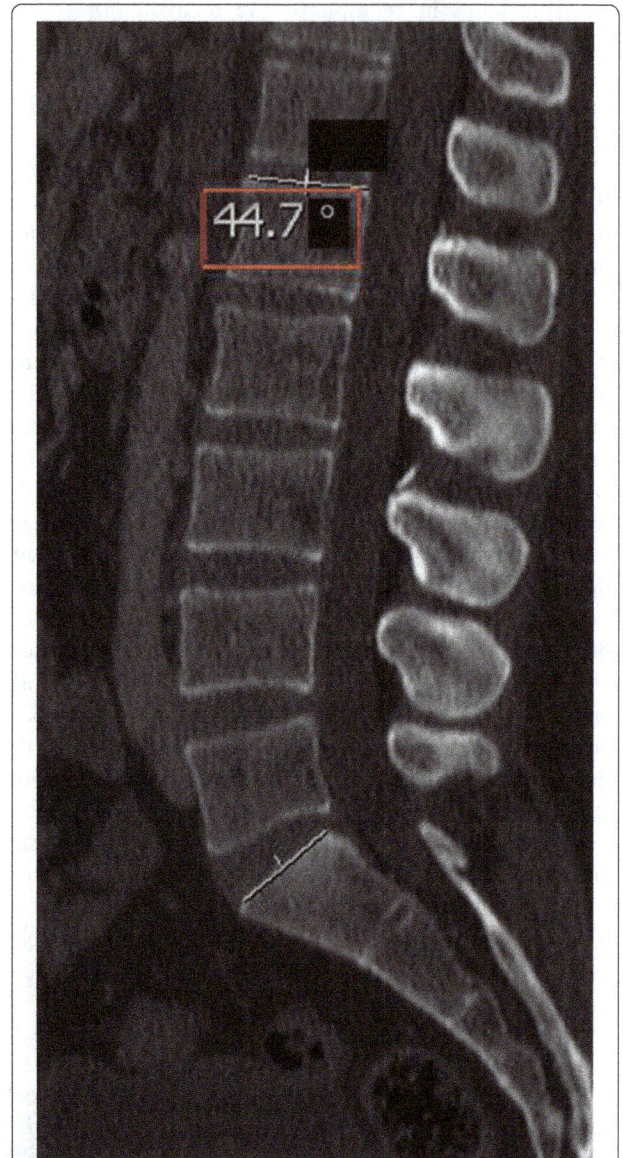

Figure 2 Lumbar Lordosis (LL): LL was evaluated on median sagittal slides by measuring the angle between the superior endplates of L1 and S1, based on the definition of Stokes and the Scoliosis Research Society [27,44]. The red box indicates the PI. The blacked out numbers were disregarded because they were created automatically by our software and contained irrelevant information.

used absolute angles, indicating that we did not consider rotation in one direction as positive nor rotation in the opposite direction as negative. The FJ orientation was labeled as coronal if angles were $> 45°$ and sagittal if angles were $\leq 45°$ [51].

All statistical analysis was performed by the Institute for Social and Preventive Medicine, Division of Biostatistics at the University of Zuerich, using the R program [52]. In a first step of the analysis, we expressed distribution of

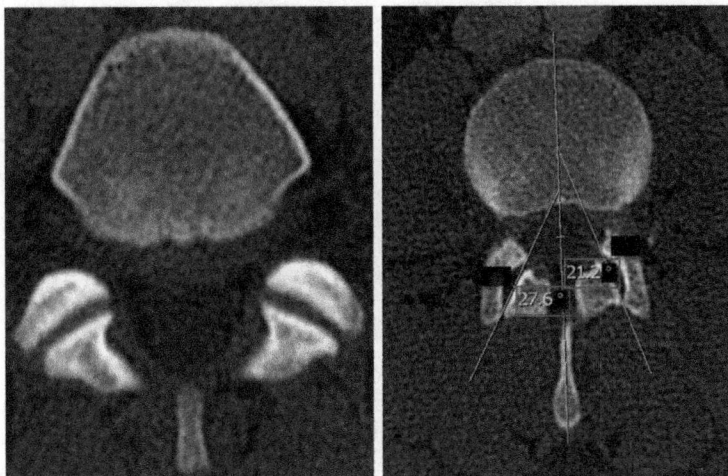

Figure 3 Facet Joints (FJs): FJ orientation was evaluated by measuring the angle between the midline of the sagittal plane and the midline of the FJ as described by Schuller and Mahato [49,50]. Coronal FJ orientation is shown on the left side, whereas sagittal orientation including measurement of FJ orientation is shown on the right side. The red box indicates the PI. The blacked out numbers were disregarded because they were created automatically by our software and contained irrelevant information.

variables using means and standard deviation (SD) for normally distributed data, and medians and interquartile ranges for non-normally distributed data. We tested data for normality with the Kolmogorow-Smirnow test and performed quantile-quantile plots of dependent variables. Several different statistical approaches were applied to test the remaining issues mentioned above and our main hypothesis [53], which assumed an association between an increased PI and FJ arthritis as well as changes in FJ orientation. (1) PI is a numerical measure without normal distribution, therefore simple linear regression models were applied. Therefore, PI was log transformed. An F-Test was used for nominal explanatory variables, such as (2) age, (3) gender and (5) FJ orientation. To compare PI with the numerical measure (4) LL, a linear regression was used. (5) FJ arthritis is an ordinal measure and in order to compare it to PI, which was not log transformed, FJ arthritis was used as an outcome and a proportional odds model was performed. This study is an observational study, which means that analysis follows a descriptive and exploratory form and p-values are interpreted as a quantitative measure of the evidence against the null hypothesis. Significant difference was assumed if $p < 0.05$.

Results

1) PI

Of our 620 individuals, who underwent a whole-body CT scan, 596 individuals yielded results for PI. 24 (3.9%) individuals could not be evaluated because the pelvis had not been imaged or reconstructed sagittally. The median for PI was 49.9° (IQR 43.2°-57.7°).

2) PI and Age

There was no significant difference for PI and age (Figure 4). In the 314 individuals of the younger age group ≤ 40 years, the mean PI (50.1°) was slightly lower than the one (51.7°) in the 282 individuals of the older age group >40 years (p = 0.07) (Table 1). These two groups are relatively equally populated and statistical analysis may be assumed to have enough power. There was no significant difference (p = 0.35) for PI when grouping individuals into age groups of ≤ 30 years, 31–50 years, 51–70 years and ≥ 71 years either (Table 1).

3) PI and Gender

We did not find a significant difference for PI and gender (p = 0.28) (Figure 5). The mean PI (50.3°) for 193 females was slightly lower than the one (51.1°) for 403 males (Table 2).

4) PI and LL

The mean value for LL was 48.9°. PI was strongly correlated with LL (p = < 0.0001, r = 0.625) (Figure 6 and Figure 7). The lower the PI, the less LL was present. The mean PI (45.5°) was lower for 307 individuals with a LL less than the mean value compared with the one (56.5°) for 287 individuals with a LL more than the mean value.

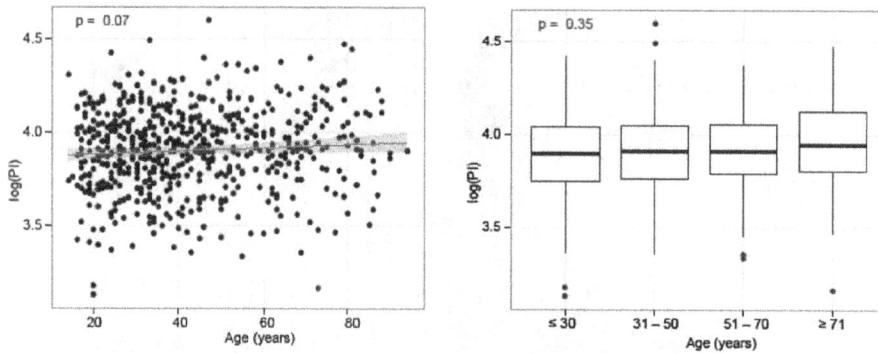

Figure 4 Pelvic Incidence (PI) and Age: There was no significant difference for PI and age.

5) PI and FJ Arthritis and Orientation

PI and FJ arthritis displayed a significant association (p = 0.0062, odds ratio 1.020 [95%-CI 1.005, 1.034]) (Figure 8 and Figure 7), whereby an increased PI was associated with increased FJ arthritis. Interestingly, the cut-off point ranged around a PI of 50°. The median PI of 49.6° (ICR 43°-56.8°) was lower in 293 individuals without FJ arthritis (grade 0) compared to the median PI of 50.4° (IQR 43.5°-59.3°) in 301 individuals with signs of FJ arthritis (grade 1–3). The unadjusted difference was 1.76° (95% CI: -0.02-3.5, p = 0.052). The median PI of 51.7° (IQR 43.2-57.0) was highest in 97 individuals with the most severe FJ arthritis (grade 3) compared to the median PI of 49.8° in individuals with a lower grade of FJ arthritis (grade 0–2). The unadjusted difference was 2.2 (95% CI: -0.18-4.59, p = 0.070). There was a significant difference in the logarithm of the mean PI and FJ orientation at the lower lumbar spine. Specifically, an increased PI was significantly associated with sagitally oriented FJs at L5/S1 (p = 0.01) (Figure 9 and Figure 7). However, comparison of the logarithm of the mean PI with FJ orientation at the upper lumbar spine did not reveal any significant differences (p = 0.71, 0.23 and 0.35 at L2/3, L3/4 and L4/5).

Discussion

Our study investigated the largest sample of CT scans from different individuals in the literature in regard to PI and (1) its physiologic values, (2) age, (3) gender, (4) LL and marks the first study to investigate its relationship with (5) FJ arthritis and orientation. We were able to show that the (1) mean value for PI on CT scans ranges around 50.8°. PI was not significantly correlated with (2) age, nor (3) gender. However, we found a significant linear relationship between PI and (4) LL, (5) FJ arthritis and sagittal FJ orientation at the lower lumbar spine, namely L5/S1. PI and FJ orientation at the upper lumbar spine were not significantly correlated.

Limitations of our study attribute to the fact that all individuals presented to a trauma department. Even though a selection bias may be assumed, we did not include individuals with a fracture of the lumbar spine or pelvis. Furthermore, we did not pay special attention to degenerative disc disease since this has been investigated in previous studies [40,54,55]. Due to the retrospective nature of this study, we were not able to investigate which individuals showed clinical signs of FJ arthritis.

Table 1 There was no significant difference for PI and age (p = 0.07)

	Overall	Females	Males	Mean PI	P Value
≤ 40 years	314	103	211	50.1°	0.07
> 40 years	282	90	192	51.7°	
≤ 30 years	185	57	128	50.0°	0.35
31-50 years	226	70	156	50.6°	
51-70 years	124	40	84	51.3°	
≥ 71 years	61	26	35	53.3°	

In the 314 individuals of the younger age group ≤ 40 years, the mean PI (50.1°) was slightly lower than the one (51.7°) in the 282 individuals of the older age group ≥ 40 years.

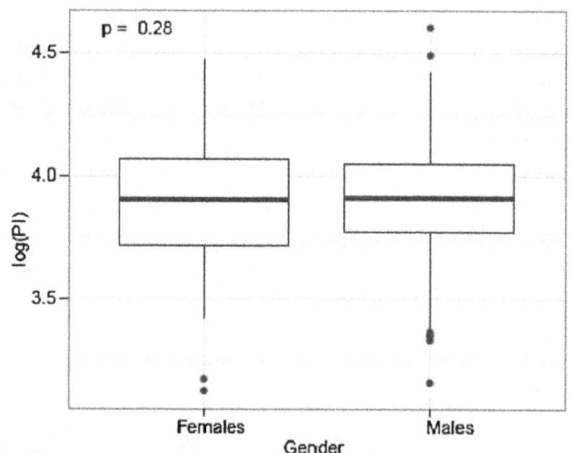

Figure 5 Pelvic Incidence (PI) and Gender: We did not find a significant difference for PI and gender.

Table 2 We did not find a significant difference for PI and gender (p = 0.28)

	Females	Males	P Value
Overall	193	403	
Mean PI	50.3°	51.1°	0.28

The mean PI (50.3°) for 193 females was slightly lower than the one (51.1°) for 403 males.

Nevertheless, radiologic proof of FJ arthritis has not been clearly associated with back pain at all times [56-58]. A recent study by Vrtovec et al. [4] came to the conclusion that computerized measurements of PI in three dimensions are less variable than manual measurements. However, our measurements were carried out before publication of this study and we applied meticulous measurement techniques in order to achieve the most accurate values. We were not able to control for intra- and interobserver reliability, but measurements were carried out by two trained specialists in this field. Furthermore, the measuring technique is based on the same concept as previous studies [7,13], where the center of the superior end plate of S1 and the midpoint of the bicoxofemoral hip axis determine the PI. It should also be noted that our measurement technique did not require complex reconstruction of 3D images, but was based on sagittal CT slides of the pelvis. We did not specify the exact level or side of FJ arthritis since all levels and sides seemed to be affected in a similar fashion, with lower levels being slightly more frequently affected [59]. Even though our study included a similar number of individuals under and over 40 years, it comprised nearly twice as many males, which may be attributed to the fact that males are injured and present to a traumatology department more often [60]. However, we do believe that statistical conclusions can be drawn from this sample

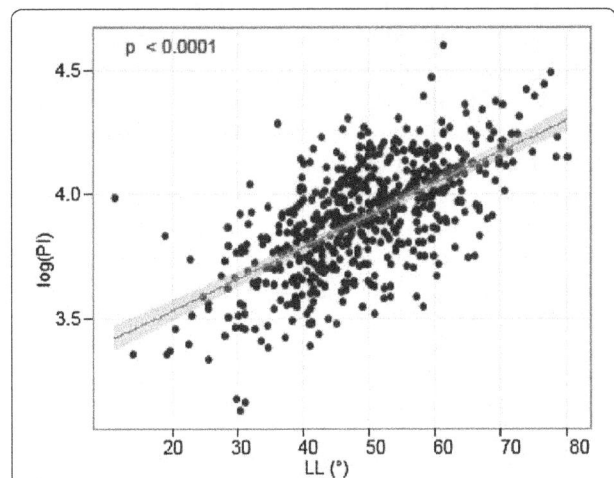

Figure 7 Pelvic Incidence and FJ Orientation at L5/S1: There was a significant difference in the logarithm of the mean PI and FJ orientation at L5/S1. The FJ orientation was labeled as coronal if angles were > 45° and sagittal if angles were ≤ 45°.

size. Furthermore, variable patient positioning in the CT scanner may lead to a misinterpretation of the exact middle of the spine and pelvis. We tried to solve this problem by choosing the same middle for the spine and sacrum. Anyhow, the same or at least very similar values can be calculated within several adjacent sagittal slides.

1) PI

Our meadian value for PI of 49.9° is in line with previous studies. A study by Peleg et al. [12,13] was the first to describe the PI in CT scans. They investigated 424 skeletons of articulated pelves as well as 20 individuals with CT scans and obtained mean values for PI of 52.8° and 57.1°. In a recent study by Vrtovec et al. [4], who successfullyevaluated CT images of 370 normal subjects, the mean value for PI was 47.1°. The large apan of values for PI indicated a relatively large natural variation. On the other hand, PI has been extensively studied on X-rays, even though overlap or magnification of structures my falsify the measured angle [7,17]. Vialle et al. [18] studied 300 lateral radiographs of volunteers and obtained a mean value for PI of 55°.

2) PI and Age

We did not find a significant difference for PI and age, even though younger (≤ 40 years) individuals had a slightly lower mean PI (50.1°) than older (≥ 40 years) individuals, who had a mean PI of 51.7°. Correspondingly, previous studies have shown that PI only increases until the age of ten and than stabilizes [19-21]. Mac-Thiong et al. [19] studied 180 healthy individuals between 4–18 years and found out that PI tends to

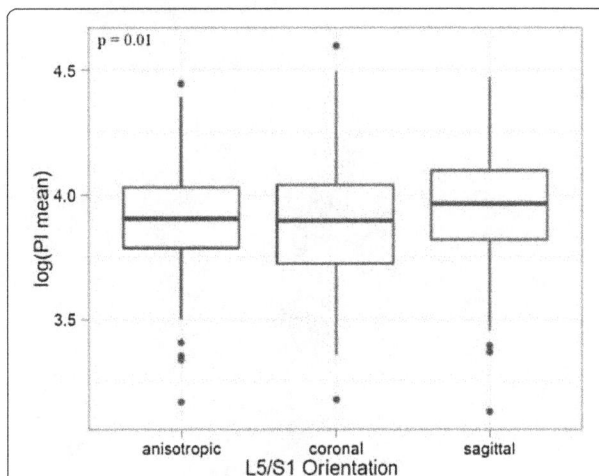

Figure 6 Pelvic Incidence (PI) and Lumbar Lordosis (LL): PI was significantly and linearly correlated with LL.

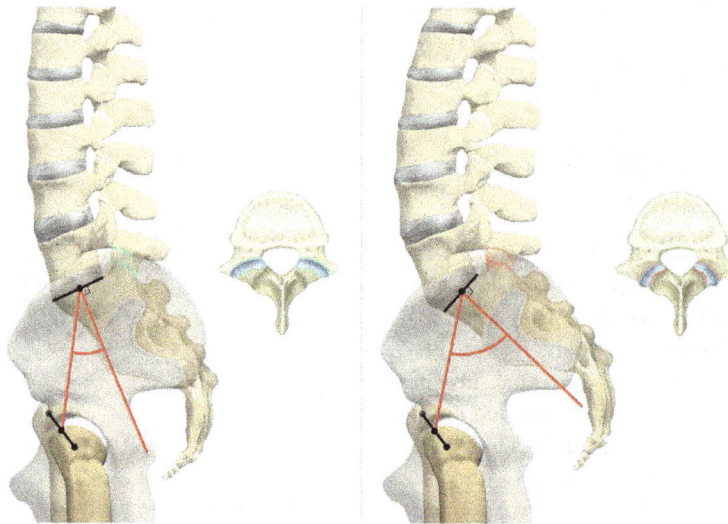

Figure 8 Pelvic Incidence (PI), Facet Joint (FJ) Arthritis and Orientation at L5/S1: **On the left side, low PI indicates a normal FJ and more coronal FJ orientation at the lower lumbar spine.** Contrarily, the right side shows increased PI with associated FJ arthritis and more sagittal FJ orientation at the lower lumbar spine.

increase until adolescence in order to keep an optimal sagittal balance and stabilizes into adulthood. Other reports mentioned an increase later on during life, especially when spondylolisthesis or sacral fractures are present [21-26]. Labelle et al. [23] studied 214 individuals with spondylolisthesis and found a linear relationship between PI and the severity of spondylolisthesis. In a study by Mendoza-Lattes et al. [25], 32 healthy teenagers were compared to 54 adults with spinal deformity and the PI was higher for the latter group. A previously mentioned study by Vrtovec et al. [4] found a linear increase of PI after skeletal maturity in normal subjects, suggesting a morphological change of the pelvis. However, our findings support the fact that PI does not

change in adults as long as there is no evidence of deformity.

3) PI and Gender

Our study did not point out a significant gender diffence for PI, even though females (50.3°) showed slighthly lower values then males (51.1°). This is in line with previous studies [4,14,27,29,61]. In a large study, Mac-Thiong et al. [14] prospectively studied the spinal balance in 709 asymptomatic adults without spinal pathology using standing lateral radiographs, and found similar mean values for PI of 52.4° for females and 52.7° for males. Similarly, Janssen et al. [27] did not find a statistical gender difference, with mean values of 50° for 30 females and 53° for 30 males. On the other hand, Vialle et al. [18] reported a significant gender difference, whereby 110 females displayed a mean PI of 56° compared to 190 males with a mean PI of 53°. However, the difference of only 3° is far less than the commonly accepted measurement error of at least 5° [25]. Overall, we don't believe that there is a significant gender difference in PI, because our study includes the largest sample size for the most accurate evaluation using CT scans, which is in line with the study with the largest last sample size for X-rays [14].

4) PI and LL

In our study, the mean value for LL was 48.9°. PI was significantly and linearly associated with LL (Figure 6 and Figure 7). Correspondingly, a predictive equation, LL = PI +9° (+/− 9°), has been recently suggested by

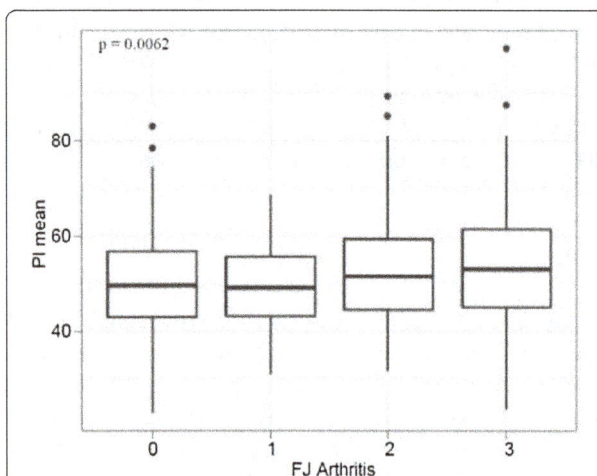

Figure 9 Pelvic Incidence (PI) and Facet Joint (FJ) Arthritis: PI and FJ arthritis displayed a significant linear correlation.

Schwab et al. [30]. Aside from this linear correlation, our study suggests a lower value for LL than for PI, so we would advocate a modified equation, such as LL = PI − 2° (+/− 11°). This is in contrast to a study by Hanson et al. [24], who postulated that PI may increase to compensate for a gradual loss in LL with age. But, the increase in PI was seen by comparing 40 patients with spondylolisthesis to a control group of 20 adults and 20 adolescents. Thus, spinal deformity might have been a confounding factor.

5) Main hypothesis: PI and FJ Arthritis and Orientation

Our study marks the first study to investigate the association of PI with FJ arthritis and orientation. According to our hypothesis and as a novel finding, PI was significantly and linearly associated with FJ arthritis and sagittally oriented FJs at the lower lumbar spine, namely L5/S1 (Figures 7, 8 and 9). However, comparison of PI with FJ orientation at the upper lumbar spine did not reveal any significant differences. This is similar to a recent study by Toy et al. [37], who investigated 120 cadaver specimen and concluded that the highest quarter of pelvic lordosis is associated with FJ arthritis at L5/S1. According to Toy et al. [37], pelvic lordosis describes the angle between the pelvic radius line and a line tangent to the upper S1 endplate that intersected at the posterior superior corner of S1. However, they did not mention an association between PI and FJ arthritis. They also used a goniometer on the osteologic specimen, which may lead to more imprecise values. This is also in line with a study by Labelle et al. [23], who found a linear association between PI and spondylolisthesis. Our results support their hypothesis that an increased PI may lead to a higher mechanical stress on the FJs. An association of FJ arthritis with sagittal FJ orientation of the lower lumbar spine has been reported in a study of CT scans with 188 individuals by Kalichman et al. [34] and a similar study by Liu et al. [35] as well as a MRI study if 111 individuals by Fujiwara et al. [36]. Considering that the lowest three lumbar FJs carry the highest loads and LL leads to higher contact force on the FJs [32], it may be postulated that increased PI may also lead to higher contact force on the lower FJs and cause FJ arthritis along with more sagittal FJ orientation. Individuals with increased PI may therefore be at high risk for FJ arthritis at the lower lumbar spine. While FJ arthritis may be considered a degenerative disease, more sagittal FJ orientation of the lower lumbar spine may be a balancing mechanism.

The establishment of a neutral upright sagittal alignment with the pelvis and spine in sync is essential in the management of spinal disorders [5,6]. Our study aids in the ongoing process [16] of defining the optimal spinal balance. It validates that PI remains a key parameter in sagittal balance and provides another mean value in a large patient population. We also present an easy method for quick and accurate evaluation of PI on sagittal slices of CT scans that does not require complicated reconstruction of 3D images. Patients with increased PI are more likely to present with FJ arthritis and possibly from associated back pain. Once these patients with increased PI (and LL) become symptomatic, orthopaedic (trauma) surgeons may consider FJ infiltration and/or establishing less lordosis with percutaneous instrumentation, where available, in order to restore spino-pelvic balance and prevent FJ arthritis if they feel that this may cause problems for the patient. In these trauma patients with increased PI (and LL), a fracture at the lumbar spine in need of spinal surgery, spondylodesis may be preferred over percutaneous instrumentation because these patients are more likely to suffer from FJ arthritis and its related pain.

Conclusion

In conclusion, our study showed that the mean value for PI on CT scans ranges around 50.8°. PI is neither significantly correlated with age nor gender. However, this is the first report showing that PI is significantly and linearly associated with LL, FJ arthritis and sagittal FJ orientation at the lower lumbar spine. Increased PI may lead to higher contact force on the lower lumbar FJs and cause FJ arthritis along with more sagittal FJ orientation. Individuals with increased PI and (and increased LL) may therefore be at high risk for FJ arthritis at the lower lumbar spine. Patients with increased PI (and increased LL) could benefit from corrective surgery and spondylodesis, once symptomatic or in the event of trauma.

Abbreviations
PI: Pelvic incidence; FJ: Facet joint; LL: Lumbar Lordosis.

Competing interests
The authors declare that they have no competing interests.

Authors' contributions
TJ: Conception and design, acquisition of data, analysis and interpretation of data, drafting the manuscript, revising the manuscript, final approval of the version to be published. JG: Acquisition of data. SB: Conception and design. KS: Revising the manuscript, statistics. DLN: Revising the manuscript. CMLW: Conception and design, analysis and interpretation of data, revising the manuscript, final approval of the version to be published. All authors read and approved the final manuscript.

Acknowledgements
We would like to thank Ms. Carol De-Simio-Hilton for her help with the preparation of the figures and Ms. Sina Rueeger from the Institute for Social and Preventive Medicine, Division of Biostatistics at the University of Zurich for her help with statistical analysis.

Author details
[1]Division of Trauma Surgery, Department of Surgery, University Hospital Zuerich, Zuerich, Switzerland. [2]Institute of Diagnostic and Interventional Radiology, University Hospital Zuerich, Zuerich, Switzerland.

References

1. Le Huec JC, Roussouly P: **Sagittal spino-pelvic balance is a crucial analysis for normal and degenerative spine.** *Eur Spine J* 2011, **20**(Suppl 5):556–557.
2. Legaye J, Duval-Beaupère G, Hecquet J, Marty C: **Pelvic incidence: a fundamental pelvic parameter for three-dimensional regulation of spinal sagittal curves.** *Eur Spine J* 1998, **7**(2):99–103.
3. Roussouly P, Gollogly S, Berthonnaud E, Dimnet J: **Classification of the normal variation in the sagittal alignment of the human lumbar spine and pelvis in the standing position.** *Spine* 2005, **30**(3):346–353.
4. Vrtovec T, Janssen MM, Pernuš F, Castelein RM, Viergever MA: **Analysis of pelvic incidence from 3-dimensional images of a normal population.** *Spine (Phila Pa 1976)* 2012, **37**(8):479–485.
5. Kuntz C, Levin LS, Ondra SL, Shaffrey CI, Morgan CJ: **Neutral upright sagittal spinal alignment from the occiput to the pelvis in asymptomatic adults: a review and resynthesis of the literature.** *J Neurosurg Spine* 2007, **6**(2):104–112.
6. Schwab F, Patel A, Ungar B, Farcy JP, Lafage V: **Adult spinal deformity-postoperative standing imbalance: how much can you tolerate? An overview of key parameters in assessing alignment and planning corrective surgery.** *Spine (Phila Pa 1976)* 2010, **35**(25):2224–2231.
7. Vrtovec T, Janssen MM, Likar B, Castelein RM, Viergever MA, Pernuš F: **A review of methods for evaluating the quantitative parameters of sagittal pelvic alignment.** *Spine J* 2012, **12**(5):433–446.
8. Duval-Beaupère G, Schmidt C, Cosson P: **A Barycentremetric study of the sagittal shape of spine and pelvis: the conditions required for an economic standing position.** *Ann Biomed Eng* 1992, **20**(4):451–462.
9. Philippot R, Wegrzyn J, Farizon F, Fessy MH: **Pelvic balance in sagittal and Lewinnek reference planes in the standing, supine and sitting positions.** *Orthop Traumatol Surg Res* 2009, **95**(1):70–76.
10. Sturesson B, Uden A, Vleeming A: **A radiostereometric analysis of movements of the sacroiliac joints during the standing hip flexion test.** *Spine (Phila Pa 1976)* 2000, **25**(3):364–368.
11. Jackson RP, Peterson MD, McManus AC, Hales C: **Compensatory spinopelvic balance over the hip axis and better reliability in measuring lordosis to the pelvic radius on standing lateral radiographs of adult volunteers and patients.** *Spine (Phila Pa 1976)* 1998, **23**(16):1750–1767.
12. Peleg S, Dar G, Medlej B, Steinberg N, Masharawi Y, Latimer B, et al: **Orientation of the human sacrum: anthropological perspectives and methodological approaches.** *Am J Phys Anthropol* 2007, **133**(3):967–977.
13. Peleg S, Dar G, Steinberg N, Peled N, Hershkovitz I, Masharawi Y: **Sacral orientation revisited.** *Spine (Phila Pa 1976)* 2007, **32**(15):397–404.
14. Mac-Thiong JM, Roussouly P, Berthonnaud E, Guigui P: **Sagittal parameters of global spinal balance: normative values from a prospective cohort of seven hundred nine Caucasian asymptomatic adults.** *Spine (Phila Pa 1976)* 2010, **35**(22):1193–1198.
15. Lazennec JY, Ramaré S, Arafati N, Laudet CG, Gorin M, Roger B, et al: **Sagittal alignment in lumbosacral fusion: relations between radiological parameters and pain.** *Eur Spine J* 2000, **9**(1):47–55.
16. Lafage V, Schwab F, Skalli W, Hawkinson N, Gagey PM, Ondra S, et al: **Standing balance and sagittal plane spinal deformity: analysis of spinopelvic and gravity line parameters.** *Spine (Phila Pa 1976)* 2008, **33**(14):1572–1578.
17. Vaz G, Roussouly P, Berthonnaud E, Dimnet J: **Sagittal morphology and equilibrium of pelvis and spine.** *Eur Spine J* 2002, **11**(1):80–87.
18. Vialle R, Levassor N, Rillardon L, Templier A, Skalli W, Guigui P: **Radiographic analysis of the sagittal alignment and balance of the spine in asymptomatic subjects.** *J Bone Joint Surg Am* 2005, **87**(2):260–267.
19. Mac-Thiong JM, Berthonnaud E, Dimar JR, Betz RR, Labelle H: **Sagittal alignment of the spine and pelvis during growth.** *Spine (Phila Pa 1976)* 2004, **29**(15):1642–1647.
20. Mangione P, Gomez D, Senegas J: **Study of the course of the incidence angle during growth.** *Eur Spine J* 1997, **6**(3):163–167.
21. Marty C, Boisaubert B, Descamps H, Montigny JP, Hecquet J, Legaye J, et al: **The sagittal anatomy of the sacrum among young adults, infants, and spondylolisthesis patients.** *Eur Spine J* 2002, **11**(2):119–125.
22. Schwab F, Lafage V, Boyce R, Skalli W, Farcy JP: **Gravity line analysis in adult volunteers: age-related correlation with spinal parameters, pelvic parameters, and foot position.** *Spine (Phila Pa 1976)* 2006, **31**(25):959–967.
23. Labelle H, Roussouly P, Berthonnaud E, Transfeldt E, O'Brien M, Chopin D, et al: **Spondylolisthesis, pelvic incidence, and spinopelvic balance: a correlation study.** *Spine (Phila Pa 1976)* 2004, **29**(18):2049–2054.

24. Hanson DS, Bridwell KH, Rhee JM, Lenke LG: **Correlation of pelvic incidence with low- and high-grade isthmic spondylolisthesis.** *Spine (Phila Pa 1976)* 2002, **27**(18):2026–2029.
25. Mendoza-Lattes S, Ries Z, Gao Y, Weinstein SL: **Natural history of spinopelvic alignment differs from symptomatic deformity of the spine.** *Spine (Phila Pa 1976)* 2010, **35**(16):792–798.
26. Hart RA, Badra MI, Madala A, Yoo JU: **Use of pelvic incidence as a guide to reduction of H-type spino-pelvic dissociation injuries.** *J Orthop Trauma* 2007, **21**(6):369–374.
27. Janssen MM, Drevelle X, Humbert L, Skalli W, Castelein RM: **Differences in male and female spino-pelvic alignment in asymptomatic young adults: a three-dimensional analysis using upright low-dose digital biplanar X-rays.** *Spine* 2009, **34**(23):E826–E832.
28. Boulay C, Tardieu C, Hecquet J, Benaim C, Mouilleseaux B, Marty C, et al: **Sagittal alignment of spine and pelvis regulated by pelvic incidence: standard values and prediction of lordosis.** *Eur Spine J* 2006, **15**(4):415–422.
29. Mac-Thiong JM, Labelle H, Berthonnaud E, Betz RR, Roussouly P: **Sagittal spinopelvic balance in normal children and adolescents.** *Eur Spine J* 2007, **16**(2):227–234.
30. Schwab F, Lafage V, Patel A, Farcy JP: **Sagittal plane considerations and the pelvis in the adult patient.** *Spine (Phila Pa 1976)* 2009, **34**(17):1828–1833.
31. Kirkaldy-Willis WH, Paine KW, Cauchoix J, McIvor G: **Lumbar spinal stenosis.** *Clin Orthop Relat Res* 1974, **99**:30–50.
32. Adams MA, Hutton WC: **The effect of posture on the role of the apophysial joints in resisting intervertebral compressive forces.** *J Bone Joint Surg Br* 1980, **62**(3):358–362.
33. Konz RJ, Goel VK, Grobler LJ, Grosland NM, Spratt KF, Scifert JL, et al: **The pathomechanism of spondylolytic spondylolisthesis in immature primate lumbar spines in vitro and finite element assessments.** *Spine (Phila Pa 1976)* 2001, **26**(4):38–49.
34. Kalichman L, Suri P, Guermazi A, Li L, Hunter DJ: **Facet orientation and tropism: associations with facet joint osteoarthritis and degeneratives.** *Spine (Phila Pa 1976)* 2009, **34**(16):579–585.
35. Liu HX, Shen Y, Shang P, Ma YX, Cheng XJ, Xu HZ: **Asymmetric Facet Joint Osteoarthritis and its Relationships to Facet Orientation, Facet Tropism and Ligamentum Flavum Thickening.** *J Spinal Disord Tech* 2012. Epub ahead of print.
36. Fujiwara A, Tamai K, An HS, Lim TH, Yoshida H, Kurihashi A, et al: **Orientation and osteoarthritis of the lumbar facet joint.** *Clin Orthop Relat Res* 2001, **385**:88–94.
37. Toy JO, Tinley JC, Eubanks JD, Qureshi SA, Ahn NU: **Correlation of sacropelvic geometry with disc degeneration in spondylolytic cadaver specimens.** *Spine (Phila Pa 1976)* 2012, **37**(1):10–15.
38. Peleg S, Dar G, Steinberg N, Masharawi Y, Been E, Abbas J, et al: **Sacral orientation and spondylolysis.** *Spine (Phila Pa 1976)* 2009, **34**(25):906–910.
39. Curylo LJ, Edwards C, DeWald RW: **Radiographic markers in spondyloptosis: implications for spondylolisthesis progression.** *Spine (Phila Pa 1976)* 2002, **27**(18):2021–2025.
40. Fujiwara A, Tamai K, Yamato M, An HS, Yoshida H, Saotome K, et al: **The relationship between facet joint osteoarthritis and disc degeneration of the lumbar spine: an MRI study.** *Eur Spine J* 1999, **8**(5):396–401.
41. Karlo C, Gnannt R, Frauenfelder T, Leschka S, Bruesch M, Wanner GA, et al: **Whole-body CT in polytrauma patients: effect of arm positioning on thoracic and abdominal image quality.** *Emerg Radiol* 2011, **18**(4):285–93. doi: 10.1007/s10140-011-0948-5. Epub 2011 Apr 7.
42. Carrera GF, Haughton VM, Syvertsen A, Williams AL: **Computed tomography of the lumbar facet joints.** *Radiology* 1980, **134**(1):145–148.
43. Kalichman L, Li L, Kim DH, Guermazi A, Berkin V, O'Donnell CJ, et al: **Facet joint osteoarthritis and low back pain in the community-based population.** *Spine (Phila Pa 1976)* 2008, **33**(23):2560–2565.
44. Stokes IA: **Three-dimensional terminology of spinal deformity. A report presented to the scoliosis research society by the scoliosis research society working group on 3-D terminology of spinal deformity.** *Spine* 1994, **19**(2):236–248.
45. Holdsworth F: **Fractures, dislocations, and fracture-dislocations of the spine.** *J Bone Joint Surg Am* 1970, **52**(8):1534–1551.
46. Pathria M, Sartoris DJ, Resnick D: **Osteoarthritis of the facet joints: accuracy of oblique radiographic assessment.** *Radiology* 1987, **164**(1):227–230.

47. Suri P, Miyakoshi A, Hunter DJ, Jarvik JG, Rainville J, Guermazi A, *et al*: **Does lumbar spinal degeneration begin with the anterior structures? a study of the observed epidemiology in a community-based population.** *BMC Musculoskelet Disord* 2011, **12**:202.

48. Masharawi YM, Alperovitch-Najenson D, Steinberg N, Dar G, Peleg S, Rothschild B, *et al*: **Lumbar facet orientation in spondylolysis: a skeletal study.** *Spine (Phila Pa 1976)* 2007, **32**(6):176–180.

49. Schuller S, Charles YP, Steib JP: **Sagittal spinopelvic alignment and body mass index in patients with degenerative spondylolisthesis.** *Eur Spine J* 2011, **20**(5):713–719.

50. Mahato NK: **Facet dimensions, orientation, and symmetry at L5-S1 junction in lumbosacral transitional States.** *Spine (Phila Pa 1976)* 2011, **36**(9):569–573.

51. Hasegawa K, Shimoda H, Kitahara K, Sasaki K, Homma T: **What are the reliable radiological indicators of lumbar segmental instability?** *J Bone Joint Surg Br* 2011, **93**(5):650–657.

52. Team RDC: *A Language and Environment for Statistical Computing*. Vienna, Austria: A Language and Environment for Statistical Computing; 2009. ISBN ISBN 3-900051-07-0 ed.

53. Kirkwood BR, Sterne JAC: *Essential Medical Statistics*. 2nd edition. Oxford: Blackwell Scientific Publications; 2003.

54. Boden SD, Riew KD, Yamaguchi K, Branch TP, Schellinger D, Wiesel SW: **Orientation of the lumbar facet joints: association with degenerative disc disease.** *J Bone Joint Surg Am* 1996, **78**(3):403–411.

55. Swanepoel MW, Adams LM, Smeathers JE: **Human lumbar apophyseal joint damage and intervertebral disc degeneration.** *Ann Rheum Dis* 1995, **54**(3):182–188.

56. Kirkaldy-Willis WH, Farfan HF: **Instability of the lumbar spine.** *Clin Orthop Relat Res* 1982, **165**:110–123.

57. Kim JS, Kroin JS, Buvanendran A, Li X, van Wijnen AJ, Tuman KJ, *et al*: **Characterization of a new animal model for evaluation and treatment of back pain due to lumbar facet joint osteoarthritis.** *Arthritis Rheum* 2011, **63**(10):2966–2973.

58. Maus T: **Imaging the back pain patient.** *Phys Med Rehabil Clin N Am* 2010, **21**(4):725–766.

59. Eubanks JD, Lee MJ, Cassinelli E, Ahn NU: **Prevalence of lumbar facet arthrosis and its relationship to age, sex, and race: an anatomic study of cadaveric specimens.** *Spine (Phila Pa 1976)* 2007, **32**(19):2058–2062.

60. American College of Surgeons CoT: *National Trauma Data Bank Annual Report*.:23. http://www.facs.org/trauma/ntdb/pdf/ntdbannualreport2010.pdf, accessed on November 4th 2013.

61. Mays S: **Spondylolysis, spondylolisthesis, and lumbo-sacral morphology in a medieval English skeletal population.** *Am J Phys Anthropol* 2006, **131**(3):352–362.

Determination of regional lung air volume distribution at mid-tidal breathing from computed tomography: a retrospective study of normal variability and reproducibility

John Fleming[1,2,4,6*], Joy Conway[1,3], Caroline Majoral[4], Michael Bennett[1], Georges Caillibotte[4], Spyridon Montesantos[4] and Ira Katz[4,5]

Abstract

Background: Determination of regional lung air volume has several clinical applications. This study investigates the use of mid-tidal breathing CT scans to provide regional lung volume data.

Methods: Low resolution CT scans of the thorax were obtained during tidal breathing in 11 healthy control male subjects, each on two separate occasions. A 3D map of air volume was derived, and total lung volume calculated. The regional distribution of air volume from centre to periphery of the lung was analysed using a radial transform and also using one dimensional profiles in three orthogonal directions.

Results: The total air volumes for the right and left lungs were 1035 +/− 280 ml and 864 +/− 315 ml, respectively (mean and SD). The corresponding fractional air volume concentrations (FAVC) were 0.680 +/− 0.044 and 0.658 +/− 0.062. All differences between the right and left lung were highly significant (p < 0.0001). The coefficients of variation of repeated measurement of right and left lung air volumes and FAVC were 6.5% and 6.9% and 2.5% and 3.6%, respectively. FAVC correlated significantly with lung space volume (r = 0.78) (p < 0.005). FAVC increased from the centre towards the periphery of the lung. Central to peripheral ratios were significantly higher for the right (0.100 +/− 0.007 SD) than the left (0.089 +/− 0.013 SD) (p < 0.0001).

Conclusion: A technique for measuring the distribution of air volume in the lung at mid-tidal breathing is described. Mean values and reproducibility are described for healthy male control subjects. Fractional air volume concentration is shown to increase with lung size.

Keywords: Regional lung volume measurement, Computed tomography, Reproducibility

Background

X-ray computed tomography (CT) is excellently suited to visualisation and accurate measurement of air volume in the airway tree [1]. CT scanning provides maps of the linear attenuation coefficient of x-rays at an average energy of 70 kV. At this energy the attenuation coefficients of low atomic number tissues such as soft tissue are closely proportional to density. Thus CT images of the lung reflect density and therefore have the advantage of providing accurate values of the air volume in the lung. They give images of the regional distribution of air volume in addition to enabling values of total lung volume to be assessed. With multi-detector high resolution CT, the whole lung field can be imaged in less than 10 s enabling images to be obtained while subjects hold their breath at a particular level of respiration. Images at total lung capacity are most common, but images at other levels of respiration can be acquired [2]. Image analysis of the CT data allows segmentation of approximately the first six generations of the airway tree, enabling accurate definition

* Correspondence: john.fleming@uhs.nhs.uk
[1]National Institute of Health Research Biomedical Research Unit in Respiratory Disease, University Hospital Southampton NHS Foundation Trust, Southampton, UK
[2]Department of Medical Physics and Bioengineering, University Hospital Southampton NHS Foundation Trust, Southampton, UK
Full list of author information is available at the end of the article

of the geometry of this section of the airway [3]. This information can be applied to derive functional parameters using computational fluid dynamics [4]. While the peripheral and alveolated airways are too small to be visualised individually, the pattern of their appearance in the images can be used to characterise typical patterns occurring in different diseases. A simple example is the assessment of the density of the peripheral area to give an emphysema score [5]. More complex pattern recognition algorithms can be used to identify the appearance of different diseases [6]. In particular, a method involving parametric response maps derived from CT data acquired at full inspiration and full expiration has been described, which is useful in distinguishing between emphysema and functional small airways disease [7].

CT-derived parameters have also been used to follow developmental and compensatory lung growth [8] and to assess structural changes in idiopathic pulmonary fibrosis [9] and emphysema [10].

Another area where measurements of regional lung volume are used is in normalisation of measurements of the regional distribution of aerosol deposition using radionuclide imaging. The relative deposition in conducting and peripheral airways is often assessed by a central to peripheral ratio. The values obtained depend quite significantly on the size of the areas chosen. This dependency can be considerably reduced by normalising the central to peripheral ratios to lung volume [11,12]. Lung volume is often estimated using transmission scanning or ventilation imaging. Both methods have disadvantages – delineation of the lungs on transmission is imprecise and ventilation does not reflect lung volume in poorly ventilated areas. The ability to use CT for this purpose overcomes these limitations. The disadvantages of CT are its relatively high radiation dose and its accessibility. Dose may be reduced using low dose protocols [13] and the use of CT in conjunction with both gamma camera tomography (Single Photon Emission Computed Tomography, SPECT) and positron emission tomography (PET) is becoming increasingly commonplace.

Measurements of lung anatomy from CT have a further application in the field of inhaled aerosol deposition. They provide anatomical information which allows improved computer modelling of the deposition pattern. In this respect images of lung volume obtained at mid-tidal breathing such as those obtained in some SPECT-CT protocols are particularly useful in that they provide information on lung anatomy at the same stage of breathing as is frequently used in experiments on aerosol inhalation.

An important disadvantage of CT, and indeed a fundamental problem of most three-dimensional imaging studies, is that the images are acquired in the horizontal position. It is known that lung anatomy varies very

significantly between supine and erect positions; the FRC of the lung is greater by around 40% with the subject erect compared to supine [13]. Therefore all information regarding lung anatomy including lung volume values have to be compared in the light of this large effect.

In addition, it has been shown that even when volume measurements in the supine position are compared, there are significant differences between values from CT and other methods, with CT values being generally lower than other techniques [14-16]. While CT scanning is now mentioned in standard texts on lung volume assessment [1], there is a shortage of reference values for expected lung volume values in control subjects. Reproducibility data is available for CT lung volumes obtained at total lung capacity and residual volume [17]. Also, some work has been done on reproducibility of lung volume values from CT in preclinical studies [13].

In this study measurements of lung volume have been made using low resolution (and therefore low dose) CT during tidal breathing in 11 healthy subjects in the supine position. This has enabled mean values of total lung volume and patterns of regional distribution to be obtained at a mid-tidal breathing position, together with measures of inter-subject variability. Each subject was imaged on two separate occasions enabling the intra-subject reproducibility of the measurements to be assessed. The results presented in this paper are derived from data acquired in a previously described experiment [18]. The prime purpose of that work was to provide data for validation of computer models of aerosol deposition by comparison with experimental measurements using medical imaging. The information on lung volume described herein is a by-product derived from that image dataset.

Methods
Subjects
The subjects described in this paper were recruited for a project to validate computer predictions of aerosol deposition by comparison with experimental measurements using medical imaging [18]. Eleven healthy, never-smoker, male subjects, between 20 and 45 years old were studied. Subjects had no evidence of respiratory disease and lung function tests within the normal range. This included being free from the common cold and rhinitis for at least four weeks before entry into the study. The study was approved by the Local Research Ethics Committee of Southampton University Hospital NHS Trust and the Administration of Radioactive Substances Advisory Committee, and patients gave written consent to participate in it. The nature of the study was explained to the subjects and each one signed a consent form. Measurements were made of height, weight, FEV1 and FRC. These are shown in Table 1.

Table 1 Subject characteristics: height, weight, FEV1, and FRC

Subject	Height (cm)	Weight (kg)	FEV$_1$ (l)	FRC ml
P00	185	91	4.82	3080
P01	180	83	5.24	3170
P02	174	56	4.27	3370
P03	171	75	4.68	3343
P04	173	80	3.88	2800
H01	174	82	4.85	2360
H02	187	88	5.57	4800
H03	177	78	4.27	3170
H04	186	87	5.48	4170
H05	173	80	3.76	3480
H06	179	N/A	4.98	2910

Acquisition of the CT scans

The CT scans were acquired as part of a combined SPECT-CT protocol on a GE Infinia dual head gamma camera with the Hawkeye 4 CT attachment (GE Medical Systems, Milwaukee, Wisconsin, USA). The participants were placed supine on the couch with the whole lung field included in the field of view. The CT scan consisted of 90 slices with an interslice separation of 4.42 mm. It used a voltage of 120 kVp and a current of 1.0 mA. The image took approximately 4 mins to acquire and therefore provided a CT image of the thorax at mean tidal breathing. The effective dose received by the subjects from the CT procedure was 0.8 mSv. The CT images have a resolution of the order of 1 mm in the transaxial plane, but this is limited in the axial (superior-inferior) direction by the inter-slice separation of 4.42 mm. The resolution in all dimensions is blurred, as the image is obtained as an average over the tidal breathing cycle.

Segmentation of the lung space

The CT images were transferred to a workstation running the Portable Imaging Computer software (PICS) processing system [19]. The analysis was carried out using a fully three dimensional approach and therefore the first step was to convert the data to 4.42 mm cubic voxels. It was next necessary to delineate the outer boundary of the lung envelope. This is straightforward in principle in that lung voxels are generally easily separated from those containing tissue by virtue of their different density and therefore different Hounsfield number. However in practice the algorithms to delineate the lung envelope are not straightforward [20,21]. In this study a semi-automatic approach has been applied; the method has been described in detail previously [22] and a brief outline is presented here.

The positions of a seed point in the trachea and the hila of the right and left lungs were defined manually

from an interactive visual display of the images. The hilum was taken as the point of the first bifurcation of the main bronchus, which was readily visible from a coronal view for the right lung or a transaxial view for the left. The software then proceeded automatically to define regions for each lung and the trachea/main bronchi using a threshold-based technique [22]. A typical segmentation of the right lung from the CT image in a transverse slice is illustrated in Figure 1.

Formation of the lung volume image

X-ray CT images consist of a map of attenuation coefficients for photons produced by the x-ray tube. For the energy used in CT, the attenuation coefficient for the soft tissue voxels in the lung can be assumed to be proportional to density. Therefore the density of the voxel, ρ_v, can be calculated using the following equation:

$$\rho_v = \frac{I_{vox} - I_{air}}{I_{tissue} - I_{air}} \tag{1}$$

where I_{air}, I_{tissue} and I_{vox} are the image intensity values for air, tissue and the voxel under consideration respectively. The fractional air volume concentration of each voxel, (FAVC) can then be calculated as:

$$FAVC = \left(1 - \frac{\rho_v}{\rho_t}\right) \tag{2}$$

where ρ_t is the average density of the tissue and blood in the lung, which is taken as 1.05 [23]. The air volume in the voxel is then FAVC.v where v is the voxel volume. It is current practice to use density as the descriptive parameter when describing CT scans. However it is considered that this new parameter, FAVC, is more appropriate to use when considering measurements of air volume. The two parameters are simply related with

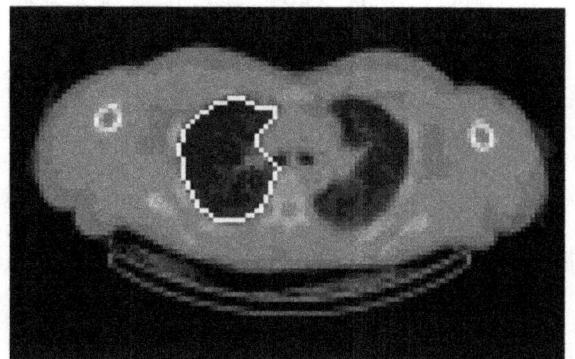

Figure 1 Example of the final segmentation of the right lung in the region of the right hilum. The outline remains close to the lung edge around the lung periphery and includes the vessels present in the area of the hilum.

FAVC being approximately one minus the density value. Two dimensional sections through a typical 3D volume image derived from CT are shown in Figure 2.

Calculation of lung volume

The lung volume is calculated by summing the air volume in all the voxels in the lung envelope [14]. This simple summation will result in a small underestimate of volume due to the partial volume effect. This occurs due to the finite resolution of the images which causes voxels on the boundary to have increased density and hence falsely low estimates of air volume. However this is exactly compensated by voxels just outside the lung having reduced density and therefore some apparent air content. To correct for this effect, the lung envelope was dilated by 1 voxel (4.42 mm) and the summation of lung air volume performed within this dilated volume. Both right and left total lung volumes were calculated.

Determination of mean volume image

It is often valuable to describe the average appearance of a particular organ of the body by forming mean images across a range of subjects. Therefore a mean image of lung volume was created for the male healthy control subjects included in this study. As the lungs in different subjects have different shapes and sizes, it was necessary to register each image to a standard template. One of the subjects with a close to average total lung volume was chosen as the template, and each of the others were registered to the template using a radial transform based on the definition of the lung outline of the subject under investigation and the standard template. This was preferred to more complicated schemes, such as active shape models, for its simplicity. The transform also required definition of a single common anatomical location in both the subject and template. The hilum of the lung is in many respects the natural choice for the centre of a spherical transform, as both airways and blood vessels branch out approximately radially from this point. However, the hilum is either on, or close to, the edge of the lung and

therefore cannot be used, as nearly half the radial paths from it have a very short or zero length within the lung. Therefore a point in the centre of the lung O (o_x, o_y, o_z) is chosen, which is related to the hilum position H (h_x, h_y, h_z) such that:

$$o_x = (h_x + p_x)/2, \quad o_y = h_y, \quad o_z = h_z \qquad (3)$$

where x, y and z represent the left/right, anterior/posterior and superior/inferior directions respectively. p_x is the x position of the lateral edge point on the lung at the same y and z co-ordinates as the hilum. The transform is illustrated in Figure 3. The purpose is to determine, for each voxel in the template shape, the corresponding position in the subject shape and then transfer the value of the CT image in the subject voxel to the equivalent template voxel. Each voxel V_t in the template shape is characterised by its direction cosines and the fractional radial distance ($f_t = OV_t / OE_t$) from the central point (O_t) to the equivalent extrapolated position on the edge (E_t). The line OE_s in the subject shape is defined as that passing through O_s with the same direction cosines as OV_t. For each voxel along this line the fractional distance to the edge ($f_s = OV_s / OE_s$) is calculated. The voxel, V_s, with the value of f_s nearest to f_t, is found. The CT image value in this voxel is transferred to voxel, V_t, in the template shape. This process is repeated for all the template voxels. Prior to registration the images were expressed in terms of the fractional air volume concentration per unit space volume, FAVC, and these absolute values were preserved in the elastic transform process.

The process was applied to the right and left lungs separately for one of the images obtained from each subject and then a combined right and left image produced. These 11 combined images were then averaged on a voxel by voxel basis to produce the mean image of fractional air volume concentrations. As the outer layers of voxels were affected by the partial volume effect resulting in a systematic reduction of the values a correction was applied. Using successive erosion of the volume outline by three

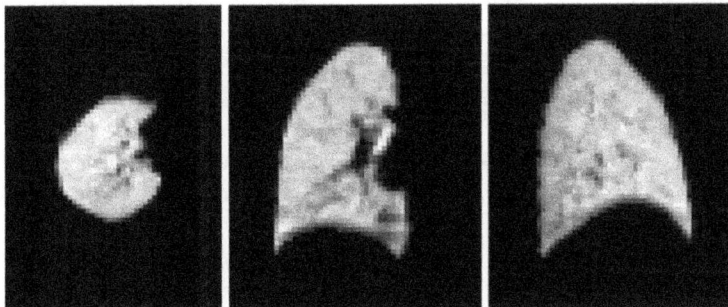

Figure 2 Example 2D transverse, coronal and sagittal sections from a 3D volume image obtained from a CT scan.

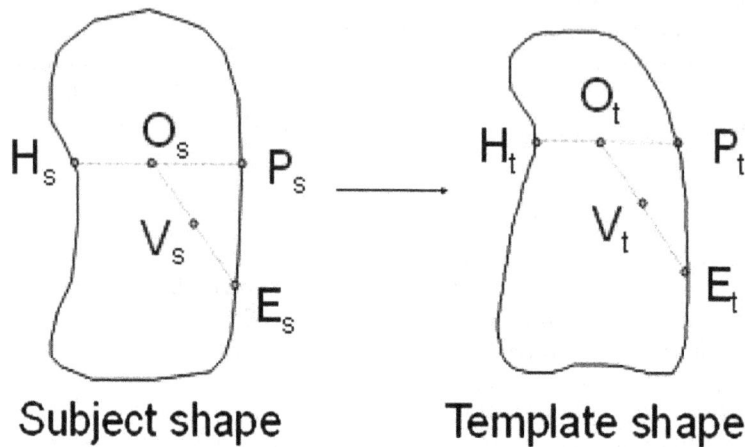

Figure 3 Schematic diagram illustrating the radial transform method of elastic registration of the images. The subject's image of fractional air volume concentration (FAVC) is transformed to the template shape by finding for each voxel in the template shape V_t. the corresponding voxel in the subject shape V_s. This is based on the direction cosines and the fractional radial distance of V_t relative to the centre of the transform O_t. The voxel in the template shape, V_t, is then filled with the FAVC value at V_s.

voxels the average air volume concentration in each was voxel layer was found. As expected the outer two layers were reduced compared to the third layer. It was then assumed that the average FAVC value in all three layers was the same and therefore all voxels in each of the outer two layers were multiplied by the appropriate factor to equalize the average FAVC.

One dimensional profiles of the average fractional air volume concentration were then derived in three orthogonal directions from the mean volume image.

Shell analysis of volume

The radial transform concept was also applied to determine the variation of fractional air volume concentration from the centre to the periphery of the airway tree. In this case the transform was carried out using the hilum as the centre of the transform with the lung being divided into ten concentric shells [24]. For each subject the total air volume per shell, V_i and mean fractional air volume concentration per shell $FAVC_i$ were calculated. The mean and standard deviation fractional air volume concentration per shell across all subjects were calculated and the intra subject reproducibility was assessed. This data was summarized as a central to peripheral ratio defined by

$$c/p = \frac{\sum_{i=1}^{5} V_i}{\sum_{i=6}^{10} V_i} \qquad (4)$$

Statistical analysis

All systematic differences between lung volume parameters were assessed using the t-test. For comparing parameters between left and right lungs and in intra-subject repeatability assessment, the paired t-test was used. Correlations between parameters were performed using linear correlation. Random differences in intra-subject variability were assessed from the standard error of the estimate of linear regression between the two sets of measurements, expressed as a percentage of the mean. Comparisons between measures of variability were performed using the F-test. The statistical analyses were performed using Microsoft Excel (Redmond, WA).

Results

Total lung volume parameters

The results of measurements of space volume, air volume, and fractional air volume concentration are summarized in Table 2. The mean values of all parameters were significantly greater for the right lung than for the left ($p < 0.0001$). The coefficient of variation of inter-subject variability of air volume was significantly greater than for the air volume concentration ($p < 0.01$). The coefficients of inter-subject variability for all parameters were greater for the left lung compared to the right, but in no case were the numbers sufficient to give statistical significance.

The total air volume in both lungs from CT correlated significantly with an erect measurement of FRC ($r = 0.67$, $p < 0.01$, COV 15%). The mean total volume (1900 ml) was significantly lower than for FRC (3332 ml). The supine volume from CT was therefore 43% reduced from the erect value obtained by helium dilution. The inter-subject coefficient of variation for FRC (19.9%) was lower than that for CT volume (31.6%) but this difference just failed to achieve significance. Fractional air volume concentration correlated significantly with space volume ($r = 0.78$, $p < 0.005$) (Figure 4).

Table 2 Summary of results of measuring global values of lung volume and fractional air volume concentration

	Mean (ml)	Standard deviation (ml)	Coefficient of variation (%)	Coefficient of variation of intra subject reproducibility (%)
Right lung space volume	1506	334	22.2	5.3
Left lung space volume	1208	375	31.0	5.8
Right lung air volume	1035	280	27.1	6.5
Left lung air volume	864	315	36.5	6.9
Fractional air volume concentration right	0.680	0.044	6.5	2.5
Fractional air volume concentration left	0.658	0.062	9.4	3.6

The coefficients of variation of repeated measurement of right and left lung space volumes and air volumes were 5.3% and 5.8%, and 6.5% and 6.9%, respectively. The correlation of repeat measurements of lung volume for both lungs is shown in Figure 5a. The corresponding Bland-Altman plot, showing the variation of the difference between the measurements and their mean is shown in Figure 5c. This suggests that the repeatability in terms of absolute volume may increase with lung size but more subjects would be required to confirm this. The coefficients of variation of intra-subject repeatability for the mean fractional air volume concentration were 2.5% and 3.6%, respectively. The correlation of repeat measurements is shown in Figure 5b and the corresponding Bland-Altman plot in Figure 5d.

Regional lung volume parameters

Transverse and coronal slices sampled through the mean air volume concentration images are shown in Figure 6. The full mean volume data is available on the departmental website. The results of shell analysis of the air volume data are shown in Figure 7. This illustrates the variation of mean total air volume and mean fractional air volume concentration for both the right and left

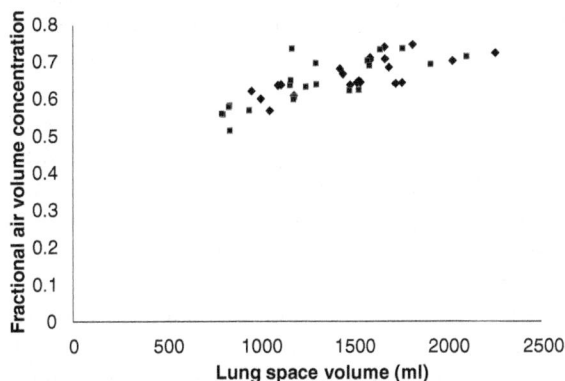

Figure 4 The variation of fraction air volume concentration with lung space volume in control subjects for the right (♦) and left (■) lungs.

lungs. The fractional concentration of air in shell 1 assumes an intermediate value for both lungs. Since the origin of the radial transform is at the hilum, which is taken as the centre of the airway where the main bronchus bifurcates, some of the voxels of shell one will contain air, while others will contain the airway wall surrounding the bronchus. These balance out to give an air volume concentration of around 0.5. The air volume concentration then decreases with shell number due to the presence of major blood vessels in shells 2 and 3. The fraction of air then increases with shell number reaching a fairly constant mean value of about 0.68 in the outer 4 shells. The concentration is slightly higher for the right lung (0.69) than for the left (0.67).

The mean value of the central to peripheral (c/p) ratio of air volume for the left lung of (0.089 +/− 0.013 SD) was significantly less than that of the right lung (0.100 +/− 0.007 SD) (p < 0.0001). The coefficient of variation of intra-subject reproducibility for repeated measurements of the c/p ratio was 8.5%.

The results of forming one dimensional profiles of the mean volume data set are shown in Figure 8. Figure 8a shows the variation of air volume concentration within the lung envelope from lateral to medial position. This demonstrates the decrease of air concentration medially due to the presence of the large blood vessels in the medial region. Figure 8b shows the variation of air volume concentration within the lung envelope from anterior to posterior position. This demonstrates the decrease of air concentration posteriorly, presumably due to the effect of gravity in the supine position. Figure 8c shows the variation of air volume concentration within the lung envelope from superior to inferior position. There is a general decrease from superior to inferior. This may be due to compression of the lower parts of the lung in the supine position due to pressure from the abdomen contents. The more rapid decrease at the lung base could be an artefact of the partial volume effect. Although a correction for the partial volume effect has been applied this is only on the basis of the average effect over the whole outer voxel layer. The lung sections at the base become very narrow, and are therefore more affected by the partial volume effect than the average for the lung.

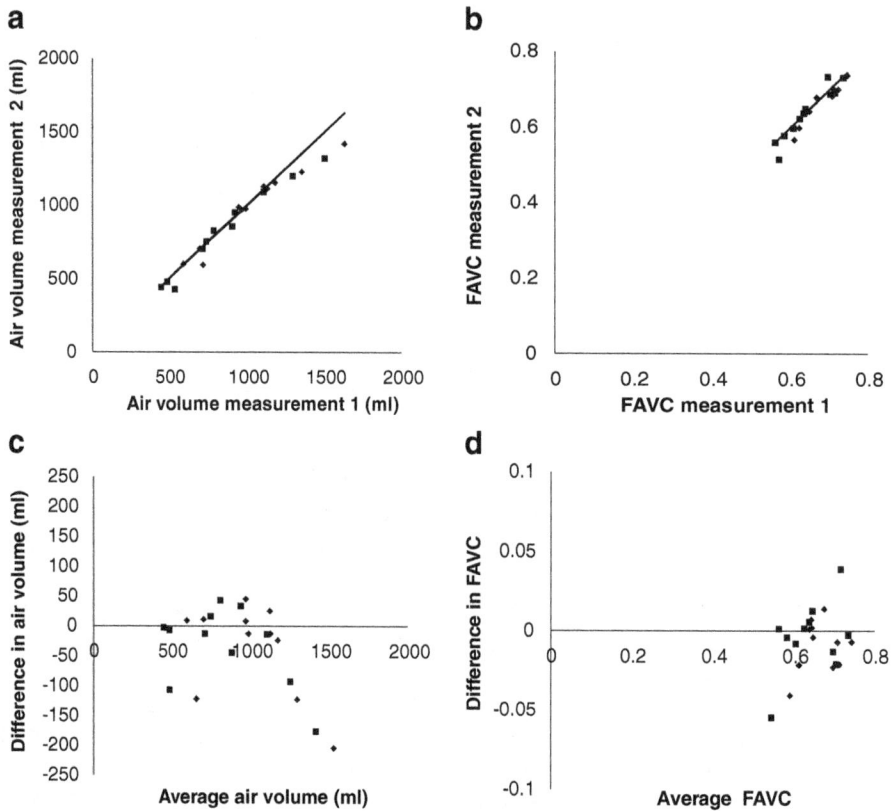

Figure 5 This illustrates the reproducibility of measuring parameters of lung volume. Graph **(a)** shows the results for total volume and **(b)** for fractional air volume concentration (FAVC) for the right lung (♦) and left lung (■). In each graph, the line is the line of identity. The corresponding Bland-Altman plots of difference in measurements against mean of measurements are shown in graphs **(c)** and **(d)**.

Discussion

This study has demonstrated that it is possible to use low resolution, and therefore low dose CT, to provide quantitative images of lung volume at approximately mid-tidal breathing. These depict the fractional lung air volume per unit space volume and they enable, among other things, the total air volume of the lungs to be obtained. A normal range for this has been defined in a set of 11 subjects and an assessment of intra-subject variability between repeat measurements has been obtained. A method for producing a mean lung volume map has been described and used to provide such a map for this group of subjects. This has been analysed to produce a description of the regional variation of fractional air volume from (i) centre to periphery of the lung using a shell analysis and (ii) as air volume profiles in three orthogonal directions. The reproducibility of the central to peripheral ratio of air volume derived from the shell analysis has also been measured.

The methodology described in this paper is not fully automated, and therefore not ideal for routine use. However algorithms are now commercially available, e.g. from VIDA Diagnostics, USA, which are capable of fully automatic segmentation of the lung and determination of lung volume. It will be interesting to see whether this software is capable of being used with low dose images such as those described in this paper and also whether the values obtained of lung volume at mid tidal breathing are similar. A key aspect of the segmentation of the lung and the subsequent analysis is the definition of the position of hilum of the lung and how much of the area around the hilum is included in the lung envelope. In this paper we have used the first bifurcation of the main bronchus to define the hilum and have used a technique involving dilation and erosion to fill in the areas in the lung envelope with high density including those around the hilum. It would be useful for the lung imaging community to make an effort to standardise these definitions so that results of different software will be comparable.

The results on total lung volume are now considered. As expected, the right lung space volume was found to be significantly higher than the left lung, contributing 53.9% of the total space volume of the lungs. The average fractional air volume concentration was also significantly higher for the right lung with the result that the fraction

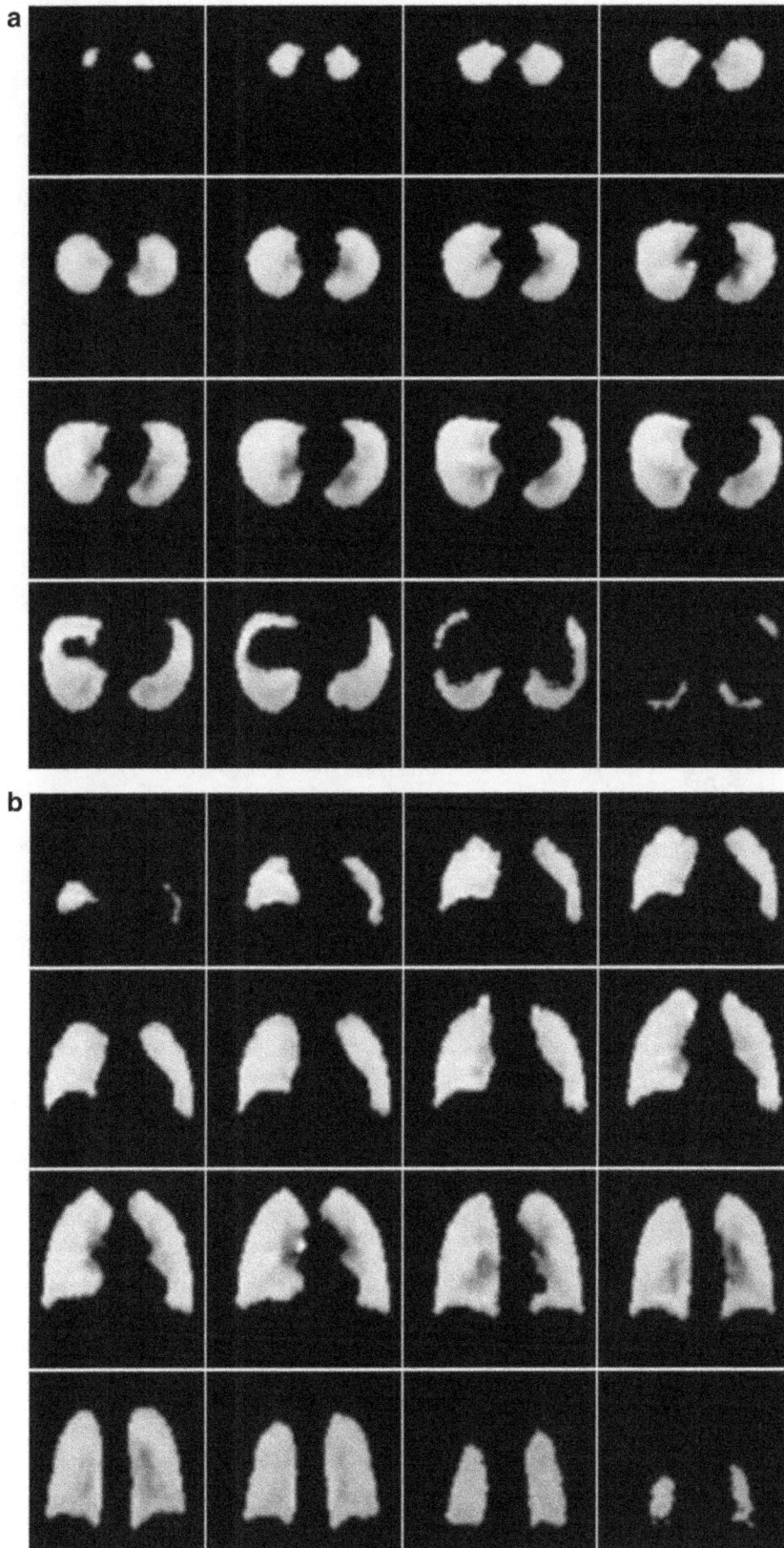

Figure 6 This illustrates the mean 3D air volume concentration dataset. Image set **(a)** shows transverse slices running from apex to base of the lung and image set **(b)** coronal slices running from anterior to posterior.

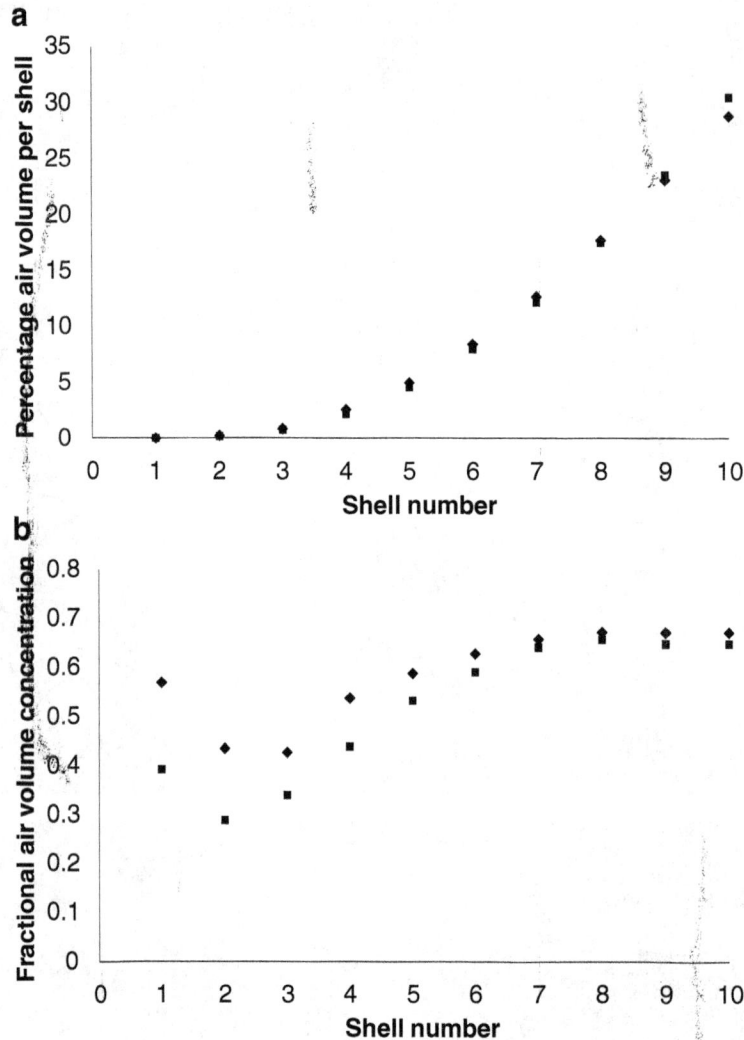

Figure 7 This illustrates the results of shell analysis of lung air volume. The graphs show the variation of **(a)** the percentage of total lung air volume and **(b)** fractional air volume concentration from the centre of the lung (shell 1) to the periphery (shell 10). Data for the right (♦) and left (■) lungs are shown separately.

of air volume from the right lung is slightly but significantly higher at 54.8%. Consistent with these findings, the averaged coefficient of inter-subject variability was found to be higher for the air volume than for the space volume, 32% compared to 27%. The inter-subject variability of fractional air volume concentration was considerably lower at 8.6%.

The average fractional air volume concentration in each lung correlated significantly with the total space volume of the lung. This is in agreement with the study by Gevenois et al. [25], who observed the fractional air volume at full inspiration in the supine position correlated with total lung capacity in healthy volunteers. This correlation may be explained by considering the gas exchange requirements of the lung. If density were to remain the same as body size increases then both the space volume

and the air volume of the lung would increase proportionately. Assuming that alveolar volume is the largest component of lung volume, the volume of alveoli will then increase in proportion to body size. However, the surface area available for gas exchange will only increase proportional to body size to the power two thirds. Therefore to allow for this, the alveolar volume will have to increase at a rate which is greater than proportional to body size to maintain the required increase in alveolar surface area. It should also be noted that the difference in FAVC between left and right lungs also followed this pattern with the larger right lung also having the higher FAVC. This variation will be important to bear in bind when interpreting results of density measurements in the assessment of emphysema. Since most diagnostic CT scanning is carried out at full inspiration or full exhalation with

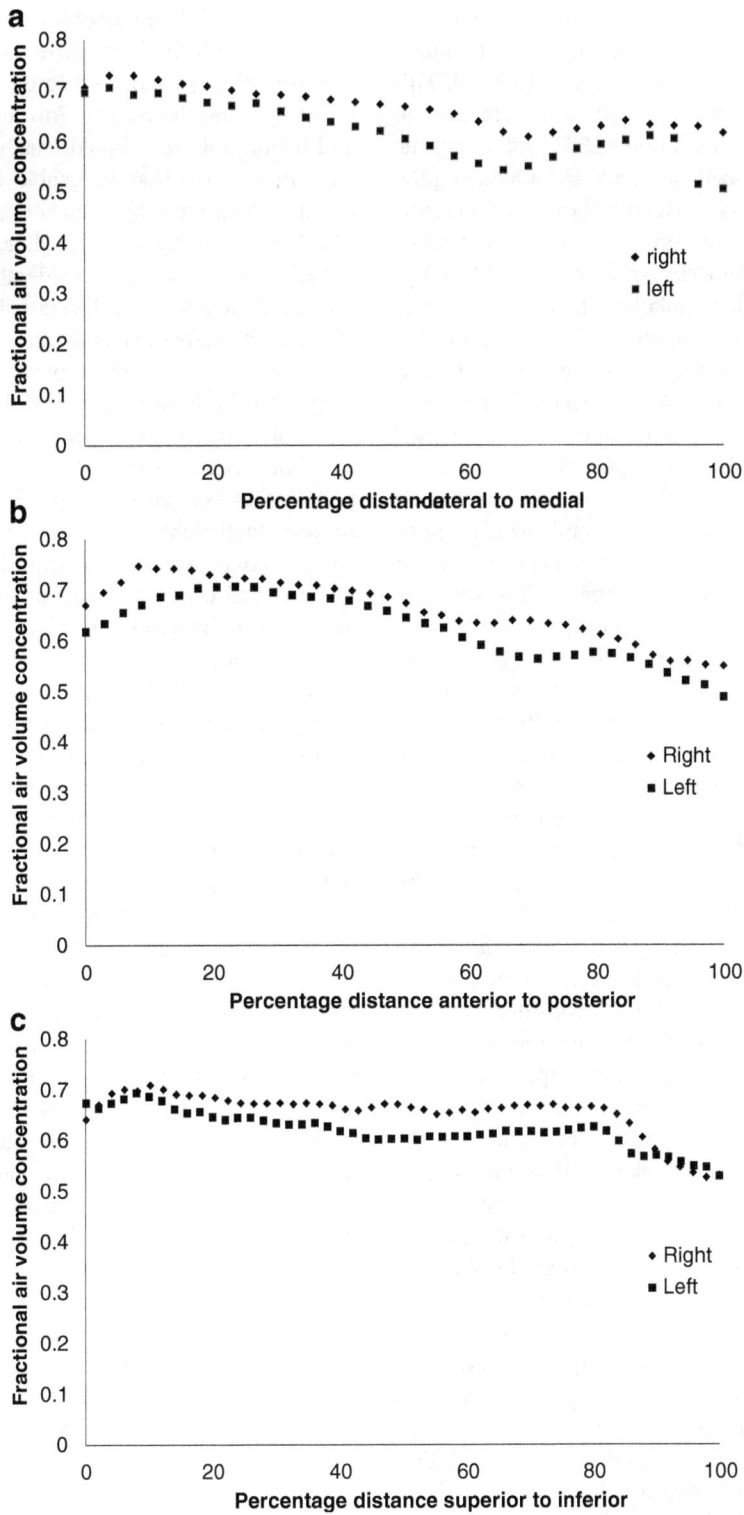

Figure 8 Variation of fractional air volume concentration within the lung envelope (a) from lateral to medial position, (b) from anterior to posterior position, and (c) from superior to inferior position.

high resolution CT, it will be important to confirm this finding in subjects imaged at these states of inhalation.

The mean total, (i.e. left plus right), mid-tidal air volume in the supine position used for imaging was 1900 ml. This is reduced by 43% from the erect FRC value obtained in these subjects using helium dilution of 3332 ml. Using the standard equation described by Stock and Quanjer [26], the mean predicted erect FRC for these subjects was found to be 3377 ml. This is very close to the mean value found, so this group of subjects can be considered to represent a typical adult male population. Ibanez and Raurich [27], found the average male supine FRC using He dilution to be 2230 ml. Therefore the CT values found in this paper are reduced by 330 ml compared to the helium dilution technique. One reason why the mean value obtained from CT will be lower is that it only describes the air volume from the lung hilum onwards. It does not include the nasopharynx, oropharynx, trachea and main bronchi. All this volume will be included in a helium dilution measurement. The mean total volume of this space in adult males is 226 ml. The components of this are nasopharynx, 138 ml [26], oropharynx, 61 ml [28], trachea, 19 ml [29] and main bronchi 8 ml [30]. This can go some way to explain the lower value obtained with CT. However, this will be balanced by the fact that a CT image obtained during tidal breathing might be expected to be higher than FRC as it should be equal to FRC plus half the tidal volume. Since the mean tidal volume is around 500 ml this means that CT values might be expected to be around 250 ml higher. This almost exactly balances out the underestimation described above due to the missing extra-pulmonary volume.

The above arguments lead us to consider whether there is any technical reason for an underestimation in the CT measurements. The most likely explanation here is due to the partial volume effect resulting from the limited spatial resolution of the scans. A first order correction for this effect has been applied as described above. However this only uses a global correction to the missing volume close to the surface of the lung and it may not apply accurately to all parts of the lung where local effects may be important. For example towards the base of the lung, the organ becomes very narrow and in some slices there is a thin section of lung volume, where no voxel may come above the threshold. The global correction applied will allow for this to some extent, but it may not be sufficient. This effect will be greater in low resolution CT studies such as those described here, particularly as mean tidal breathing has been used as compared to a breath hold. Investigation of the magnitude of this effect using image simulation techniques will be the subject of further study.

The correlation of CT lung air volume with FRC was reasonably good (COV 15%) and comparable with previously described results [31]. CT imaging might be considered as an alternative method for measuring FRC, although the large difference in supine compared to erect values would need to be taken into consideration in interpreting the results. Further studies comparing CT and helium dilution should ideally measure a supine FRC with helium dilution to enable a direct comparison of results. The inter-subject variability of CT lung air volume (32%) was not significantly different from that of FRC (20%). However it was considerably larger than for FRC. Increased number of subjects will enable clarification of whether this difference is significant.

There was good intra-subject reproducibility for total lung air volume in these control subjects, with a coefficient of variation of repeat measurements on separate occasions being 6.5%. This compares favourably with previous assessments of reproducibility [13]. The intra-subject coefficient of variation of average fractional air volume concentration was even lower at 3.1%. However this reduced variation might be expected given the lower inter-subject variation for this parameter compared to total air volume.

CT scans of the lung give the opportunity of investigating the three dimensional distribution of air volume in the lung at various stages of respiration. Most work to date has centred on looking at the number of voxels with very high air volume concentration at full inspiration as a measure of emphysema [5]. The values obtained for this parameter will be dependent on the precise imaging protocol [32] and analysis of these low resolution scans of the airway tree at average tidal breathing are not likely to be useful for this purpose. The elastic registration of each image to a standard template has enabled a mean image of the distribution of air volume to be obtained. This provides a database of the normal distribution of air volume against which air volume distributions of subjects with suspected lung diseases might be compared using techniques such as statistical parametric mapping [33]. The method of non-rigid registration described in this paper uses a simple global spatial transformation, suitable for the relatively low resolution spatial images acquired. More sophisticated techniques would be required for high resolution images where fiducial markers such as the bifurcation points can be identified using commercially available software (e.g. Apollo, VIDA Diagnostics, USA). These would allow a more precise local deformation to be applied.

Two methods of analysing the spatial distribution of air volume in terms of one-dimensional vectors have been described in this paper. The first is the radial transform or shell analysis technique which allows a description of the variation of air volume concentration from centre to periphery of lungs. The different shells defined in the analysis correlate approximately with airway generation number and therefore provide a first order approximation to distribution of air volume concentration with airway generation. This form of analysis has been used in describing the three dimensional spatial variation of inhaled aerosol deposition from the centre to the periphery of the lung [24]. In both two dimensional [11] and three dimensional [34] imaging of aerosol deposition, it has been found valuable to normalise the shell data to the distribution of either ventilation or lung volume. Normalisation to ventilation has the disadvantage that it may not be valid in diseases of the lung with abnormal ventilation. Normalisation to lung air volume seems a more robust method and, as CT provides the best imaging of lung air volume distribution available, it could be regarded as the gold standard method for this type of normalisation. The finding that the central to peripheral ratio of lung air volume was different for the left and right lungs shows that normalisation of aerosol deposition should be carried out separately for each lung. The intra-subject reproducibility for the c/p ratio of 8.5% was considered to be reasonably good, although more variation was found for this parameter compared to measures of the total air volume in the lung.

The other method of analysis described is the one dimensional analysis of fractional air volume concentration in three orthogonal directions. This has provided some interesting observations on the trends of this parameter in three dimensions in the supine position. The data provides a baseline against which other measurements of these profiles can be compared and it will be interesting to observe how consistently the variation described in this paper is found in future studies.

There were also differences in the distribution of air volume between the left and right lungs. The one dimensional profiles illustrated the lower values of FAVC for the left lung but the variations in the three orthogonal directions all showed similar patterns of variation for both lungs. The variation of FAVC with shell number again showed the consistently lower value for the left lung, but the relative difference was much greater for the inner shells resulting in a significantly lower central to peripheral ratio for the left lung. This is presumably as a result of the relatively higher proportion of major vessels in the reduced space volume of the lung envelope on the left side, due to the presence of the heart.

The results described in this paper on lung volume in the mid-tidal position are a by-product of a study carried out for a different purpose. For this reason not all aspects of the experimental design are optimised for lung volume measurement. Nevertheless, it is considered that useful novel results on the use of CT scanning to measure total and regional lung volume have been obtained. The number of subjects studied for example was not particularly optimised for this study. However from the repeat measurements on the 11 subjects studied, reasonably precise measures of average parameters of lung volume and repeatability have been calculated. In addition statistically significant conclusions on differences between parameters and correlations have been made. Comparison of the mid-tidal volume measurements obtained in the supine position with erect measurement of FRC was not ideal. In principle FRC would have ideally been carried out supine at the same time as the CT scan was being acquired, so that direct comparison of the measurements could be made.

Further work required on the spatial analysis of the distribution of volume is a description of the fractional air volume concentration by lobe and by segment. Since it is now possible to delineate lobes directly from CT images, and estimate the outline of the segments, lung volume parameters can be expressed per lobe and per segment. Initial work has shown that airway volume does vary regionally [35] and this will be the subject of future study.

The determination of regional lung volume at a particular point in the respiratory cycle using CT gives the possibility of looking at change in lung volume between different points of the cycle. The recent development of four dimensional CT (4DCT) enables dynamic CT imaging to be carried out over the respiratory cycle [36]. This would enable visualization of regional changes in volume, leading to high resolution quantitative ventilation imaging. This could potentially give important new information on lung physiology.

The potential of magnetic resonance imaging in providing information on lung volume needs also to be considered, as this provides three dimensional image data without incurring any risk due to ionizing radiation. Conventional proton MR does not provide images that are easily related to air volume, and so are unlikely to compete with CT for this purpose. However, measurements of regional lung volume would be clearly possible using hyperpolarised gas imaging [37]. If this were to become readily available then it could find an important role in this area.

Conclusions

In conclusion a method of delineating the lung outline from CT images of the thorax has been described. This has been applied to low resolution CT scans obtained in control subjects at mean supine tidal volume. Average measurements of total lung volume and its regional distribution are described together with the inter-subject variability and the intra-subject variability of repeated measurements. The values obtained are reproducible and are in good agreement with previous results where such a comparison is possible. Fractional air volume concentration is shown to increase with lung size, a result which has important implications for the quantitative interpretation of measurements of lung density.

Competing interests
This work was part of study (EudraCT # 2007-003563-43) which was sponsored by Air Liquide. JF acts as a consultant to Air Liquide. The University of Southampton has received funding from Astra Zeneca, Sweden for a study in which JF, JC and MB were involved.

Authors' contributions
JF designed the study, developed the image analysis software used in the study and drafted the manuscript. JC was the principal investigator of the overall project of which the current study was a part, and oversaw the clinical acquisition of the imaging data. CM performed the image analysis. MB and SM contributed to the design of the software. GC contributed to the study design. IK contributed to the study design and helped to draft the manuscript. All authors read and approved the final manuscript.

Acknowledgements
We thank the members of the Department of Nuclear Medicine at the University Hospital NHS Foundation Trust Southampton who performed the imaging studies and in particular Dr Livia Tossici-Bolt who was responsible for management of the image data. We also acknowledge the work of Leslie Collier in managing the visits of the subjects.
This work was part of study (EudraCT # 2007-003563-43) was sponsored by Air Liquide. JF was employed by Air Liquide to write the paper. JF, JC and MB are employed by the National Institute of Health Research Biomedical Research Unit in Respiratory Disease, Southampton. CM, GC, SM and IK are employed by Air Liquide Santé International.

Author details
[1]National Institute of Health Research Biomedical Research Unit in Respiratory Disease, University Hospital Southampton NHS Foundation Trust, Southampton, UK. [2]Department of Medical Physics and Bioengineering, University Hospital Southampton NHS Foundation Trust, Southampton, UK. [3]Faculty of Health Sciences, University of Southampton, Southampton, UK. [4]Medical R&D, Air Liquide Santé International, Centre de Recherche Claude-Delorme, Les Loges-en-Josas, France. [5]Department of Mechanical Engineering, Lafayette College, Easton, PA, USA. [6]Department of Nuclear Medicine, Southampton General Hospital, Mail Point 26, Southampton SO166YD, UK.

References
1. Wanger J, Clausen JL, Coates A, Pedersen OF, Brusasco V, Burgos F, Casaburi R, Crapo R, Enright P, van der Grinten CPM, Gustafson P, Hankinson J, Hensen R, Johnson D, MacIntyre N, McKay R, Miller MR, Navajas D, Pellegrino R, Viegi G: **Standardisation of the measurement of lung volumes.** *Eur Respir J* 2005, **25:**511–522.
2. Hoffman EA: **Effect of body orientation on regional lung expansion: a computed tomographic approach.** *J Appl Physiol* 1985, **59:**468–480.
3. Sauret V, Halson PH, Brown IW, Fleming JS, Bailey AG: **Study of the three-dimensional geometry of the central conducting airways in man using computed tomographic (CT) images.** *J Anat* 2002, **200:**123–134.
4. De Backer LA, Vos WG, Salgado R, De Backer JW, Devolder A, Verhulst SL, Claes R, Germonpré PR, De Backer WA: **Functional imaging using computer methods to compare the effect of salbutamol and ipratropium bromide in patient-specific airway models of COPD.** *Int J Chron Obstruct Pulmon Dis* 2011, **6:**637–646.
5. Kim WJ, Silverman EK, Hoffmann E, Criner GJ, Mosenifar Z, Sciurba FC, Make BJ, Carey V, Estepar RSJ, Diaz A, Reilly JJ, Martinez FJ, Washko GR, and the NETT Research Group: **CT metrics of airway disease and emphysema in severe COPD.** *Chest* 2009, **136:**396–404.
6. Zavaletta VA, Bartholmai BJ, Robb RA: **High resolution multi-detector CT-aided tissue analysis and quantification in lung fibrosis.** *Acad Radiol* 2007, **14:**772–787.
7. Galban CJ, Han MK, Boes JL, Chughtai KA, Mater CR, Johnson TD, Galban S, Rehemtulla A, Kazerooni EA, Martinez FJ, Ross BD: **Computed tomography- based biomarker provides unique signature for diagnosis of COPD phenotypes and disease progression.** *Nat Med* 2012, **18**(11):1711–1715.
8. Ravikumar P, Yilmaz C, Danc DM, Johnson RI Jr, Estrera AS, Hsia CC: **Developmental signals do not further accentuate nonuniform postpneumonectomy compensatory lung growth.** *J Appl Physiol* 2007, **102:**1170–1177.
9. Yilmaz C, Watharkar SS, de LA D, Garcia CK, Patel NC, Jordam KG, Hsia CC: **Quantification of regional interstitial lung disease from CT-derived fractional tissue volume – a lung tissue research consortium study.** *Acad Radiol* 2011, **18:**1014–1023.
10. Grydeland TB, Dirksen A, Coxson HO, Eagan TML, Thorsen E, Pillai SG, Sharma S, Eide GE, Gulsvik A, Bakke PS: **Quantitative computed tomography measures of emphysema and airway wall thickness are related to respiratory symptoms.** *Am J Respir Crit Care Med* 2010, **181:**353–359.
11. Biddiscombe MF, Meah SN, Underwood SR, Usmani OS: **Comparing lung regions of interest in gamma scintigraphy for assessing inhaled therapeutic aerosol deposition.** *J Aerosol Med* 2011, **24:**165–173.
12. Fleming JS, Sauret V, Conway JH, Holgate ST, Bailey AG, Martonen TB: **Evaluation of the accuracy and precision of lung aerosol deposition measurements from SPECT using simulation.** *J Aerosol Med* 2000, **13:**187–198.
13. Reske AW, Rau A, Reske AP, Kozoi M, Gottwald B, Alel M, Ionita J-C, Spieth P, Hepp P, Seiwerts M, Beda A, Bormn S, Scheuermann G, Amato MBP, Wrigge H: **Extrapolation in the analysis of lung aeration by computed tomography: a validation study.** *Crit Care* 2011, **15:**R279.
14. Hsia CCW, Hyde DM, Weibel ER OM: **An official research policy statement of the American Thoracic Society/ European Respiratory Society: standards for quantitative assessment of lung structure.** *Am J Respir Crit Care Med* 2010, **181:**394–418.
15. Patroniti N, Bellani G, Manfio A, Maggioni E, Giuffrida A, Foti G, Pesenti A: **Lung volume in mechanically ventilated patients: measurement by simplified helium dilution compared to quantitative CT scan.** *Intensive Care Med* 2004, **30:**282–289.
16. Takeda S, Wu EY, Epstein RH, Estrera AS, Hsia CC: **In-vivo assessment of changes in air and tissue volumes after pneumonectomy.** *J Appl Physiol* 1997, **82:**1340–1348.
17. Brown MS, Kim HJ, Abtin F, Da Costa I, Pais R, Ahmad S, Angel E, Ni C, Kleerup EC, Gjertson DW, McNitt-Gray MF, Goldin JG: **Reproducibility of lung and lobar volume measurements using computed tomography.** *Acad Radiol* 2010, **17:**316–322.
18. Conway J, Fleming J, Majoral C, Katz I, Perchet D, Peebles C, Tossici-Bolt L, Collier L, Caillibotte G, Pichelin M, Sauret-Jackson V, Martonen T, Apiou-Sbirlea G, Muellinger B, Kroneberg P, Gleske J, Scheuch G, Texereau J, Martin A, Montesantos S, Bennett M: **Controlled, parametric, individualized 2-D and 3-D imaging measurements of aerosol deposition in the respiratory tract of healthy human subjects for model validation.** *J Aerosol Sci* 2012, **52:**1–17.
19. Fleming JS, Britten AJ, Perring S, Keen AC, Howlett PJ: **A general software package for the handling of medical images.** *J Med Eng Technol* 1991, **15:**162–169.
20. De Nunzio G, Tommasi E, Agrusti A, Cataldo R, De Mitri I, Favetta M, Maglio S, Massafra A, Quarta M, Torsello M, Zecca I, Belotti R, Tangaro S, Calvini P, Camarlinghi N, Falaschi F, Cerello P, Oliva P: **Automatic lung segmentation in CT images with accurate handling of the hilar region.** *J Digit Imaging* 2011, **24:**11–27.
21. Hu S, Hoffman EA, Reinhardt JM: **Automatic lung segmentation for accurate quantitation of volumetric x-ray CT images.** *IEEE Trans Med Imaging* 2001, **20:**490–498.
22. Fleming JS, Conway JH, Bennett MJ, Majoral C, Katz I, Caillibotte G: **A technique for determination of lung outline and regional lung air volume distribution from computed tomography.** *J Aerosol Med Pulm Drug Deliv* 2014, **27:**35–42.
23. Diem K, Lentner C (Eds): *Documenta Geigy Scientific Tables.* Seventhth edition. Basle, Switzerland: Geigy Pharmaceuticals; 1970.
24. Perring S, Summers Q, Fleming JS, Nassim MA, Holgate ST: **A new method of quantification of the pulmonary regional distribution of aerosols using combined CT and SPECT and its application to nedocromil sodium administered by metered dose inhaler.** *Brit J Radiol* 1994, **67:**46–53.
25. Gevenois PA, Scillia P, de Maertelaer V, Michils A, De Vuyst P, Yernault J-C: **The effects of age, sex, lung size and hyperinflation on CT lung densitometry.** *Am J Roentgenol* 1996, **167:**1169–1173.
26. Stocks J, Quanjer PH: **Reference values for residual volume, functional residual capacity and total lung capacity.** *Eur Respir J* 1995, **8:**492–506.

Determination of regional lung air volume distribution at mid-tidal breathing from computed...

55

27. Ibanez J, Raurich JM: Normal values of functional residual capacity in the sitting and supine positions. *Intensive Care Med* 1982, **8**:173–177.

28. Porter MJ, Maw AR, Kerridge DH, Williamson IM: Manometric rhinometry: a new method of measuring the volume of air in the nasal cavity. *Acta Otolaryngol* 1997, **117**:298–301.

29. Burnell PKP, Asking L, Borgstrom L, Nichols SC, Olsson B, Prime D, Shrubb I: Studies of the human oropharyngeal airspaces using magnetic resonance imaging IV – the oropharyngeal retention effect for four inhalation delivery systems. *J Aerosol Med* 2007, **20**:269–281.

30. ICRP (International Commission for Radiological Protection) Publication 66: *Human Respiratory Tract Model for Radiological Proection*. Oxford UK: Pergamon Press; 1994.

31. Graf J, Santos A, Dries D, Adams AB, Marini JJ: Agreement between functional residual capacity estimated via automated gas dilution versus via computed tomography in a pleural effusion model. *Respir Care* 2010, **55**:1464–1468.

32. Boedeker KL, McNitt-Gray MF, Rogers SR, Truong BS, Brown MS, Gjesrtson DW, Goldin JG: Emphysema: effect of reconstruction algorithm on CT imaging measures. *Radiology* 2004, **232**:295–301.

33. Friston KJ, Holmes AP, Worsley KJ, Poline JP, Frith CD, Frackowiak RSJ: Statistical parametric maps in functional imaging: a general linear approach. *Hum Brian Mapp* 1995, **2**:189–210.

34. Fleming JS, Conway JH, Majoral C, Tossici-Bolt L, Katz I, Caillibotte G, Perchet D, Pichelin M, Muellinger B, Martonen TB, Kroneberg P, Apiou-Sbirlea G: The use of combined single photon emission computed tomography and x-ray computed tomography to assess the fate of inhaled aerosol. *J Aerosol Med* 2011, **24**:49–60.

35. Montesantos S, Fleming JS, Tossici-Bolt L: A spatial model of the human airway tree: the hybrid conceptual model. *J Aerosol Med* 2010, **23**:59–68.

36. McClelland JR, Blackall JM, Tarte S, Chandler AC, Hughes S, Ahamd S, Landau DB, Hawkes DJ: A continuous 4D motion model from multiple respiratory cycles for use in lung radiotherapy. *Med Phys* 2006, **33**:3348–3358.

37. Liu Z, Araki T, Okajima Y, Albert M, Hatabu H: Pulmonary hyperpolarized nobel gas MRI: recent advances and perspectives in clinical application. *Eur J Radiol* 2014, **83**:1282–1291.

7

Masked smoothing using separable kernels for CT perfusion images

David S Wack[1*], Kenneth V Snyder[2], Kevin F Seals[3] and Adnan H Siddiqui[2]

Abstract

Background: CT perfusion images have a high contrast ratio between voxels representing different anatomy, such as tissue or vessels, which makes image segmentation of tissue and vascular regions relatively easy. However, grey and white matter tissue regions have relatively low values and can suffer from poor signal to noise ratios. While smoothing can improve the image quality of the tissue regions, the inclusion of much higher valued vascular voxels can skew the tissue values. It is thus desirable to smooth tissue voxels separately from other voxel types, as has been previously implemented using mean filter kernels. We created a novel Masked Smoothing method that performs Gaussian smoothing restricted to tissue voxels. Unlike previous methods, it is implemented as a combination of separable kernels and is therefore fast enough to consider for clinical work, even for large kernel sizes.

Methods: We compare our Masked Smoothing method to alternatives using Gaussian smoothing on an unaltered image volume and Gaussian smoothing on an image volume with vascular voxels set to zero. Each method was tested on simulation data, collected phantom data, and CT perfusion data sets. We then examined tissue voxels for bias and noise reduction.

Results: Simulation and phantom experiments demonstrate that Masked Smoothing does not bias the underlying tissue value, whereas the other smoothing methods create significant bias. Furthermore, using actual CT perfusion data, we demonstrate significant differences in the calculated CBF and CBV values dependent on the smoothing method used.

Conclusion: The Masked Smoothing is fast enough to allow eventual clinical usage and can remove the bias of tissue voxel values that neighbor blood vessels. Conversely, the other Gaussian smoothing methods introduced significant bias to the tissue voxels.

Background

CT perfusion imaging uses many high resolution scans in a dynamic series to determine parametric image maps of Cerebral Blood Flow (CBF), Cerebral Blood Volume (CBV), and Time to Peak (TTP), among other data types. A characteristic of CT image volumes is the high contrast ratio of voxel intensity values located in skull (or calcified regions) versus tissue regions, which can exceed 15:1. Furthermore, with the injection of a tracer, voxels representing vascular regions may have intensity values greater than four times higher than neighboring tissue regions. Kudo et al. demonstrated that the inclusion of vascular voxels could overestimate CBF [1]. The

SNR within tissue regions is relatively low. Spatial smoothing is often applied to trade high spatial resolution for improved SNR characteristics. However, regular smoothing overestimates many tissue voxels due to nearby, high-valued vascular voxels.

While the importance of smoothing has been noted in the literature, it usually receives little discussion [2-4]. Klotz and König gave a brief but important description of their smoothing method as a "running mean smoothing procedure that operates separately on brain and vascular pixels" [5] (pg 173). As such, their approach operated in 2D and avoided blurring from smoothing high valued vascular pixels into tissue regions. Our method also operates separately on brain and vascular pixels, however we use a Gaussian kernel. Furthermore, our Masked Smoothing method can execute quickly, even when applied as 3D, by utilizing a combination of

* Correspondence: dswack@buffalo.edu
[1]Dept. of Nuclear Medicine and Center for Positron Emission Tomography, The University at Buffalo, State University of New York, Buffalo, NY, USA
Full list of author information is available at the end of the article

separable kernels. This offers an improvement in execution time of a few orders of magnitude relative to what could be achieved otherwise.

A "separable" 3D smoothing kernel can be expressed as the outer product of three vectors, and 3D smoothing can be applied as three successive 1D smoothings in the x, y, and z directions. While Gaussian kernels and mean kernels are separable, they do not remain separable if they must exclude vascular voxels. Our method overcomes this hurdle.

Related methods

Many smoothing methods are "adaptive" [6] and arrive at an optimal solution through the progressive refinement of an initial solution. Some methods preserve edges [7,8], similar to our desire to separate vessel and tissue voxels. Other methods consider the first or second spatial derivatives [9-12] or use the Discreet Cosine Transform [13]. A strength is these methods do not need a priori knowledge, such as voxel classifications [8]. A 4D extension of bilateral filters varies the weight of neighboring voxels according to distance and intensity, or "similarity" differences [14,15], and has been applied to CT perfusion scans [16]. The TIPS (Time Intensity Profile Similarity) bilateral filter method [17] calculates the similarity of neighboring pixels across all image frames. While this reduces processing time to some degree, the TIPS bilateral smoothing kernel is not strictly separable. While TIPS offers great flexibility in expressing the smoothing formulation, its execution time [17], even applied as a 2D filter, is much slower than what can be achieved using separable 3D kernels.

There are two advantages of CT perfusion imaging over most other image smoothing problems. First, there are multiple image volumes such that voxels in the same spatial location will have the same classification. The second is that there are extreme voxel intensity differences between voxels of different classifications for some image volumes. While thresholding the mean image and the difference of the maximum and minimum images is a simple but powerful way of identifying vascular voxels, more sophisticated methods have been presented for the identification of arteries and veins [18]. Hence Masked Smoothing makes use of the easy access to a mask image of the tissue regions that adaptive smoothing or bilateral filters fail to utilize.

Masked smoothing algorithm

Smoothing methods typically use a weighted sum of voxels within the smoothing neighborhood of a given tissue voxel, V_x, to assign a new value to V_x. The weights are all nonnegative and sum to one. The smoothing neighborhood for a given tissue voxel will, in general, include voxels of different segmentation classes—such as a

high valued vessel voxel. This inclusion will have a tendency to artificially increase the smoothed value found at V_x from the true underlying tissue value. Our goal is to apply smoothing by only using voxels of like classes. Excluding voxels of a different class could be achieved by setting their weight values to zero, while rescaling the weights of same class voxels so they sum to one.

We define sum of weights (SW) for V_x as the sum of all weights of voxels that are both within the area of the smoothing kernel and the mask of the same tissue region (without rescaling). SW will equal one if the all the voxels within the smoothing neighborhood of V_x are all of the same class as V_x. Otherwise SW will be less than one. The reciprocal of SW (1/SW) can be used to rescale the weights so that they sum to one.

Setting some weights to zero and rescaling the remaining weights associated with each voxel within the smoothing neighborhood of Vx is computationally cumbersome. We can simplify the computation by making two changes: 1) Rather than resetting the smoothing kernel weight values of voxels outside of our tissue mask to zero, we instead set voxel values outside of our tissue mask to zero. 2) Rather than rescaling the individual weights within our mask by 1/SW, we rescale the weighted sum of voxel values by (1/SW), employing the distributive property. That is, if SW is known for each voxel, then smoothing the image with non-tissue voxels set to zero and dividing voxel by voxel by SW will result in the desired with-in class masked smoothing. Post-smoothing, non-tissue voxels can be set to zero, replaced by their original values, or smoothed separately.

Fortunately, calculating SW for each tissue voxel is easy. *SW for each tissue voxel is the result of applying the smoothing kernel to the binary mask that designates voxels classified as tissue with a 1 and non-tissue voxels with 0.* This is true since the within-tissue class weights get multiplied by the mask image value of one, whereas the weights for voxels outside our mask are multiplied by zero. Smoothing the binary image is then simply the sum of the weights that are within class, i.e. SW. While we made the above argument for voxels classified as tissue, the same argument can be made in general for any classification.

To summarize, the smoothing process for a given image, Im_{orig}, is: 1) create an image mask, Msk, with 1 values at voxel locations representing tissue, and 0 otherwise; 2) Create Im_{masked} by setting all non-tissue voxels of Im_{orig} to zero; 3) Apply the desired smoothing to Im_{masked} and Msk, creating $Sm(Im_{masked})$ and $Sm(Msk)$; 4) Create the "Masked Smoothing" image by setting tissue voxels to the voxel-wise quotient $Sm(Im_{masked})/Sm(Msk)$, and non-tissue voxels to their original values. By using a separable smoothing kernel in Step 3) the Masked Smoothing method will be orders of magnitude faster than directly using the 3D kernel for the calculation.

Masked smoothing assertions

We developed Masked Smoothing as an alternative to basic Gaussian smoothing, which we term "Simple Smoothing", and a method where the vessel voxels are set to zero prior to smoothing in an attempt to minimize the impact on tissue voxels, which we term "Removed Smoothing". We believe that if Simple Smoothing, Removed Smoothing, and Masked Smoothing are used to process the same image, then tissue voxels that neighbor vessel voxels will best maintain their true value with Masked Smoothing. Furthermore, we believe that the differences between smoothing methods can lead to meaningful consequences in the determination of critical CT perfusion parameters. That is, if each smoothing method is applied to the individual time frames of a CT perfusion scan, then tissue voxels that are located near vessel voxels will have significant and meaningful differences in the resulting values of CBF, CBV and TTP depending on the smoothing method used.

Methods

The Masked Smoothing method was tested against two smoothing methods (Simple and Removed Smoothing) that are similar, but which do not limit the smoothing to tissue voxels. The smoothing methods were tested using simulated data, phantom data, and anonymized CT perfusion data from patients. The simulations provide a framework for determining the noise reduction and bias for each method. The phantom data allows us to test for bias using real scanner data. The CT perfusion data from 23 patients allows an assessment of the impact of bias caused by smoothing the CT Perfusion time series images on the calculation of CBF, CBV, and TTP.

Smoothing methods

The three smoothing methods were implemented in Matlab (Mathworks, Natick, MA) using Gaussian smoothing kernels:

1) Simple Smoothing: The unmodified image volume is smoothed using a Gaussian kernel.
2) Removed Smoothing: The vascular voxels are set to zero, and the image is smoothed as in (1) above.
3) Masked Smoothing: First, Simple Smoothing is performed on the binary tissue mask. Second, the voxel-by-voxel ratio of the Removed Smoothing image and the smoothed tissue mask image (i.e. the result of the first step of this method) is returned as the Masked Smoothing image. Voxel values outside of the tissue mask are assigned the original image value, except for the phantom experiment. We used this case to also demonstrate that Masked

Smoothing can be used to separately smooth both the object and object background.

Simulation experiment
Parameters

We created a simulated volume that included a tissue region; a long thin vascular region, which could be varied in intensity and width; and a border that was set to zero. The dimension of the simulated volume was $100 \times 100 \times 100$, and used voxel sizes of $0.4 \times 0.4 \times 0.4$ mm. Each simulation used the following parameters:

1) Intensity ratio: The intensity ratio is the ratio between the value assigned to vascular voxels and the tissue region. The tissue value was set to 50. The simulations used intensity ratios of: 2 to 1, 3 to 1, and 4 to 1, which correspond to vascular voxel values of 100, 150, and 200.
2) SNR: Gaussian noise was added to all simulation iterations. The standard deviation for the noise generator was set to 50, 25, and ~16.6, which corresponded to SNR values 1, 2, and 3 (lowest noise).
3) Vessel width: Is the cross-sectional width of the vascular region. Values used were: .8, 1.6, 2.4 mm.
4) Smoothing kernel –FWHM: The isotropic Gaussian smoothing kernel size was set to Full Width Half Max (FWHM) values of 1, 2, and 4 mm.

Iteration

For each iteration of a simulation run:

1) The simulated volume was formed with intensity values of tissue voxels set to 50. Vascular voxels were selected according to "Vessel Width", and assigned an intensity value according to the variable "Intensity Ratio".
2) Gaussian noise was added at a level determined by the Signal to Noise Ratio (SNR), Figure 1, image a.
3) All three smoothing methods were applied. All methods used the same Gaussian kernel with the kernel size determined from the variable "Kernel FWHM", Figure 1, images b-d.
4) The value at a tissue location located midway along, and directly next to, the vascular voxels was selected and the value with noise and smoothing applied was recorded. Figure 2 shows the intensity profile for the different smoothing methods for a vertical line passing through the images of Figure 1.

Assessment

500 iterations were used to determine the mean and standard deviation for a selected tissue voxel that neighbored the vessel voxels for different settings of parameters. Since in-tissue values in all cases were set to 50, the

parameter set allowing for examination of deviation from the expected tissue value of 50 for each smoothing method.

CT phantom experiment

Thirty image volumes of a CT phantom were collected using a Phillips Gemini PET/CT; 0.5 mm thickness, 0 increment, 80 kV, 125 mAs, collimation: 32×1.25 l, rotation time: 0.5 sec, FOV 250, 512 matrix, with voxel size 0.49 × 0.49 × 0.5 mm. All three methods of smoothing, using a 5 × 5 × 5 mm Gaussian kernel, were applied to the first image volume. Additionally, the mean across images volumes was calculated, which was used as the reference because of the reduced noise characteristics. One slice is shown for each smoothing method, and the mean (Figure 3). Two lines were chosen that passed through a large and small object identified on the CT. The line profiles for these lines are shown in Figures 4 and 5. Finally a line of 41 pixels in length was identified directly above of the larger object. The mean and standard deviation was calculated for this set of voxels across all 30 image volumes (i.e. 30 × 41 voxels), for the Simple and Masked smoothing methods, and compared to the mean and standard deviation calculated from the 41 voxels of the mean image. To demonstrate a variation from the simulation experiment, we performed masked smoothing, separately, to both the non-object region and object region.

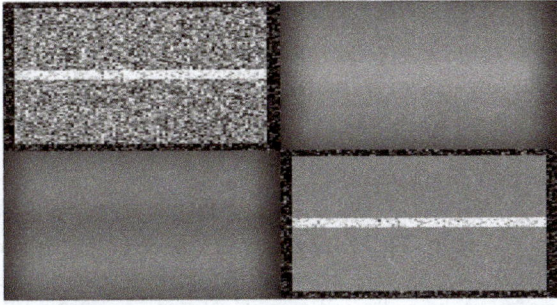

Figure 1 Simulation vessel with tissue background – raw and smoothed images. Top Left rectangle is the raw image from the simulation. Top Right rectangle is of Simple Smoothing applied to the raw image. Bottom Left rectangle is of Removed Smoothing applied to the raw image and the Bottom Right rectangle is of Masked Smoothing applied to the raw image. A smoothing kernel of 2 mm was used for each, with a vessel size of 2 mm and a raw image Signal to Noise level of 2.

calculated mean value from 500 iterations even if a high level of noise is added is expected to be very close to 50 unless a bias is present. The four parameters (Intensity Ratio, SNR, Vessel Width, and Smoothing Kernel FWHM) were individually varied using the values given above for each. When one parameter was varied the other values were set to default values (Intensity Ratio = 2 to 1, SNR = 2, Vessel Width = 1.6 mm, and FWHM = 2 mm). One simulation run (500 iterations) was performed for each

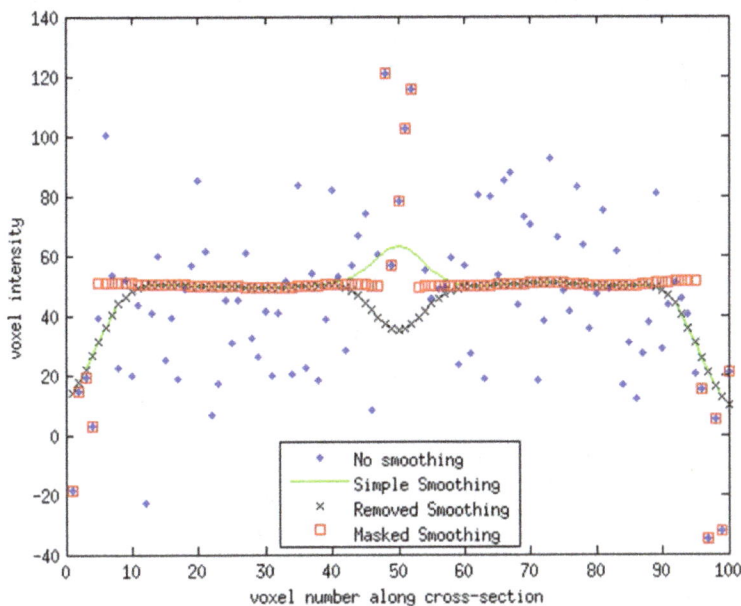

Figure 2 Vertical line profile for smoothing methods from Figure 1. The boundary and vessel voxels are identical for the Masked Smoothing and original values, since Masked Smoothing was only applied to the tissue values. The Simple and Removed smoothing methods had identical results except near the vessel voxels. The Simple Smoothing method over estimates the true value of the tissue near the vessel and underestimates the true value near the boundary. The Removed Smoothing methods underestimates the true value both near the boundary and vessel. For points away from both the boundary and vessel the three smoothing methods gave identical results. The smoothing kernel applied was 2 x 2 x 2 mm for all methods.

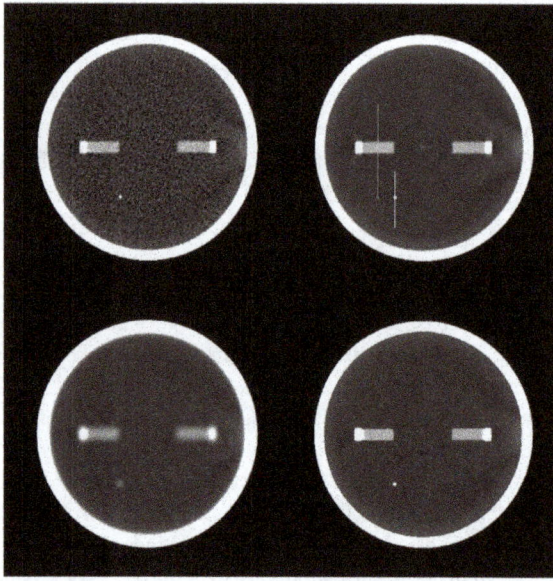

Figure 3 Image slice from phantom study: raw, mean, and smoothed images. Top left image is a slice from the first of 30 image volumes. Top right image is the mean of the same slice across all image volumes. Lower left image is the same slice as the upper left but with Gaussian smoothing applied. Lower right image is the same slice as the upper left but with Masked Smoothing applied.

Influence of smoothing method on CBF, CBV, and TTP values

Twenty-three CT perfusion studies were selected from the Neurosurgery department's stroke research database, at the University at Buffalo. Each dataset consisted of nineteen CT perfusion volumes from a Toshiba Aquilion ONE, 320 slice scanner (with voxel sizes of .42×.42×.5 mm) which were collected from patients presenting with symptoms of a stroke. Images were converted from Dicom to NifTI format, and corrected for motion using SPM8 (www.fil.ion.ucl.ac.uk/spm). Image volumes were "skull striped", and vascular voxels were identified using in-house software written in Matlab. The middle cerebral artery was automatically identified and a center portion was segmented and used for the arterial input function. A similar procedure was used to select the sagittal sinus, and these values were used to ensure the proper scaling of the arterial input function. A parametric image of CBF values was calculated using the maximum slope method, while a CBV image was calculated using the integral of tracer activity divided by the integral of arterial activity.

Tissue voxels immediately adjacent to a selected artery were selected by performing a voxel-wise dilation of the voxels representing a selected artery followed by an intersection with the tissue masks resulting in the elimination of the vascular voxels. For each smoothing method we calculated CBF, CBV, and TTP values for the selected neighboring tissue voxels, using a Gaussian kernel size of 4 × 4 × 4 mm, FWHM. Mean and voxel-wise

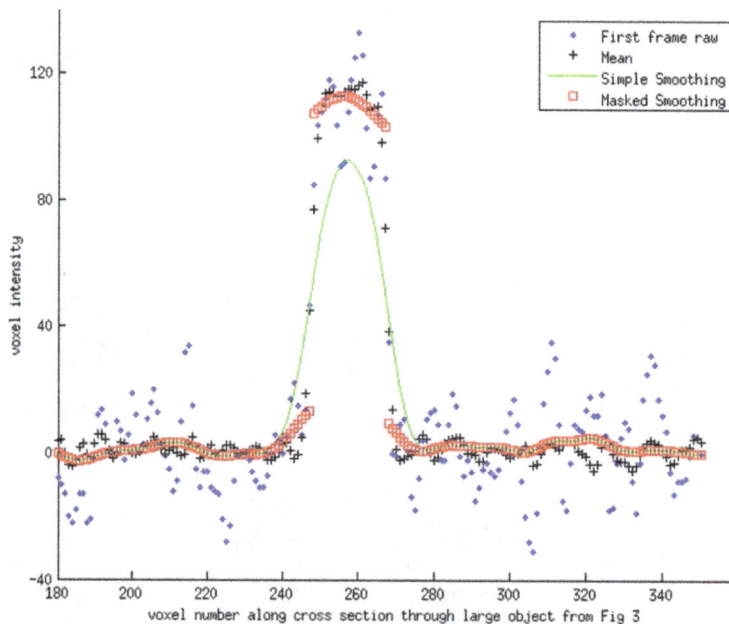

Figure 4 Intensity profile for line passing through the large object seen in Figure 3. Simple Gaussian smoothing underestimates the raw values for the object, but overestimates the values neighboring the object. Values neighboring the object have a small increase in value, which is related to the underlying neighboring voxels being correlated as a result of the reconstruction process. Notice that Masked Smoothing was applied both to the background and the object.

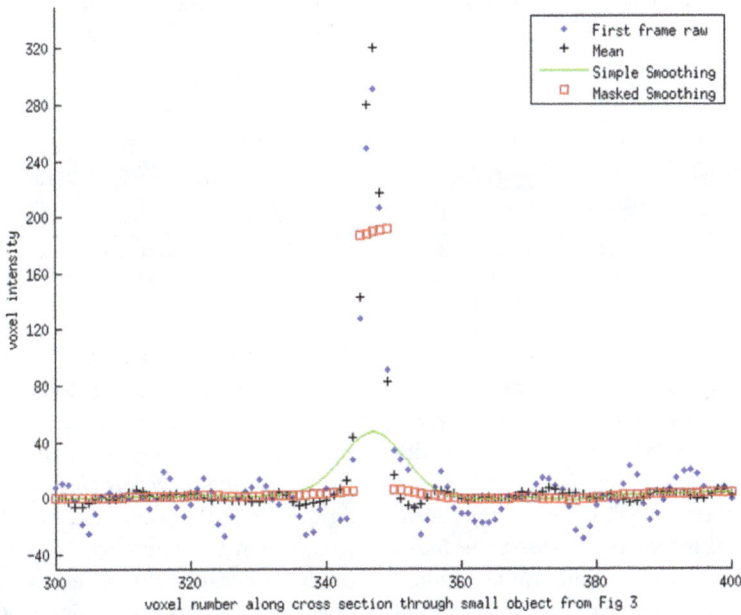

Figure 5 Intensity profile for line passing through the small object seen in Figure 3. The line profile has similar behavior near the object as in Figure 4. Likewise, it can be seen that both smoothing methods give identical results away from the object.

statistics were calculated to examine differences in CBF, CBV, and TTP due to the smoothing method used.

Ethics
This project is approved by the University at Buffalo Health Sciences Institutional Review Board.

Results
Simulation experiment
Figure 2 displays line profiles, each corresponding to a vertical line across each image of Figure 1, to demonstrate the effects of the Simple, Removed, and Masked Smoothing methods.

Simulation experiment intensity ratio
Tissue mean and standard deviation results for different Intensity Ratios are provided in Table 1. When the

intensity ratio was varied and the other variables were fixed, all smoothing methods provided over a 10 fold decrease of the standard deviation (Table 1). For the Simple Smoothing method the tissue mean increased with an increase in intensity of the neighboring vessel voxels. The Simple Smoothing method has a 100% increase (bias) for the tissue mean for the highest level of vessel voxel intensity (4 to 1). The Removed Smoothing method showed a bias which lowered the value (~28% decrease) and was unaffected by changes in the intensity of neighboring vessel voxels. The Masked Smoothing method did not show any significant bias in the calculation of the mean tissue value. The standard deviation resulting from the Removed Smoothing was slightly lower than the standard deviation of from the Simple and Masked Smoothing approaches.

Simulation experiment – SNR
Tissue mean and standard deviation results for different SNRs are provided in Table 2. The Simple Smoothing method showed an upward bias, while the Removed Smoothing method exhibited a downward bias. The biases were essentially identical for all three noise conditions. The standard deviation decreased with a decrease in the level of noise (increase of SNR) used in the simulation for all smoothing methods. The standard deviation was markedly smaller for all smoothing methods compared to the non-smoothed images. The Masked Smoothing method did not show a bias in the calculation of the mean tissue value.

Table 1 Simulation—intensity ratio: mean values and (standard deviation)

Method\Intensity ratio	1.5 to 1	2 to 1	4 to 1
Noise – No smoothing	49.7 (25.1)	50.3 (25.0)	49.0 (25.7)
Simple smoothing	58.2 (1.6)	66.3 (1.6)	99.3 (1.7)
Removed smoothing	33.6 (1.3)	33.5 (1.3)	33.5 (1.4)
Masked smoothing	50.0 (1.9)	50.0 (1.9)	50.0 (2.1)

As the ratio of the intensity of the arterial voxels compared to tissue voxels increased, the values from Masked Smoothing and Removed Smoothing held constant. However, the removed smoothing values were significantly reduced compared to their true underlying value of 50. Masked Smoothing values were equal to their true underlying value in all cases. Tissue voxels for the Simple Smoothing method increased with the increase in the arterial ratio.

Table 2 Simulation—SNR: mean values and (standard deviation)

Method\SNR	1	2	3 (least noise)
Noise – No smoothing	53.6 (49.0)	49.9 (27.1)	50.8 (16.9)
Simple smoothing	66.4 (3.3)	66.4 (1.6)	60.4 (1.1)
Removed smoothing	33.6 (2.6)	33.6 (1.3)	33.6 (0.8)
Masked smoothing	50.0 (3.9)	49.9 (1.9)	50.0 (1.3)

The standard deviation values were lower for low SNR than for high SNR. Standard deviation values were slightly poorer for the Masked Smoothing method, which is explained by fewer voxels being averaged because non-tissue voxels were excluded.

Simulation experiment: change of vessel diameter

Tissue mean and standard deviation results for different vessel widths are provided in Table 3. When the width of the simulated vessel increased, the Simple Smoothing method biased the mean tissue value to greater levels, while the Removed Smoothing method biased the mean value to lesser values. The Masked Smoothing method did not show any bias associated with the mean tissue value. All smoothing methods greatly reduced the standard deviation of the results.

Simulation experiment: change of smoothing kernel FWHM

The Simple Smoothing method yielded an upward bias for tissue mean values, while the Removed Smoothing method yielded a downward bias. The magnitude of the bias decreased with increased filter size. Masked Smoothing displayed no significant bias of the tissue mean value. For all methods, the standard deviation of the smoothed tissue value decreased when the Smoothing Kernel FWHM increased. Mean and standard deviation values for our three FWHM values and three smoothing methods is provided in Table 4.

All reported biases

For all simulations the number of iterations was 500, and the standard deviation was relatively small compared to the size of the bias. Hence, all biases reported above were strongly significant ($p < 0.0001$).

Table 3 Simulation—vessel width: mean values and (standard deviation)

Method\Vessel diameter	1	2	3 mm
Noise – No smoothing	51.2 (26.0)	50.2 (24.5)	48.5 (25.5)
Simple smoothing	61.3 (1.6)	66.5 (1.7)	68.6 (1.6)
Removed smoothing	38.8 (1.4)	33.6 (1.4)	31.6 (1.3)
Masked smoothing	50.0 (1.8)	50.1 (2.0)	50.1 (2.1)

Masked Smoothing is much closer to the true value of 50 than either of the other smoothing methods. The standard deviation values are markedly better for all smoothing methods than the No Smoothing data. A clear bias is evident for the Simple and Removed Smoothing methods.

Table 4 Simulation—smoothing kernel FWHM: mean values and (standard deviation)

Method\kernel FWHM	1	2	4 mm
Noise – No smoothing	51.7 (25.1)	49.9 (25.9)	50.0 (24.0)
Simple smoothing	64.6 (4.1)	66.4 (1.6)	60.4 (0.6)
Removed smoothing	35.7 (3.6)	33.6 (1.3)	39.6 (0.5)
Masked smoothing	50.2 (5.1)	50.0 (2.0)	50.0 (0.7)

Only the Masked Smoothing method had mean values close to the true underlying value of 50. Standard deviation values decreased as the kernel size increased.

Phantom data experiment

The line profiles passing through the small and large object show that each smoothing method is essentially identical for voxels away from the object (Figures 4 and 5). However, where the profiles cross through the object, the Simple Smoothing method has significantly lower valued voxels than the reference, i.e. mean across all image volumes. In contrast, for several voxels on either side of the object, the Simple Smoothing method has higher intensity values than the reference. The Masked Smoothing method has values close to the reference both for voxels located within the object, and outside of the object. We notice that there are a few voxels at either side of the object where the reference values lay between central values for the object and background. This is an indication of the limitation in the scanner resolution and reflects partial volume and an inherent smoothness of the raw data. Similar effects are seen for the line profile passing through the smaller object.

The mean and standard deviation for the 41 voxel line parallel and adjacent to the large object, for all 30 collected image volumes was 6.90 (13.08) HU. With Simple Smoothing, using $5 \times 5 \times 5$ mm Gaussian kernel, the mean increased to 29.78 HU, but the standard deviation decreased to 1.76. With the corresponding Masked Smoothing applied the mean equaled 8.26 HU, i.e. much closer to the original. Further, the standard deviation equaled 1.96 HU, close to same value seen with Simple Smoothing.

Patient CT perfusion data – calculation of CBF, CBV, and TTP values

The ROIs of the tissue voxel that neighbored vascular voxels, formed for each of the 23 datasets had a mean size of 376,575 voxels, and was used for determining the mean parameter values. The calculated values for CBF, CBV, and TTP, for the three smoothing methods are reported in Table 5. Mean values for CBV were greater than 50% higher, and CBF were greater than 100% higher, for the Simple Smoothing method than the Masked Smoothing method. Mean values for both CBV and CBF were both more than 30% lower for the Removed Smoothing method than the Masked Smoothing method. The mean TTP values for all smoothing methods were similar.

Table 5 Mean Parametric values for subjects' CT perfusion scan data

Method\Parameter	CBF (ml/(cc x min))	CBV (ml/cc)	TTP (min)
Simple smooth	1.48	.112	.52
Removed smooth	.35	.029	.54
Masked smooth	.67	.048	.54

CBF and CBV values were higher and lower than would be expected physiologically for the Simple and Removed Smoothing methods, respectively. Time to Peak (TTP) values were similar for all methods.

All voxel-by-voxel comparisons for CBF, CBV, and TTP were significantly different (p << .0001, paired t-test) for all pairwise comparisons of Simple Smoothing, Removed Smoothing, and Masked Smoothing methods, with the exception of TTP calculated from Removed and Masked Smoothing. Identical results (voxel by voxel) were found in comparing TTP calculated from volumes smoothed with the Removed Smoothing and Masked Smoothing methods. Despite finding a significant difference between TTP calculated with Simple Smoothing and either Removed or Masked Smoothing, the magnitude of the difference was very small (1.14 seconds, while the time between volumes was 3 seconds). For illustration, we display the results of the three smoothing methods for one slice using an 8 × 8 × 8 mm kernel (Figure 6).

Execution time of the Masked Smoothing method was 66 seconds for the 512×512×320×19 voxel CT perfusion image volume using a Gaussian Filter with size 2 × 2 × 2 mm FWHM, which required a 25 × 25 × 21 voxel kernel. Execution time using an 8 × 8 × 8 mm FWHM Gaussian filter, which required a kernel of 99×99×93 voxels, was 81 seconds. Execution time was measured using "tic" and "toc" Matlab functions, on a multi-user Dell PowerEdge R710 server with Dual 2.4 GHz processors, and 48 GB RAM.

Discussion

Our simulation and phantom data show that the Simple (i.e. ordinary Gaussian smoothing) and Removed Smoothing introduce a significant bias to tissue voxels that neighbor vessels, whereas our Masked Smoothing method did not introduce a bias. Our experiment using patient data revealed that the bias of the Simple and Removed Smoothing methods had a large impact on the calculation of CBF and CBV. The Removed Smoothing method had the lowest values for CBF and CBV and were influenced by factoring in zero values in the place of neighboring vascular values. The Simple Smoothing method had increased CBF and CBV values for tissue voxels that neighbor vessels that were not physiologically reasonable. The Masked Smoothing method had physiologically reasonable values for CBF and CBV, between the extremes returned by the Removed and Simple smoothing methods (Table 5). Given that the Masked Smoothing method does not introduce bias (as opposed to the Removed and Simple Smoothing methods), is easy to implement, and executes fast enough to allow clinical use, we advocate its use over the other methods for the smoothing of CT perfusion images.

Study design

We used simulated data to test the performance characteristics of the three smoothing methods in situations where the smoothing neighborhood for a tissue voxel included the much higher valued vessel voxels. In all simulations the tissue and vessel intensity values remained constant, allowing us to measure the effect of varying vessel characteristics (both vessel size and tracer concentration), the effect of varying SNR, and influence of the smoothing kernel FWHM. Using phantom imaging we were able to further show potential biases caused by the different smoothing methods. Using real world data from 23 patients, we also compared Simple, Masked, and Removed Smoothing to examine whether the theoretical improvement seen on simulations can have a real life impact in the calculation of CBF, CBV, and TTP. Using this approach we not only showed that Masked Smoothing did not have the bias of the other methods, but we also demonstrated the large practical impact this has on determining physiological parametric images for CBF and CBV.

Change of intensity ratio/vessel width

Our simulation experiments indicate that the Simple Smoothing method has a large upward bias for tissue voxels surrounding a vessel that increases as the intensity of the vessel voxel increases. By setting the vessel voxels to zero for the purpose of smoothing, the Removed Smoothing method has a downward bias for tissue voxels neighboring a vessel voxel that is both fixed and independent of the vessel voxel's intensity level. The Masked Smoothing method avoided bias by compensating for voxels set to zero. Increasing the vessel width increased the bias for the Simple Smoothing method, which reflects that a greater number of high intensity vessel voxels are within the smoothing neighborhood of the tissue voxel. The Removed Smoothing method also increased its bias (downward) with an increase in vessel size. This is reasonable, since for a given smoothing neighborhood the Removed Smoothing method would have a greater number of vascular voxels set to zero as the vessel width increases. Again, by compensating for voxels that were set to zero the Masked Smoothing method did not exhibit a bias.

Change of SNR/smoothing kernel FWHM

All smoothing methods provided a large decrease in the noise level. Increasing the noise level caused an increase in the standard deviation measured for all methods, but

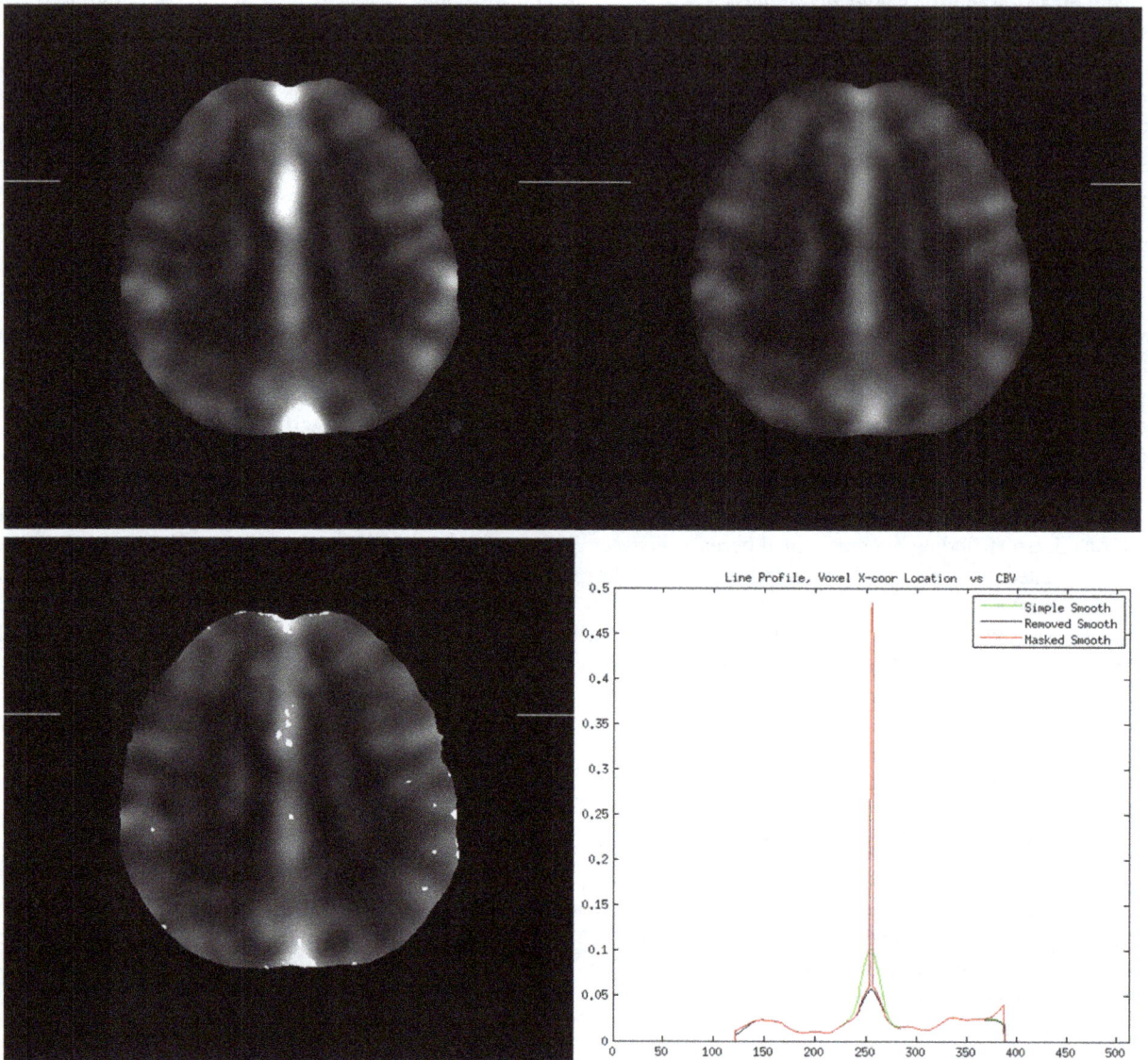

Figure 6 Simple, Removed, and Masked Smoothing images, with sample line profile. Top row: Simple and Removed Smoothing images; Bottom row: Masked Smoothing image and the line profile of each along the line connecting the edge marks of the images. The line profile of the Masked Smoothing image preserves the high intensity value for a vessel that is crossed near the line center, whereas the peak is much smaller for the Simple Smoothing method, and smallest for the Removed Smoothing method. The Simple Smoothing method has much higher values around the peak, due to the smoothing of the vessel's intensity into neighboring tissue. Along the right edge the Masked Smoothing method maintained the higher intensity values of the tissue, whereas the Simple and Removed Smoothing methods have lower values that are influenced by surrounding zero values. An 8x8x8 mm smoothing kernel was selected for this illustration to simplify the line profile.

had no effect on the calculated mean value. Increasing the filter kernel for all methods reduced the measured standard deviation. Increasing the filter size from 1 mm to 2 mm increased the bias for both Simple and Removed Smoothing. However, increasing the smoothing kernel further to 4 mm resulted in the smallest bias. The change in bias reflects the weighted proportion of voxels that are within the smoothing neighborhood. With the 4 mm smoothing kernel, the smoothing is incorporating a significant number of voxels from the "other-side" of

the vessel, hence lessening the influence of the vessel itself. As in all cases, the Masked Smoothing exhibited no significant bias.

Influence of smoothing method on the calculation of CBF, CBV, and TTP

Smoothing is a critical noise reduction pre-processing step prior to the calculation of physiologic parameters as we have demonstrated previously using simulations [19-21]. The CBF and CBV derived from the Simple and

Removed Smoothing methods differed, approximately, by a factor of four for tissue voxels close to vessels, thus demonstrating the critical importance of the smoothing method. The CBF and CBV values, calculated using the Masked Smoothing method, were in-between and significantly different from the other smoothing methods, and closest to physiologically expected values. Since the Masked Smoothing approach showed no bias on the simulated data, we believe these CBF and CBV values are the most accurate. The TTP values for the Removed and Masked Smoothing were identical because the time activity curves for a given voxel will only differ by a scaling multiple, and were close to the Simple Smoothing method.

Filter selection

We used a Gaussian smoothing kernel for our implementation because it is commonly used for medical images, and allows for fast implementations because it is separable. Our 3D execution times for an entire volume was significantly faster than a 2D TIPs bilateral filter on a single slice. Klotz and König [5] also applied smoothing separately on brain and vascular voxels. Their approach used multiple applications of a mean filter, whereas we utilized a Gaussian kernel. Our approach would also work with mean filters, since they are also separable. There are very fast methods for implementing mean filters; and furthermore, multiple passes of a mean filter can be used to approximate a Gaussian filter. However, internal timings during development favored our approach.

Segmentation and segmentation

The Masked Smoothing method assumes that satisfactory segmentation is available. However, if the thickness between planes is high then partial volume effects may hinder segmentation. If a vessel voxel were to be classified as a tissue voxel, then neighboring tissue voxels will be biased upward, especially as the tracer concentration peaks in the vessel. However, this bias cannot exceed the bias from using Simple Smoothing. Because of the quantitation, some voxels partially represent both underlying tissue and vessel. This is not a problem in practice. If this voxel is excluded, the estimate for a nearby tissue voxel proceeds without using the value. If the voxel is included, then a neighboring voxel may be biased upward, but the effect will be minimal since the voxel partially represents tissue and thus will not reach especially high intensity levels. This is similar to the situation seen with the phantom data, where the mean of the raw data shows a gradual increase to the higher intensity object. In this case the Masked Smoothing best approximated the best estimate of the true value found by calculating the mean across 30 image volumes. Finally, our method allows both the arterial and tissue regions to be smoothed separately.

Conclusion

We demonstrated that the Masked Smoothing method executes rapidly and can readily integrate into existing smoothing kernels. The Masked Smoothing method does not introduce a bias in situations where nearby voxels have a different classification and a large difference in intensity values. This accuracy, coupled with speed, gives the Masked Smoothing method the potential to significantly improve the clinical processing of perfusion imaging.

Competing interests
The authors declare they have no competing interests.

Authors' contributions
DSW developed the algorithm and developed software for the experiments. DSW and KFS drafted the manuscript. KFS, KVS, and AHS set criteria for and identified appropriate scans for inclusion. All authors participated in the experimental design, and have read and approved the final manuscript.

Acknowledgements
The authors wish to thank Carmen Mieles, RTCT at WNY PET/CT, for her technical expertise and assistance for the phantom data collection.

Author details
[1]Dept. of Nuclear Medicine and Center for Positron Emission Tomography, The University at Buffalo, State University of New York, Buffalo, NY, USA. [2]Dept. of Neurosurgery and Toshiba Stroke and Vascular Research Center, The University at Buffalo, State University of New York, Buffalo, NY, USA. [3]School of Medicine, The University at Buffalo, State University of New York, Buffalo, NY, USA.

References
1. Kudo K, Terae S, Katoh C, Oka M, Shiga T, Tamaki N, Miyasaka K: Quantitative cerebral blood flow measurement with dynamic perfusion CT using the vascular-pixel elimination method: comparison with H215O positron emission tomography. *AJNR Am J Neuroradiol* 2003, 24(3):419–426.
2. König M, Bültmann E, Bode-Schnurbus L, Koenen D, Mielke E, Heuser L: Image quality in CT perfusion imaging of the brain. *Eur Radiol* 2007, 17(1):39–47.
3. Kudo K, Sasaki M, Yamada K, Momoshima S, Utsunomiya H, Shirato H, Ogasawara K: Differences in CT Perfusion Maps Generated by Different Commercial Software: Quantitative Analysis by Using Identical Source Data of Acute Stroke Patients1. *Radiology* 2010, 254(1):200.
4. Sasaki M, Kudo K, Oikawa H: *CT perfusion for acute stroke: current concepts on technical aspects and clinical applications.* Elsevier; 2006:30–36.
5. Klotz E, Konig M: Perfusion measurements of the brain: using dynamic CT for the quantitative assessment of cerebral ischemia in acute stroke. *Eur J Radiol* 1999, 30(3):170–184.
6. Saint-Marc P, Chen J, Medioni G: Adaptive smoothing: a general tool for early vision. *IEEE Trans Pattern Anal Mach Intell* 1991, 13(6):618–624.
7. Nagao M, Matsuyama T: Edge preserving smoothing. *Computer graphics and image processing* 1979, 9(4):394–407.
8. Fang M, Qian J: Adaptive edge-preserving smoothing filter. In *Google Patents*. 1998. US Patent: 08/672,194, Publication date: June 23.
9. Alvarez L, Guichard F, Lions PL, Morel JM: Axioms and fundamental equations of image processing. *Archive for rational mechanics and analysis* 1993, 123(3):199–257.
10. Alvarez L, Lions PL, Morel JM: Image selective smoothing and edge detection by nonlinear diffusion. II *SIAM Journal on numerical analysis* 1992, 29(3):845–866.
11. Angenent S, Pichon E, Tannenbaum A: Mathematical methods in medical image processing. *Bulletin of the American Mathematical Society* 2006, 43(3):365–396.
12. Chan TF, Shen J, Vese L: Variational PDE models in image processing. *Notices AMS* 2003, 50:14–26.

13. Garcia D: **Robust smoothing of gridded data in one and higher dimensions with missing values.** *Computational Statistics & Data Analysis* 2010, **54**(4):1167–1178.

14. Paris S, Durand F: **A fast approximation of the bilateral filter using a signal processing approach.** *International Journal of Computer Vision* 2009, **81**(1):24–52.

15. Paris S, Kornprobst P, Tumblin J: **Bilateral filtering.** *Theory and applications, Foundations and Trends in Computer Graphics and Vision* 2009, **4**(1):1–73.

16. Mendrik A, Vonken E, Dankbaar JW, Prokop M, Van Ginneken B: *Noise filtering in thin-slice 4D cerebral CT perfusion scans.* SPIE Proceedings; 2010. 7623.

17. Mendrik AM, Vonken E, van Ginneken B, de Jong HW, Riordan A, van Seeters T, Smit EJ, Viergever MA, Prokop M: **TIPS bilateral noise reduction in 4D CT perfusion scans produces high-quality cerebral blood flow maps.** *Phys Med Biol* 2011, **56**:3857.

18. Mendrik A, Vonken E, van Ginneken B, Smit E, Waaijer A, Bertolini G, Viergever MA, Prokop M: **Automatic segmentation of intracranial arteries and veins in four-dimensional cerebral CT perfusion scans.** *Med Phys* 2010, **37**:2956.

19. Fisher J: *Improvements in Computed Tomography Perfusion Output using Complex Singular Value Decomposition and the Maximum Slope Algorithm.* Master's Thesis, Boston University, School of Medicine; 2014.

20. Wack DS, Badgaiyan RD: **Complex singular value decomposition based noise reduction of dynamic PET images.** *Current Medical Imaging Reviews* 2011, **7**(2):113–117.

21. Snyder K, Seals K, Wack D: **Using simulations to explore the characteristics of CT perfusion calculations in the assessment of stroke.** *Current Medical Imaging Reviews* 2014, **10**(3). In press.

8

Influence of trigger type, tube voltage and heart rate on calcified plaque imaging in dual source cardiac computed tomography

Tobias Penzkofer[1,2,3]*, Eva Donandt[1], Peter Isfort[1,3], Thomas Allmendinger[4], Christiane K Kuhl[1],
Andreas H Mahnken[1,3,5] and Philipp Bruners[1,3]

Abstract

Background: To investigate the impact of high pitch cardiac CT vs. retrospective ECG gated CT on the quantification of calcified vessel stenoses, with assessment of the influence of tube voltage, reconstruction kernel and heart rate.

Methods: A 4D cardiac movement phantom equipped with three different plaque phantoms (12.5%, 25% and 50% stenosis at different calcification levels), was scanned with a 128-row dual source CT scanner, applying different trigger types (gated vs. prospectively triggered high pitch), tube voltages (100-120 kV) and heart rates (50–90 beats per minute, bpm). Images were reconstructed using different standard (B26f, B46f, B70f) and iterative (I26f, I70f) convolution kernels. Absolute and relative plaque sizes were measured and statistically compared. Radiation dose associated with the different methods (gated vs. high pitch, 100 kV vs. 120 kV) were compared.

Results: Compared to the known diameters of the phantom plaques and vessels both CT-examination techniques overestimated the degrees of stenoses. Using the high pitch CT-protocol plaques appeared larger (0.09 ± 0.31 mm, 2 ± 8 percent points, PP) in comparison to the ECG-gated CT-scans. Reducing tube voltage had a similar effect, resulting in higher grading of the same stenoses by 3 ± 8 PP. In turn, sharper convolution kernels lead to a lower grading of stenoses (differences of up to 5%). Pairwise comparison of B26f and I26f, B46f and B70f, and B70f and I70f showed differences of $0-1 \pm 6-8$ PP of the plaque depiction. Motion artifacts were present only at 90 bpm high pitch experiments. High-pitch protocols were associated with significantly lower radiation doses compared with the ECG-gated protocols (258.0 mGy vs. 2829.8 mGy $CTDI_{vol}$, $p \leq 0.0001$).

Conclusion: Prospectively triggered high-pitch cardiac CT led to an overestimation of plaque diameter and degree of stenoses in a coronary phantom. This overestimation is only slight and probably negligible in a clinical situation. Even at higher heart rates high pitch CT-scanning allowed reliable measurements of plaque and vessel diameters with only slight differences compared ECG-gated protocols, although motion artifacts were present at 90 bpm using the high pitch protocols.

Background

Cardiac computed tomography (CT) is an established non-invasive method of assessing coronary artery morphology both in emergency and routine settings [1]. It is superior to magnetic resonance based methods of coronary angiography with respect to temporal and spatial resolution. However, continuous motion of the heart makes cardiac cross-sectional imaging a challenging task [1,2]. Different methods have been developed to overcome this problem, many of them rely on the uniformity of the cardiac cycle by imaging different sections of the heart over several consecutive heart beats. To date the vast majority of current CT systems uses either a prospectively ECG-triggered or retrospectively ECG-gated scanning protocol for this purpose. Since all these methods are associated with ionizing radiation applied to the patient, the risks and benefits need to be carefully weighted [3].

* Correspondence: tpenzkofer@ukaachen.de
[1]Department of Diagnostic and Interventional Radiology, Aachen University Hospital, RWTH Aachen University, Pauwelsstr. 30, 52074 Aachen, Germany
[2]Surgical Planning Laboratory, Department of Radiology, Brigham and Women's Hospital, 75 Francis Street, 02115 Boston, USA
Full list of author information is available at the end of the article

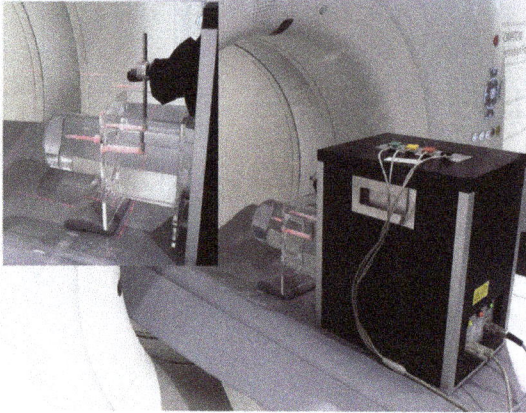

Figure 1 Cardiac movement phantom setting during the scans.
(inlay) the coronary artery phantom (CAP) was placed in a water
filled container. The cardiac phantom provides 4D motion with
ECG-syncing over the scanners standard ECG-interface (ECGI).

the need for gating or multi-step triggering, i.e. acquisition techniques that are inherently associated with
redundant scan ranges leading to increased radiation
doses.

The goal of this study was to evaluate the quantification
of calcified stenosis in high pitch cardiac CT-scans versus
an ECG-gated scan protocol in a controlled phantom environment. Secondary goal was to evaluate the influence
of tube current, convolution kernel and heart rate on the
different acquisition protocols.

Methods
Coronary movement phantom
A 4D coronary movement simulator (Sim4Dcardiac,
QRM GmbH, Möhrendorf, Germany, Figure 1) was used
for the study performing coronary artery movement patterns with heart rates of 50, 70 and 90 beats per minute
(bpm). Three custom made dedicated coronary artery
phantoms (QRM GmbH, Möhrendorf, Germany) each
with defined calcified (high, medium and low calcification
at 796, 401 and 197 mgHA/cm^3 at densities of 1.58, 1.30
and 1.16 g/cm^3) coronary stenoses of various degrees
(50%, 25% and 12.5%) were used in a simulated 4.0 mm
vessel. The absolute stenosis sizes were 0.5 mm (12.5%),

Recent advances in CT technology led to the development of dual source based high pitch (pitch up
to 3.4) scanning protocols with table speeds of up to
46 cm/sec [4-6], or even higher [7,8]. These protocols
promise to image the heart within one heartbeat, obviating

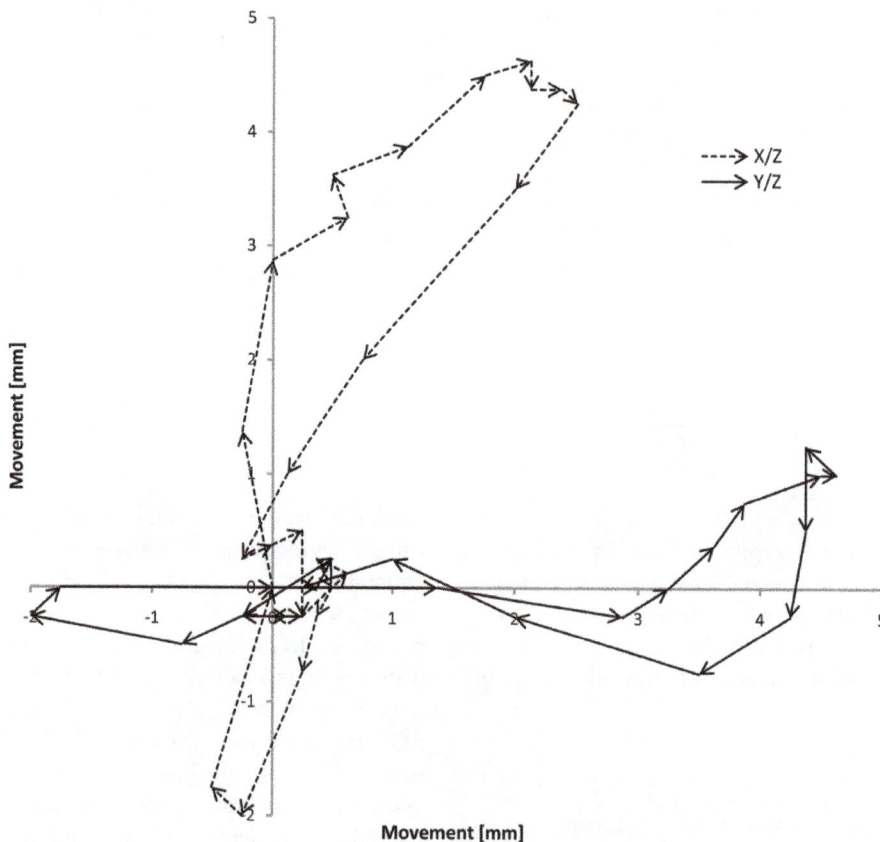

Figure 2 Cardiac movement as performed by the coronary movement simulator. The solid line represents the movement in the Y/Z plane,
while the dashed line shows the path in the X/Z plane. Arrow length corresponds to movement speed.

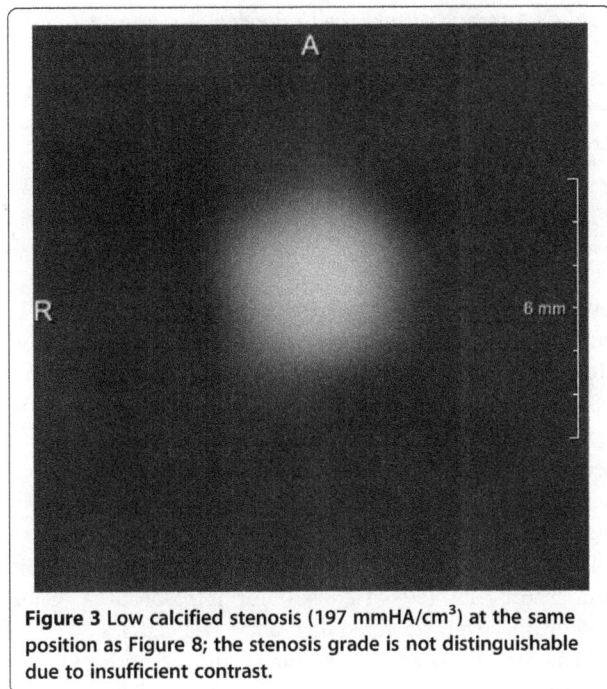

Figure 3 Low calcified stenosis (197 mmHA/cm^3) at the same position as Figure 8; the stenosis grade is not distinguishable due to insufficient contrast.

1 mm (25%) and 2 mm (50%). The movement protocol was derived from an electron beam scan (Figure 2) [9]. The coronary simulator provides an ECG output mapping the movement pattern to an ECG signal readable by the scanner's ECG analysis module.

CT examination protocols

A 128 slice high pitch capable dual source computed tomography scanner (Siemens Somatom Flash, Siemens Healthcare, Forchheim, Germany) was used for all experiments. The high pitch scans were performed using a dedicated high pitch cardiac protocol (dual source, 100 and 120 kV, 320 mAs/rot, pitch 3.4, prospective ECG trigger, collimation 128 × 0.6 mm, FoV 190 × 190 mm, scan length 90.0 mm, rotation time 0.28s) and a retrospectively ECG gated protocol (100 and 120 kV, 320 mAs/rot, retrospective ECG gating after pulsing at 50-100%, collimation 128 × 0.6 mm, pitch 0.19, rotation time 0.28s). Reconstructions were performed according to the vendor's specifications, identically for both modes with B26f, B46f, B70f standard kernels and iterative I26f and I70f kernels with a field of view of 190 × 190 mm and slice thicknesses of 0.6 mm (B26f, B46f, B70f) and 0.75 mm (I26f, I70f) avoiding undersampling of the acquired data.

Measurements

Measurements were performed manually using dedicated DICOM viewer software (Synedra View, Version 3.1, Synedra GmbH, Aachen, Germany) by one observer, and checked for validity by two others with 3 and 5 years of experience in thoracic imaging. For each combination of Kernel/Method/kV/plaque phantom three repeated measurements of plaque diameter and three repeated measurements of total vessel diameter were

Table 1 Absolute calcified stenosis diameters (true diameters: 12.5%: 0.5 mm, 25%: 1.0 mm, 50%: 2.0 mm), measured total vessel diameters (true diameter 4.0 mm) as measured for the different protocol types per phantom type

Density [mmHA/cm^3]	True stenosis size	Method	Plaque diameter [mm]	Vessel diameter [mm]	Measured stenosis [%]
197	12,5 %	High pitch	-	-	-
	(0.5 mm/4.0 mm)	Gating	-	-	-
	25%	High pitch	-	-	-
	(1.0 mm/4.0 mm)	Gating	-	-	-
	50%	High pitch	-	-	-
	(2.0 mm/4.0 mm)	Gating	-	-	-
401	12,5%	High pitch	0.97 ± 0.1	3.96 ± 0.1	24.6 ± 2.7
	(0.5 mm/4.0 mm)	Gating	0.88 ± 0.1	3.95 ± 0.1	22.4 ± 3.3
	25%	High pitch	1.48 ± 0.2	4.13 ± 0.2	35.8 ± 4.3
	(1.0 mm/4.0 mm)	Gating	1.40 ± 0.2	4.00 ± 0.1	34.9 ± 4.6
	50%	High pitch	1.98 ± 0.2	4.08 ± 0.2	48.6 ± 4.3
	(2.0 mm/4.0 mm)	Gating	1.98 ± 0.2	4.00 ± 0.1	49.6 ± 4.6
796	12,5%	High pitch	1.27 ± 0.1	4.35 ± 0.4	29.2 ± 2.4
	(0.5 mm/4.0 mm)	Gating	1.18 ± 0.1	4.52 ± 0.4	26.2 ± 2.6
	25%	High pitch	1.80 ± 0.4	4.52 ± 0.4	39.7 ± 5.9
	(1.0 mm/4.0 mm)	Gating	1.71 ± 0.4	4.70 ± 0.5	36.1 ± 5.0
	50%	High pitch	2.39 ± 0.4	3.99 ± 0.3	59.6 ± 7.1
	(2.0 mm/4.0 mm)	Gating	2.22 ± 0.3	3.93 ± 0.2	56.3 ± 5.9

The lowest density plaque phantoms (197 mmHA/cm^3) were not measurable as no sufficient contrast could be established between the lumen and the plaque mimic.

performed resulting in a total of 2,880 data points. The repeated measurements were averaged and used for statistical analyses.

Statistical analyses

Statistical analysis was performed using SPSS 19 (SPSS Inc., Chicago, Illinois, USA) and MedCalc (MedCalc Software, Mariakerke, Belgium). Tests performed were Analysis of Variances with post-hoc testing and Bland-Altman as well as Mountain plot method comparisons. P-values of 0.05 or lower were considered statistically significant, multiple testing correction (Bonferroni) was performed where applicable. Additional tests were performed using non-parametric Mann–Whitney-U analyses.

Results

The plaque phantom featuring the lowest calcification level (197 mmHA/cm^3) was not measureable with the applied methods due to low contrast between plaque and vessel lumen (Figure 3). The following data result from the measurements of the intermediately (401 mmHA/cm^3) and heavily (796 mmHA/cm^3) calcified plaque phantoms.

Comparison to phantom dimensions

In comparison to the phantom vessel dimensions retrospectively ECG-gated and prospectively ECG-triggered high pitch scanning provided vessel diameters of between 3.93 ± 0.2 mm and 4.70 ± 0.5 mm with a tendency to a slight

Table 3 Average difference in degree of stenosis (Δ percentage) and measured plaque diameter (Δ diameter) between the two cardiac CT methods and tube voltages (first vs. second mentioned)

Comparison	Δ Percentage	Δ Diameter
Gated/high pitch	2 ± 8 PP	0.09 ± 0.31 mm
100 kV/120 kV	3 ± 8 PP	0.14 ± 0.32 mm

(PP: percent points).

overestimation (Table 1). The plaque thickness was measured at between 0.88 ± 0.1 mm and 1.27 ± 0.1 mm (0.5 mm/12.5%), 1.40 ± 0.2 mm and 1.80 ± 0.4 mm (1 mm/25%) and 1.98 ± 0.2 mm and 2.39 ± 0.4 mm (2 mm/50%) again showing an overestimation for both cardiac CT techniques which was more pronounced for high-pitch scanning. These findings led to the following degrees of stenoses: 22.4 ± 3.3% and 29.2 ± 2.4% (12.5% stenoses), 34.9 ± 4.6% and 39.7 ± 5.9% (25% stenoses) and 48.6 ± 4.3% and 59.6 ± 7.1% (50% stenoses) for retrospectively gated and prospectively triggered high pitch, respectively.

Separated by heart rate of the phantom, both examination protocols showed an overestimation of vessel diameter, plaque diameter and degree of stenosis which was more pronounced for the 12.5% in comparison to the 50% stenosis and for the high pitch protocol in comparison to ECG-gated scanning. Diameter measurements for the same degree of stenosis at different heart rates did not show relevant differences (Table 2).

Table 2 Absolute plaque/stenosis diameters (true diameters: 12.5%: 0.5 mm, 25%: 1.0 mm, 50%: 2.0 mm), measured vessel diameters (true diameter 4.0 mm) per heart rate and cardiac CT method

True stenosis [%]	Heart rate [bpm]	Method	Plaque diameter [mm]	Vessel diameter [mm]	Stenosis [%]	Deviation [PP]
12.5%	50	High pitch	1.13 ± 0.19	4.17 ± 0.35	27.0 ± 3.5	14.5
		Gating	1.03 ± 0.19	4.23 ± 0.45	24.4 ± 3.7	11.9
	70	High pitch	1.12 ± 0.18	4.14 ± 0.35	27.1 ± 3.4	14.6
		Gating	1.03 ± 0.19	4.26 ± 0.41	24.1 ± 3.6	11.6
	90	High pitch	1.11 ± 0.19	4.15 ± 0.30	26.7 ± 3.5	14.2
		Gating	1.03 ± 0.19	4.22 ± 0.40	24.4 ± 3.4	11.9
25%	50	High pitch	1.63 ± 0.34	4.35 ± 0.38	37.2 ± 5.7	12.2
		Gating	1.53 ± 0.33	4.35 ± 0.49	35.0 ± 4.6	10.0
	70	High pitch	1.65 ± 0.33	4.33 ± 0.36	37.8 ± 5.1	12.8
		Gating	1.53 ± 0.34	4.35 ± 0.51	34.8 ± 4.6	9.8
	90	High pitch	1.66 ± 0.35	4.29 ± 0.39	38.4 ± 5.8	13.4
		Gating	1.61 ± 0.36	4.36 ± 0.51	36.7 ± 5.2	11.7
50%	50	High pitch	2.19 ± 0.37	4.06 ± 0.20	53.9 ± 8.0	3.9
		Gating	2.08 ± 0.28	3.95 ± 0.18	52.7 ± 6.2	2.7
	70	High pitch	2.16 ± 0.36	4.00 ± 0.23	54.0 ± 7.9	4.0
		Gating	2.11 ± 0.27	3.99 ± 0.14	52.9 ± 6.1	2.9
	90	High pitch	2.20 ± 0.38	4.05 ± 0.21	54.4 ± 8.4	4.4
		Gating	2.11 ± 0.32	3.96 ± 0.19	53.1 ± 6.7	3.1

Deviations are given in percentage difference to the true diameters as specified by the phantom manufacturer. (PP: percent points).

Comparison of trigger types

High pitch scanning resulted in a larger depiction of the plaques in comparison to the ECG-gated scan method (0.09 ± 0.31 mm). This difference accounted for an additional overestimation of the stenoses by 2 ± 8 percent points (PP) (Table 3). Bland-Altman plotting (Figure 4) revealed this systematic difference, while mountain plotting additionally revealed no outliers and a narrow distribution profile.

Trigger type and heart rate

Comparing the two CT imaging methods with respect to their plaque depiction depending on heart rate, a descending difference of the measured plaque diameter was found with increasing heart rate (50 bpm: 0.1 ± 0.28 mm, 70 bpm: 0.09 ± 0.31 mm and 90 bpm: 0.07 ± 0.35 mm, Table 4). However, the difference was so small at all heart rates that no clinically relevant effect on the degree of stenosis (2 ± 7–8 PP) was observed (Table 4).

Tube voltage

In comparison to 120 kV tube voltage 100 kV CT imaging resulted in a difference of 0.14 ± 0.32 mm regarding plaque diameters. This led to a 3 ± 8 PP overestimation of the stenosis diameter using 100 kV scan protocols (Figure 5, Table 4).

Reconstruction kernels

Smooth reconstruction kernels (B26f, I26f) showed a higher deviation from the true plaque diameters in comparison to the sharp kernels (B70f, I70f). This result was even more pronounced for the heavily calcified plaques which were significantly overestimated regarding their diameter when smooth kernels were used for image reconstruction. The B46f kernel exhibited a intermediate

Table 4 Average difference in degree of stenosis (Δ percentage) and measured plaque diameter (Δ diameter) per heart rate between the two cardiac CT examination protocols (PP: percent points)

Heart rate	Δ Percentage (gating vs. high pitch)	Δ Diameter
50 bpm	2 ± 7 PP	0.10 ± 0.28 mm
70 bpm	2 ± 8 PP	0.09 ± 0.31 mm
90 bpm	2 ± 8 PP	0.07 ± 0.35 mm

performance, with the least deviation in the less calcified plaque and a deviation between the standard and iterative kernels in the heavily calcified setting. The comparison between corresponding standard and iterative reconstruction kernels (B26f vs. I26f; B70f vs. I70f) did not reveal any relevant difference (Table 5, Figure 6).

Radiation dose comparison

Radiation doses were significantly lower for high pitch CT in comparison to ECG gated scanning (258.0 mGy vs. 2829.8 mGy for CTDIvol, 36.3 mGycm vs. 341.2 mGycm for the dose-length-product, DLP), and lower for 100 kV vs. 120 kV scan protocols (962.6 mGy vs. 2125.2 mGy CTDIvol and 115.1 mGycm vs 262.4 mGycm DLP). All these differences were statistically significant ($p \leq 0.0001$ for trigger type and $p \leq 0.0005$ for tube voltage, Tables 6, 7).

Motion artifacts

Coronal reconstruction revealed motion artifacts, present at the proximal end of the coronal phantom for the 90 bpm high pitch prospectively gated scans (Figure 7), which were not present in retrospectively gated scanning or the 50 or 70 bpm high pitch experiments. No other occurrences of motion artifacts were observed.

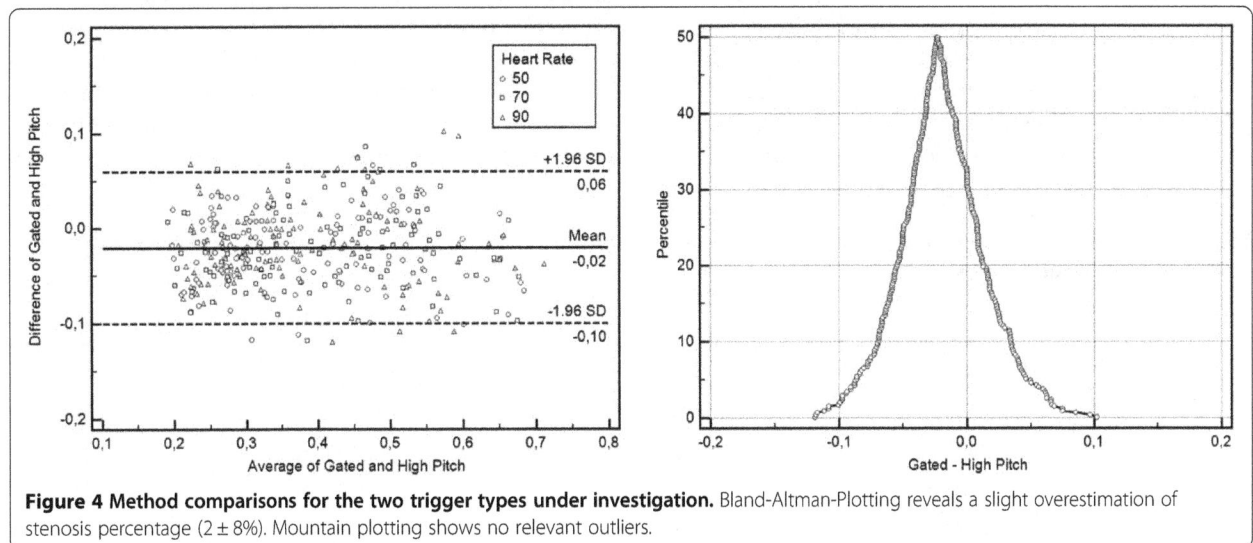

Figure 4 Method comparisons for the two trigger types under investigation. Bland-Altman-Plotting reveals a slight overestimation of stenosis percentage (2 ± 8%). Mountain plotting shows no relevant outliers.

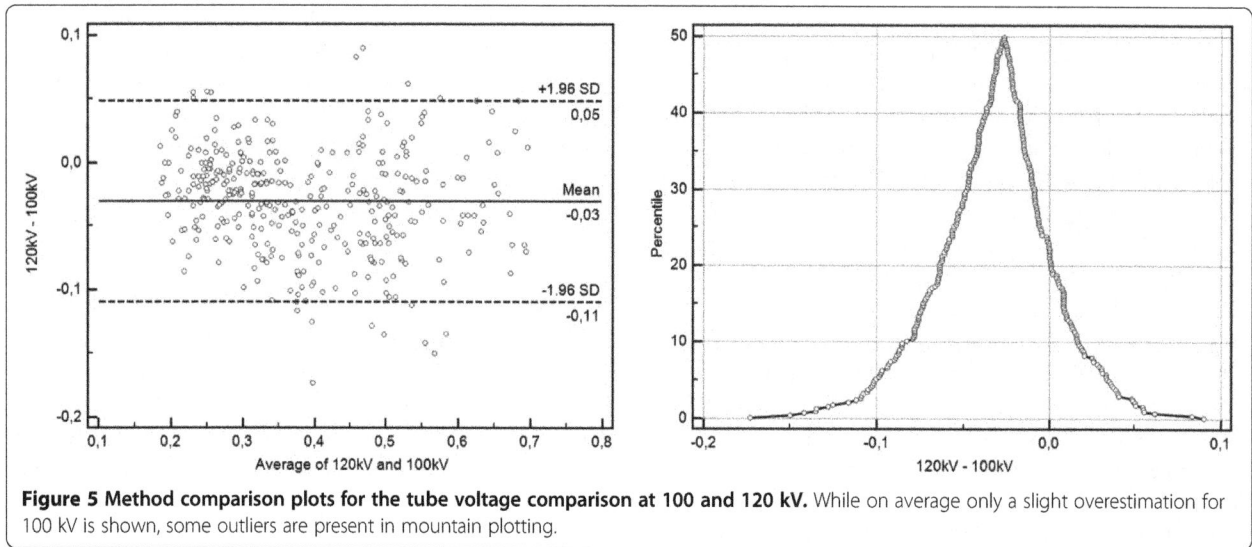

Figure 5 Method comparison plots for the tube voltage comparison at 100 and 120 kV. While on average only a slight overestimation for 100 kV is shown, some outliers are present in mountain plotting.

Discussion

Despite the fact that coronary CTA has found its way into the clinical workup of patients with suspected coronary artery disease, there are still major concerns regarding the applied radiation dose, which was determined to be in the typically order of 12 mSv (8–18 mSv) [10]. In comparison the effective radiation doses applied during invasive coronary angiography are reported to be approximately 5 mSv [11] with ranges from 2.3 to 22.7 mSv [3]. Because of its ability to rule out hemodynamically relevant coronary stenoses with a high negative predictive value, coronary CTA is especially suited for patients presenting with typical symptoms but having a low pre-test likelihood for coronary artery disease [12]. During the last few years different technical developments have been introduced in clinical routine practice in order to significantly reduce radiation dose of coronary CTA. These techniques include the use of lower tube voltage (e.g. 100 instead of 120 kV) [13] and the application of ECG-dependent tube current modulation. The latter bases upon the reduction of tube current of up to 80% during systolic phase and full dose is only applied during diastolic phase. This approach allows for dose reduction of up to

50% [14]. Another technique resulting in substantial reduction of radiation dose is realized by the use of prospective ECG-triggered transverse data acquisition (also known as "step and shot acquisition") instead of retrospective gated spiral scanning [15].

With the introduction of a modern dual-source CT scanner with simultaneous acquisition of 64 slices and a gantry rotation time of 330 ms a temporal resolution of 83 ms became technically feasible [16]. Latest generation of dual-source scanners reduced the rotation time to 0.28 s. Furthermore, due to the ca. 95° offset of both x-ray tubes within the gantry of dual source CT in combination with fast and precise table movement the use of high-pitch (>3.0) scan protocols for coronary CTA could be performed. The result was the ability to cover the whole heart within a single cardiac cycle [17]. Since then, different studies showed the diagnostic value of prospectively ECG-triggered high-pitch spiral coronary CTA [18,19].

The aim of the presented study was to investigate influence of scan protocol in combination with ECG-synchronization (prospective triggered high-pitch vs. retrospective ECG-gated spiral CT), tube voltage (100

Table 5 Pairwise comparisons of the average difference in degree of stenosis (Δ percentage) and measured plaque diameter for all used kernels

| | 796 mmHA/cm³ | | 401 mmHA/cm³ | |
	Δ Diameter	Δ Percentage	Δ Diameter	Δ Percentage
B26f	0.88 ± 0.26 mm	15.9 ± 4.2%	0.39 ± 0.27 mm	8.6 ± 6.8%
I26f	0.86 ± 0.25 mm	10.8 ± 5.0%	0.38 ± 0.26 mm	4.3 ± 6.5%
B46f	0.53 ± 0.27 mm	9.2 ± 6.6%	0.18 ± 0.26 mm	6.9 ± 6.9%
B70f	0.36 ± 0.33 mm	15.3 ± 4.0%	0.26 ± 0.27 mm	8.5 ± 6.6%
I70f	0.34 ± 0.33 mm	8.9 ± 6.7%	0.21 ± 0.26 mm	5.8 ± 6.6%

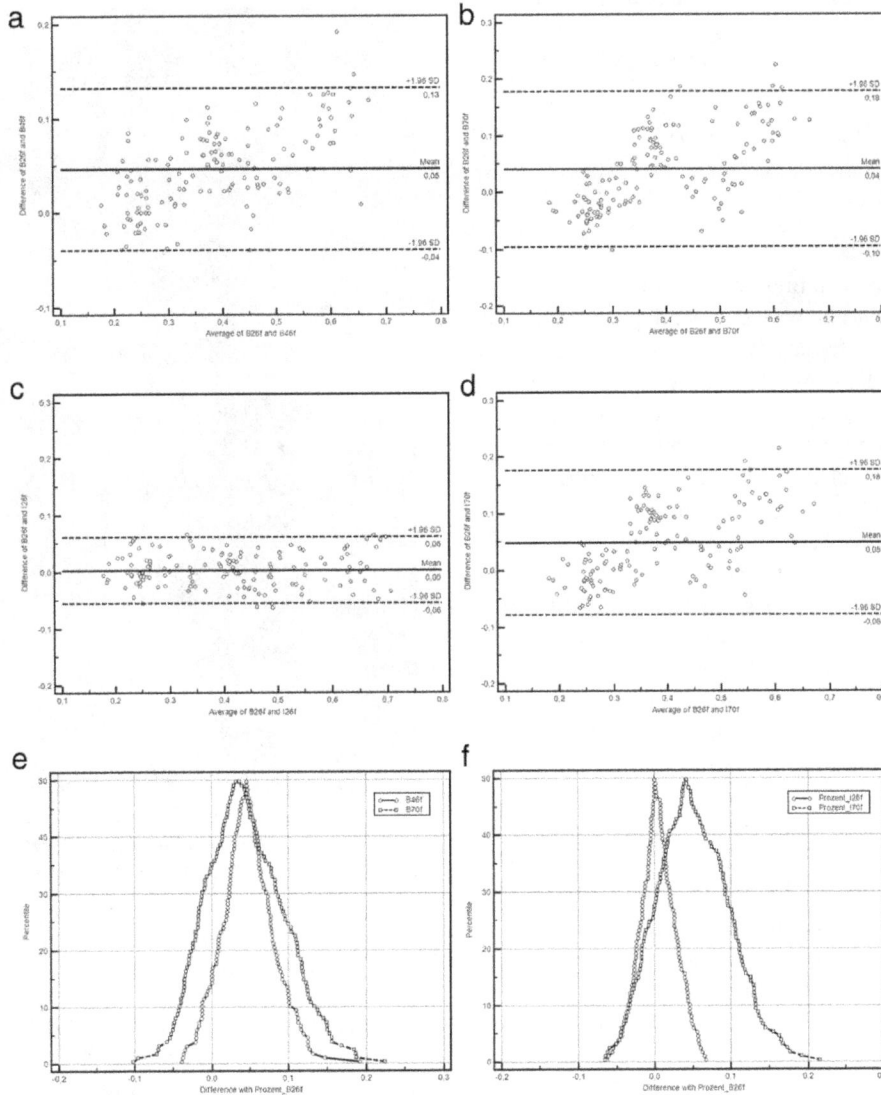

Figure 6 Method comparison plots for kernel comparisons (a-d Bland-Altman plots, e-f mountain plots). Shown are the differences between the standard B26f and the other kernels under investigation (**a**, **e**: B46f, **b**, **e**: B70f, **c**, **f**: I26f, **d**, **f**: I70f). While for B26f and I26f align perfectly, skewed distributions with outliers are visible for all other comparisons.

vs. 120 kV) and heart rate (50, 70, 90 bpm) on quantification of coronary artery stenosis due to plaques with different calcification levels. In general, all used CT examination protocols resulted in an overestimation of stenoses which increased with increasing calcium content and decreased with increasing grade of stenoses. This overestimation was slightly higher for the high pitch examination protocols in comparison to the retrospective ECG-gated technique. Both observations (overestimation of small lesions, which are highly calcified) are mainly due to blooming artifacts which occur when sharp edges with high attenuation differences are encountered in the scan volume [20,21]. A reason for the slight worsening of this phenomenon, when high pitch examination protocols are

used, may be the fact that attenuation data of two separate detectors are used for image reconstruction. However, in the clinical situation this finding may be of little relevance due to a maximum difference of 3 percent points regarding grade of stenosis (small, highly calcified plaque).

In most of the recently published clinical studies on prospective ECG-triggered high pitch cardiac CT a heart rate more than 60 bpm was defined as an exclusion criterion [4,18]. In our experimental setup there were no significant differences regarding vessel diameter, plaque diameter and grade of stenoses between the different heart rates (50, 70, 90) although we found a slight trend to larger deviations of the measured parameters comparing the 50 and the 90 bpm data (Table 2). The motion artifacts observed at

Table 6 Dose comparison between the two used cardiac CT methods

Trigger	Gated	High pitch	Statistics
CTDIvol [mGy]	2829.8 ± 1539.4	258.0 ± 66.3	p < 0.0001
DLP [mGycm]	341.2 ± 150.7	36.3 ± 9.6	p < 0.0001

Both DLP and CTDIvol are significantly lower for high pitch cardiac CT protocols in comparison to gating.

90 bpm high pitch scanning should however raise concerns about the applicability of the technique at such heart rates (Figure 8). This finding is at least to some degree in contrast to clinical findings which were recently published [22]. Scharf et al. reported about a cohort of 111 consecutive patients who underwent prospectively ECG-triggered high-pitch spiral CT of the chest for non-cardiac reason. The evaluation of image quality showed a significant difference of mean heart rate and mean heart rate variability between patients with diagnostic and non-diagnostic images of the coronary arteries. The optimal values were calculated with a heart rates lower than 64 bpm and heart rate variabilities of less than 13 bpm. With respect to this result it needs to be discussed that we used an extremely reliable experimental setup providing an absolutely stable heart rate. Nevertheless, our results may be a hint that prospectively ECG-triggered high-pitch cardiac CT may also be suited for patients presenting stable heart rates > 60 bpm and a low heart rate variability. This hypothesis is supported by the results of Feuchtner et al. who found significantly higher diagnostic image quality in patients with stable sinus rhythm but without premedication for heart rate control in comparison to patients with arrhythmia using a prospective triggered "step and shoot" CT-examination mode [23]. In this study a mean heart rate of 66.2 ± 8 bpm in patient group with stable sinus rhythm was associated with only 0.5% non-diagnostic coronary segments whereas 4% of coronary segments were scored non-diagnostic in the arrhythmia group with a mean heart rate of 70 ± 15 bpm.

In our experimental setting the use of a prospectively ECG-triggered high-pitch spiral examination protocol resulted in a reduction of radiation exposure of approximately 90% in comparison to a retrospective ECG-gated cardiac CT-examination (Table 6). This finding is mainly due to the significant oversampling using a pitch of 0.19 for retrospective ECG-gating in order to acquire enough data in all

Table 7 Dose comparison between the two used tube voltages

kV	100	120	Statistics
CTDIvol [mGy]	962.6 ± 862.9	2125.2 ± 2082.3	p = 0.0005
DLP [mGycm]	115.1 ± 93.4	262.4 ± 225.2	p = 0.0002

Both DLP and CTDIvol are significantly lower for 100 kV in comparison to 120 kV.

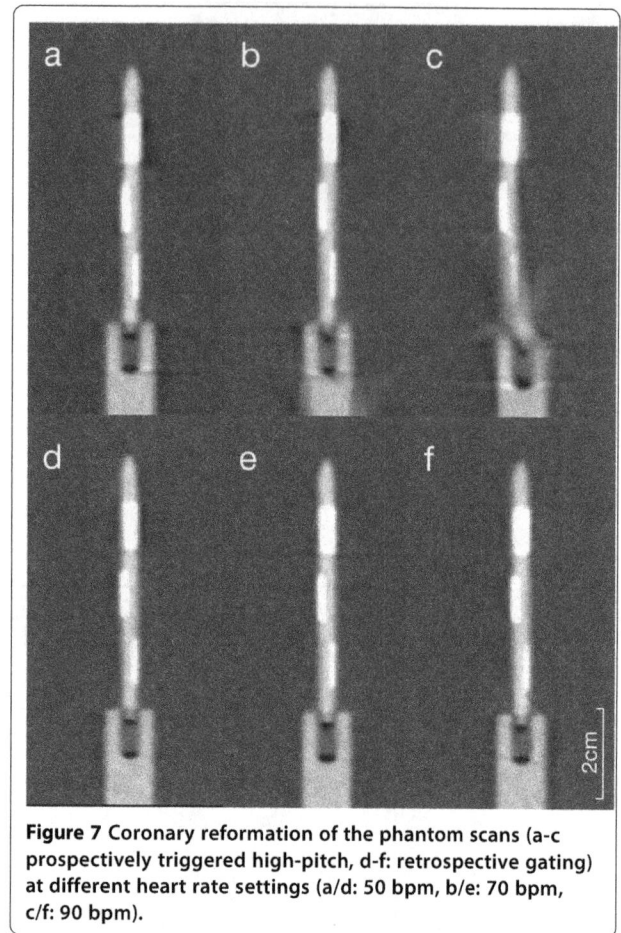

Figure 7 Coronary reformation of the phantom scans (a-c prospectively triggered high-pitch, d-f: retrospective gating) at different heart rate settings (a/d: 50 bpm, b/e: 70 bpm, c/f: 90 bpm).

cardiac phases. On the other hand this allows quantification of cardiac function in addition to the evaluation of coronary arteries. Comparing the measured diameters for the 100 and 120 kV examination modes we found a slight overestimation for the 100 kV CT-protocol (Table 3). However, we consider the differences (3 ± 8%) clinically not relevant whereas reduction of tube voltage results in further reduction of radiation dose applied to the patient. Due to the fact that lower tube voltage leads to increased image noise some authors used 100 kV scan protocols in patients < 100 kg body weight and 120 kV for > 100 kg, respectively [24].

Due to the experimental design of the study our results cannot be directly transferred into the clinical situation. The employed phantom provides a stable sinus rhythm without any variability due to arrhythmia or respiration. Furthermore, motion of the patient is not an issue in this setup. Another limitation that needs to be discussed is the fact that we did not really measure the applied radiation dose but simply compared the dose indices derived from the CT-scanner's software. Moreover, regarding the different tube voltages (100 vs. 120 kV) we cannot make conclusion regarding image quality in obese patients due to

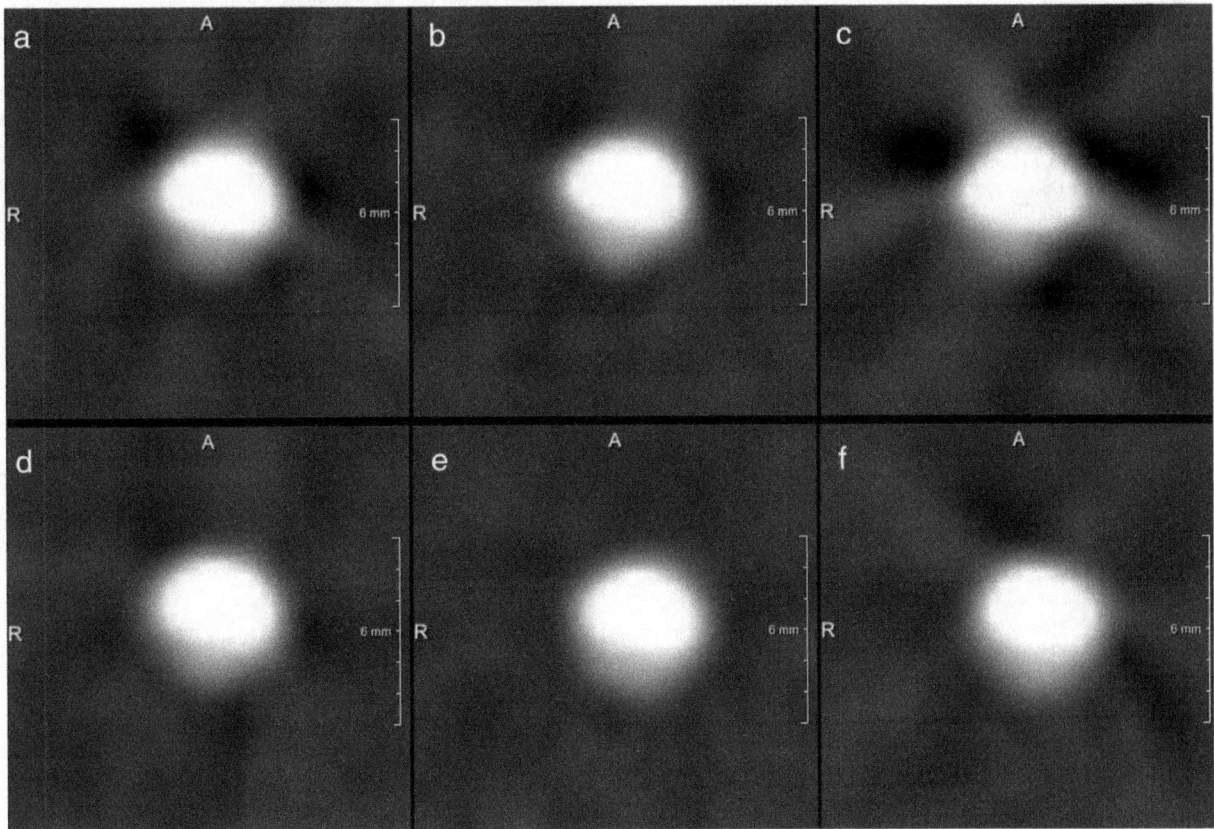

Figure 8 Image data reconstructed in different heart rate settings (a/d: 50 bpm; b/e: 70 bpm; c/f: 90 bpm, B26f) using either prospectively ECG-triggered high-pitch scanning (a – c) or retrospectively ECG-gated cardiac CT (d – f).

the fact that the phantom does not account for different subject weight. Further experiments should include these factors, for instance by applying different attenuation phantoms in the setup.

Conclusion

In conclusion, the presented results do not reveal any relevant differences in vessel diameter, plaque diameter and grade of stenoses between prospectively ECG-triggered high-pitch spiral CT in comparison to retrospectively ECG-gated spiral data acquisition in differently calcified plaques using a motion phantom. While there was reasonable agreement even at higher heart rates (90 bpm) between both examination modes, the presence of motion artifacts at 90 bpm questions the full applicability of the high pitch technique under these circumstances.

Competing interests
The study was carried out as part of a research agreement with Siemens Healthcare – CT Division -, Forchheim, Germany. TA is an employee of Siemens Healthcare, Forchheim, Germany.

Authors' contributions
Study design: TP, ED, PI, TA, CKK, AHM, PB, experiments, measurements: TP, ED, PI, TA, PB, manuscript draft: TP, PI, TA, CKK, AHM, PB. All authors read and approved the final manuscript.

Author details
[1]Department of Diagnostic and Interventional Radiology, Aachen University Hospital, RWTH Aachen University, Pauwelsstr. 30, 52074 Aachen, Germany. [2]Surgical Planning Laboratory, Department of Radiology, Brigham and Women's Hospital, 75 Francis Street, 02115 Boston, USA. [3]Applied Medical Engineering, Helmholtz-Institute Aachen, RWTH Aachen University, Pauwelsstr. 20, 52074 Aachen, Germany. [4]Siemens Healthcare, CT Division, Forchheim, Germany. [5]Department of Diagnostic and Interventional Radiology, University Hospital Marburg, Philipps University of Marburg, Marburg, Germany.

References
1. Vorobiof G, Achenbach S, Narula J: **Minimizing radiation dose for coronary CT angiography.** *Cardiol Clin* 2012, **30**(1):9–17.
2. Alkadhi H: **Radiation dose of cardiac CT–what is the evidence?** *Eur Radiol* 2009, **19**(6):1311–1315.
3. Einstein AJ, Moser KW, Thompson RC, Cerqueira MD, Henzlova MJ: **Radiation dose to patients from cardiac diagnostic imaging.** *Circulation* 2007, **116**(11):1290–1305.
4. Achenbach S, Marwan M, Ropers D, Schepis T, Pflederer T, Anders K, Kuettner A, Daniel WG, Uder M, Lell MM: **Coronary computed tomography angiography with a consistent dose below 1 mSv using prospectively electrocardiogram-triggered high-pitch spiral acquisition.** *Eur Heart J* 2010, **31**(3):340–346.
5. Flohr TG, Leng S, Yu L, Allmendinger T, Bruder H, Petersilka M, Eusemann CD, Stierstorfer K, Schmidt B, McCollough CH: **Dual-source spiral CT with pitch up to 3.2 and 75 ms temporal resolution: image reconstruction and assessment of image quality.** *Med Phys* 2009, **36**(12):5641–5653.

6. Flohr TG, McCollough CH, Bruder H, Petersilka M, Gruber K, Suss C, Grasruck M, Stierstorfer K, Krauss B, Raupach R, Primak AN, Kuttner A, Achenbach S, Becker C, Kopp A, Ohnesorge BM: **First performance evaluation of a dual-source CT (DSCT) system.** *Eur Radiol* 2006, **16**(2):256–268.

7. Morsbach F, Gordic S, Desbiolles L, Husarik D, Frauenfelder T, Schmidt B, Allmendinger T, Wildermuth S, Alkadhi H, Leschka S: **Performance of turbo high-pitch dual-source CT for coronary CT angiography: first *ex vivo* and patient experience.** *Eur Radiol* 2014, **24**(8):1889–1895.

8. Gordic S, Husarik DB, Desbiolles L, Leschka S, Frauenfelder T, Alkadhi H: **High-pitch coronary CT angiography with third generation dual-source CT: limits of heart rate.** *Int J Cardiovasc Imaging* 2014, **30**(6):1173–1179.

9. Ulzheimer S, Kalender WA: **Assessment of calcium scoring performance in cardiac computed tomography.** *Eur Radiol* 2003, **13**(3):484–497.

10. Hausleiter J, Meyer T, Hermann F, Hadamitzky M, Krebs M, Gerber TC, McCollough C, Martinoff S, Kastrati A, Schomig A, Achenbach S: **Estimated radiation dose associated with cardiac CT angiography.** *JAMA* 2009, **301**(5):500–507.

11. Coles DR, Smail MA, Negus IS, Wilde P, Oberhoff M, Karsch KR, Baumbach A: **Comparison of radiation doses from multislice computed tomography coronary angiography and conventional diagnostic angiography.** *J Am Coll Cardiol* 2006, **47**(9):1840–1845.

12. Hoffman U, Venkatesh V, White RD, Woodard PK, Carr JJ, Dorbala S, Earls JP, Jacobs JE, Mammen L, Martin ET, Ryan T, White CS: *ACR Appropriateness Criteria: Acute Nonspecific Chest Pain - low Probability of Coronary Artery Disease.* Reston, VA, USA: American College of Radiology; 2011. ACR Appropriateness Criteria.

13. Pflederer T, Rudofsky L, Ropers D, Bachmann S, Marwan M, Daniel WG, Achenbach S: **Image quality in a low radiation exposure protocol for retrospectively ECG-gated coronary CT angiography.** *AJR Am J Roentgenol* 2009, **192**(4):1045–1050.

14. Paul JF, Abada HT: **Strategies for reduction of radiation dose in cardiac multislice CT.** *Eur Radiol* 2007, **17**(8):2028–2037.

15. Maruyama T, Takada M, Hasuike T, Yoshikawa A, Namimatsu E, Yoshizumi T: **Radiation dose reduction and coronary assessability of prospective electrocardiogram-gated computed tomography coronary angiography: comparison with retrospective electrocardiogram-gated helical scan.** *J Am Coll Cardiol* 2008, **52**(18):1450–1455.

16. Flohr TG, Bruder H, Stierstorfer K, Petersilka M, Schmidt B, McCollough CH: **Image reconstruction and image quality evaluation for a dual source CT scanner.** *Med Phys* 2008, **35**(12):5882–5897.

17. Achenbach S, Marwan M, Schepis T, Pflederer T, Bruder H, Allmendinger T, Petersilka M, Anders K, Lell M, Kuettner A, Ropers D, Daniel WG, Flohr T: **High-pitch spiral acquisition: a new scan mode for coronary CT angiography.** *J Cardiovasc Comput Tomogr* 2009, **3**(2):117–121.

18. Achenbach S, Goroll T, Seltmann M, Pflederer T, Anders K, Ropers D, Daniel WG, Uder M, Lell M, Marwan M: **Detection of coronary artery stenoses by low-dose, prospectively ECG-triggered, high-pitch spiral coronary CT angiography.** *JACC Cardiovasc Imaging* 2011, **4**(4):328–337.

19. Kropil P, Rojas CA, Ghoshhajra B, Lanzman RS, Miese FR, Scherer A, Kalra M, Abbara S: **Prospectively ECG-triggered high-pitch spiral acquisition for cardiac CT angiography in routine clinical practice: initial results.** *J Thorac Imaging* 2012, **27**(3):194–201.

20. Dey D, Slomka P, Chien D, Fieno D, Abidov A, Saouaf R, Thomson L, Friedman JD, Berman DS: **Direct quantitative *in vivo* comparison of calcified atherosclerotic plaque on vascular MRI and CT by multimodality image registration.** *J Magn Reson Imaging* 2006, **23**(3):345–354.

21. Joseph PM, Spital RD: **The exponential edge-gradient effect in x-ray computed tomography.** *Phys Med Biol* 1981, **26**(3):473–487.

22. Scharf M, Bink R, May MS, Hentschke C, Achenbach S, Uder M, Lell MM: **High-pitch thoracic CT with simultaneous assessment of coronary arteries: effect of heart rate and heart rate variability on image quality and diagnostic accuracy.** *JACC Cardiovasc Imaging* 2011, **4**(6):602–609.

23. Feuchtner G, Goetti R, Plass A, Baumueller S, Stolzmann P, Scheffel H, Wieser M, Marincek B, Alkadhi H, Leschka S: **Dual-step prospective ECG-triggered 128-slice dual-source CT for evaluation of coronary arteries and cardiac function without heart rate control: a technical note.** *Eur Radiol* 2010, **20**(9):2092–2099.

24. Lell M, Marwan M, Schepis T, Pflederer T, Anders K, Flohr T, Allmendinger T, Kalender W, Ertel D, Thierfelder C, Kuettner A, Ropers D, Daniel WG, Achenbach S: **Prospectively ECG-triggered high-pitch spiral acquisition for coronary CT angiography using dual source CT: technique and initial experience.** *Eur Radiol* 2009, **19**(11):2576–2583.

9

The accuracy of a designed software for automated localization of craniofacial landmarks on CBCT images

Shoaleh Shahidi[1], Ehsan Bahrampour[2*], Elham Soltanimehr[3], Ali Zamani[4], Morteza Oshagh[5], Marzieh Moattari[6] and Alireza Mehdizadeh[4]

Abstract

Background: Two-dimensional projection radiographs have been traditionally considered the modality of choice for cephalometric analysis. To overcome the shortcomings of two-dimensional images, three-dimensional computed tomography (CT) has been used to evaluate craniofacial structures. However, manual landmark detection depends on medical expertise, and the process is time-consuming. The present study was designed to produce software capable of automated localization of craniofacial landmarks on cone beam (CB) CT images based on image registration and to evaluate its accuracy.

Methods: The software was designed using MATLAB programming language. The technique was a combination of feature-based (principal axes registration) and voxel similarity-based methods for image registration. A total of 8 CBCT images were selected as our reference images for creating a head atlas. Then, 20 CBCT images were randomly selected as the test images for evaluating the method. Three experts twice located 14 landmarks in all 28 CBCT images during two examinations set 6 weeks apart. The differences in the distances of coordinates of each landmark on each image between manual and automated detection methods were calculated and reported as mean errors.

Results: The combined intraclass correlation coefficient for intraobserver reliability was 0.89 and for interobserver reliability 0.87 (95% confidence interval, 0.82 to 0.93). The mean errors of all 14 landmarks were <4 mm. Additionally, 63.57% of landmarks had a mean error of <3 mm compared with manual detection (gold standard method).

Conclusion: The accuracy of our approach for automated localization of craniofacial landmarks, which was based on combining feature-based and voxel similarity-based methods for image registration, was acceptable. Nevertheless we recommend repetition of this study using other techniques, such as intensity-based methods.

Background

Cephalometric analysis is one of the key tools for arriving at an accurate diagnosis, planning treatment, evaluating growth, and research [1-3]. Landmark-based analysis is the most common method for cephalometric analysis [4]. Detection of landmarks plays an essential role in medical diagnosis and treatment planning [5].

Two-dimensional (2D) projection radiographs have been traditionally considered the modality of choice for orthodontic cephalometric analysis [6]. However, plain radiography has many shortcomings, such as superimposition of

structures of the left and right sides of the skull, unequal magnification of bilateral structures [4], the possibility of distortion of mid-facial structures [7], and random errors that arise as a result of variations in positioning the patient in the cephalostat [8].

To overcome these shortcomings, three-dimensional (3D) computed tomography (CT) has been used to evaluate craniofacial structures with less distortion than plain-film views [4]. The introduction of cone beam computed tomography (CBCT) during the past decade offers advantages over plain CT, such as smaller machines, reduced costs, and increased accessibility [9]. With the development of CBCT, 3D assessment of the craniofacial region has become an alternative for patient imaging [10].

* Correspondence: e.bahrampour@gmail.com
[2]Department of Oral and Maxillofacial Radiology, School of Dentistry, Shiraz University of Medical Sciences, Shiraz, Iran
Full list of author information is available at the end of the article

The accuracy and reliability of landmark detection and cephalometric measurements using 3D data gathered using the CBCT technique have been confirmed [1,4,9,11,12]. For example, it has been shown that 3D images are more accurate and reliable than traditional cephalographic projections for both landmark detection [4] and measurements [11]. However, using 3D landmark identification is more time-consuming than using conventional 2D cephalographic tracings [12].

Landmark detection can be performed manually or automatically. Manual landmark detection depends on medical expertise [13]. In addition to the necessity of previous experience, the process is time-consuming and tedious [14]. Hence, there have been efforts to computerize and automate cephalometric analysis based on 2D data [13] and 3D data [5,14]. For 2D images, four approaches are available when designing software that can locate cephalometric landmarks (image filtering plus knowledge-based landmark search, model-based approaches, soft-computing approaches, hybrid approaches). Leonardi et al. concluded that the errors in landmark detection using these methods were greater than those experienced with manual tracing, concluding that these systems are not accurate enough for clinical purposes [15].

To the best of our knowledge, few studies have focused on 3D data. Those that are available were limited to studying 3D surface-rendered models. For example, Mestiri and Hamrouni designed software using Reeb graphs [5]. Pan Zheng et al. used a Visualization Toolkit (VTK) and wrapper language Tcl/tk as a computer-assisted method. They suggested that automatic localization of 3D craniofacial landmarks should be studied in the future [14].

Although there are problems with manual detection, developing a fully automated system for identifying landmarks remains challenging [14]. We have found no published studies that have attempted to develop software that can detect landmarks based on image registration. Presumably, such an automated system would result in more convenient and accurate measurements. The present study was designed to produce software capable of automated localization of craniofacial landmarks based on image registration. We then evaluated its accuracy.

Methods
Study design
A total of 28 CBCT images were imported into our newly designed software. After three experts localized 14 landmarks, 8 of the 28 CBCT images were used as reference images to create a head atlas. The remaining 20 CBCT images were used as test images to evaluate our software.

This study was performed in accordance with the Declaration of Helsinki and was approved by the ethics committee of Shiraz University of Medical Sciences (ECSUMS) issued on 07 July 2013 (reference code EC-P-92-5479).

Written informed consent was obtained from each patient for the publication of this report and any accompanying images.

Subjects
To create the atlas, 8 CBCT images that came from patients with ideal cephalometric measurements (ages 10–45 years, distributed in intervals of about 5 years) were selected from an archive of 500 previously acquired images at one of the two main private oral and maxillofacial radiology centers in Shiraz.

For testing our system, 20 CBCT images were randomly selected from the same archive. They were randomized using a random numbers table. The number selected from the table showed the CBCT code that would be selected from the archive. The inclusion criteria for test images were large field-of-view (FOV) CBCT images of orthodontic patients. Exclusion criteria included images with significant fractures or severe skeletal anomalies. All of the subjects were aged between 10 and 43 years.

Each patient was positioned in the NewTom VGi Cone Beam CT machine (QR SRL Company, Verona, Italy) with the aid of a guide light. The Frankfort horizontal plane (FHP) was parallel to the floor, and the mid-sagittal plane passed through the glabella. The examinations were performed at 4.71 mA and 110 kVp, with a scan time of 3.6 s. The FOV was 15 × 15 cm for all images.

The raw images from the CBCT scan were converted to digital information and communication in medicine (DICOM) three multifiles using the NNT viewer software version 2.21 (Quantitative Radiology, Verona, Italy). The DICOM images were loaded into our new software for localizing the landmarks manually and then automatically.

Software
Technical experts designed the software using MATLAB programming language. This system is capable of presenting images that allow us to locate landmarks manually, reporting the coordinates of landmarks in x, y, and z planes, and detecting landmarks in its automated mode.

Localizing landmarks manually
A total of 14 cephalometric landmarks were located based on the description of the landmarks provided by Zamora et al. [1]. The 14 landmarks were at point A, point B, anterior nasal spine (ANS), posterior nasal spine (PNS), pogonion (Pog), nasion (N), sella (S), gnathion (Gn), menton (Me), right gonion (Go), tip of the right upper central incisor (U1T), apex of the right upper central incisor (U1A), tip of the right lower central incisor (L1T), and apex of the right lower central incisor (L1A).

Three experts (two orthodontists and one maxillofacial radiologist) were trained to locate landmarks using a set of three CBCT images not included in this study. Working independently after calibration and using the software, each of the three experts located the landmarks twice in all 28 CBCT images during two examinations separated by an interval of 6 weeks. Image presentation was in a four-panel window containing axial, coronal, and sagittal slices beside the 3D rendered model (Figure 1). Image enhancement features such as zoom in/out and changes of brightness and contrast were available for finding the landmarks more accurately. Landmarks were identified using a mouse-driven graphical cursor on the displayed 3D surface-rendered model, followed by adjusting the landmark using multiplanar reconstruction (MPR) images. This method was described by Bassam Hassan as the most precise method for localizing craniofacial landmarks [9]. The mean of the coordinates of six manual identifications of each landmark was defined as the baseline.

Creating a 3D cephalometric head atlas

We needed to create a 3D cephalometric head atlas that contained the 14 normal landmarks as a reference model. For accurate registration, it was better to reduce the scaling, translation, and rotation among images. More similarity among the images would eliminate these factors, rendering the registration more accurate. We used each patient's age as a criterion for the size of his or her head (older patients would have larger heads because of the natural growth process). We then used the eight CBCT images to create the atlas. When the software was presented with a test image, it automatically selected the reference image from among those eight samples based on age-matched data for the test subject and the reference subject.

Automated landmark detection

We used image registration to transfer the landmarks from our atlas images to the test images. For this purpose, we used a method proposed by Too et al. that has the benefits of both feature-based and voxel similarity-based methods [16]. Briefly, transformation parameters are calculated based on the centroid and the principal axes of the two CBCT images (Figure 2). The method uses the whole 3D volume to provide reliable registration results. Extraction of the principal axis of the 3D object is accomplished in three steps: feature extraction, centroid calculation, and principal axis calculation. A binary volume is used as the feature to represent the 3D geometric shape to extract the principal axes. Gray-scale CBCT images were changed to binary images using adaptive thresholding.

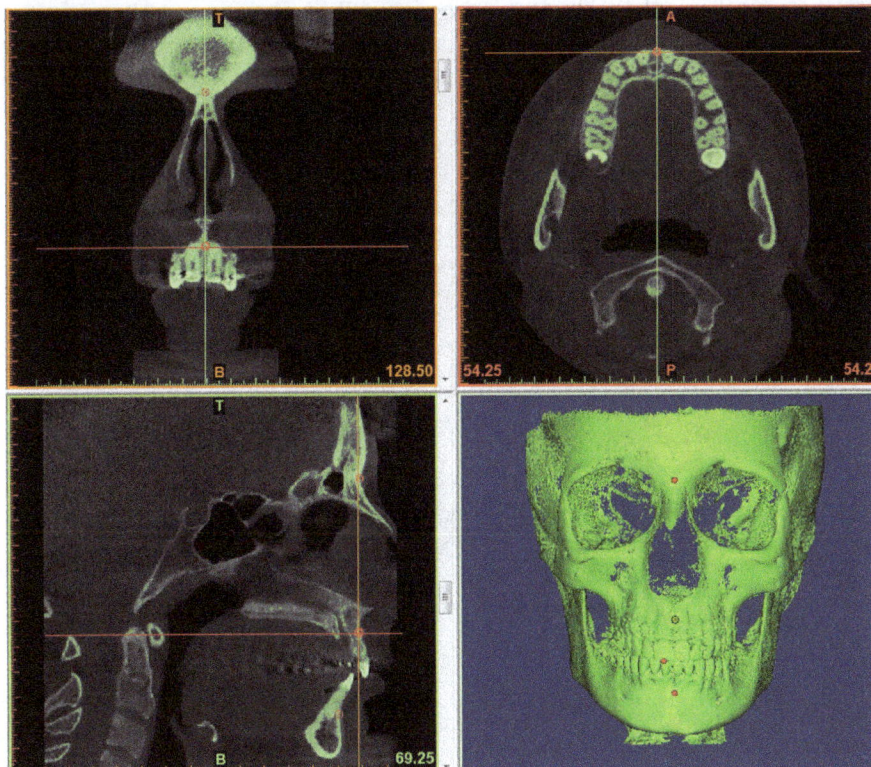

Figure 1 Landmark localization window displaying coronal, sagittal, and axial MPR views beside the 3D surface rendered skeletal volume.

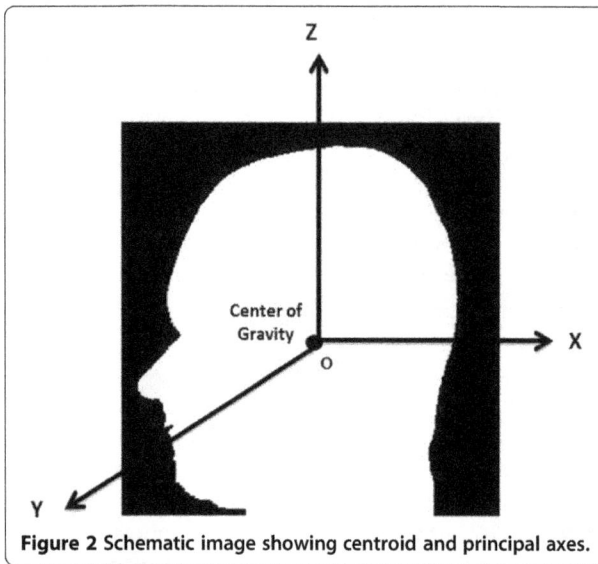

Figure 2 Schematic image showing centroid and principal axes.

Statistical analysis

All variables and measurements were introduced into a version 12.0 Excel spreadsheet (Microsoft Corp., Redmond, WA, USA) and were then analyzed using version 20.0 of the statistical package SPSS for Windows (IBM Corp., Somers, NY, USA). Intraclass correlation coefficients (ICCs) were used to determine intraobserver and interobserver agreement. To compare the values generated by the software to the values provided by experts, distances of coordinates of each landmark on each image between manual and automated detection methods were calculated with a 3D Euclidian distance formula,

$$\text{Distance} = \sqrt{(x_1 - x_2)^2 + (y_1 - y_2)^2 + (z_1 - z_2)^2},$$

where x_1, y_1, z_1 are coordinates for manual detection and x_2, y_2, z_2 are coordinates for automated detection.

Results

The ICCs and 95% confidence intervals (95% CI) for intraobserver reliability on measurements were 0.86 (0.81 to 0.95) for observer 1; 0.89 (0.83 to 0.96) for observer 2; 0.93 (0.88 to 0.96) for observer 3. The combined ICC for intraobserver reliability was 0.89. The ICC and 95% CI for interobserver reliability were 0.87 and 0.82–0.93.

The minimum error, maximum error, mean error, standard error of the mean, and percentage of cases with <3 mm mean error from the baselines for the manually and automatically identified landmarks are summarized in Tables 1 and 2. According to Table 1, the most precisely identified landmark was the pogonion, with a 3 mm mean error. The least precisely identified landmark was point B, which had a mean error of 3.86 mm.

Discussion

This study was performed to assess the accuracy of new software that had been specifically designed based on

During this process, a threshold is calculated for each pixel in the image. The output is thus a binary image representing the segmentation. Principal axes and the centroids for both images were computed with respect to equations explained by Too et al. [16]. We completed the registration by scaling, rotation, and translation of the test image (Figures 3 and 4). After scaling, the test image vector was as long as the reference image vector in all directions (axial, coronal, sagittal). For the last step, the landmark was transferred between images. The flowchart of our algorithm is shown in Figure 5.

Evaluation of the software

To evaluate the accuracy of the software regarding its automated detection of landmarks, we compared each landmark's coordinates generated from the 20 CBCT images by the software to the mean values that experts had determined previously as the reference.

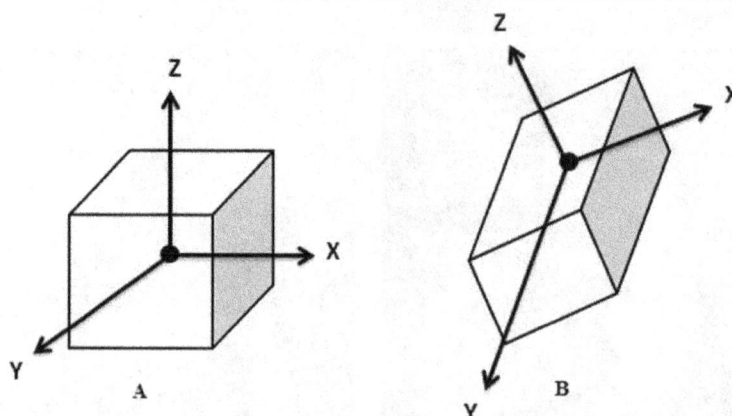

Figure 3 Schematic image showing scaling function and image registration, A is the reference image and B is the test image.

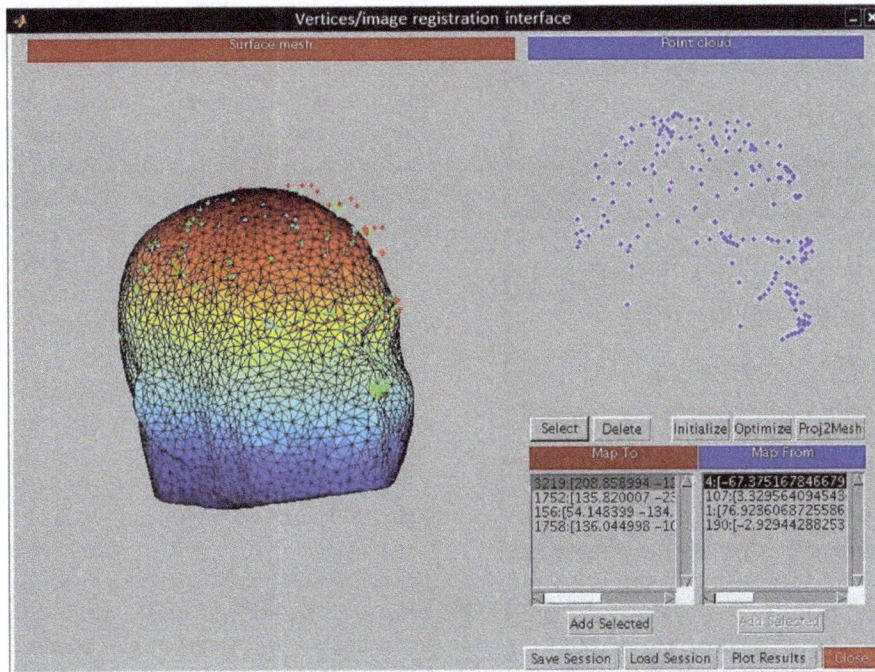

Figure 4 Image registration interface. The 3D image in the left side illustrating the test image and the blue points on the right side are the landmarks of the reference image used for registration process. These landmarks are different from the craniofacial landmarks.

image registration. Its purpose was automated localization of craniofacial landmarks. Our approach was based on volume matching using the whole 3D volume. The mean errors of all 14 landmarks were <4 mm. Also, 63.57% of the landmarks had a mean error of <3 mm compared to manual detection (gold standard method). The mean error for all of the automatically identified landmarks in our study was higher than the mean error for the manually detected landmarks. However, in some studies on 2D images, a distance of ≤4 mm was considered acceptable [17,18]. De Oliveira et al. stated that the clinical significance of the accuracy of the landmark identification error depends on the level of accuracy required [12]. However, it seems that the acceptability of this error should be further evaluated. Mestiri and Hamrouni proposed a system that was designed to use Reeb graphs for automatic localization of cephalometric landmarks. The authors reported that 18 of 20 landmarks related to just one case were recognized successfully, with errors from baseline of 0.5 to 2.8 mm [5]. Pan Zheng et al. tried to visualize craniofacial landmarks and identify them using a Visualization Toolkit (VTK) and wrapper language Tcl/tk. Their method was not completely automated [14].

In this study, we used 28 CBCT images from an archive of 500 CBCTs. All the subjects had been positioned in the CBCT machine with the FHP parallel to the floor and the mid-sagittal plane passing through the

glabella. Bassam Hassan et al. considered that 3D images were preferred to 2D images because of the higher accuracy they offered in regard to head position. They stated that small variations in the patient's head position do not influence the measurement accuracy in 3D images, whereas there was a significant difference between the ideal and rotated scan positions for the 2D images [6].

In our study, three experts manually identified all landmarks in our 28 CBCT images at two separate sessions, ensuring the validity of the coordinates against our gold standard values. We asked them to use 3D surface-rendered models in addition to MPR images because the addition of MPR images to the 3D model can increase the precision of landmark detection. Research performed in 2009 showed that the use of MPR images takes full advantage of the 3D CBCT information, whereas locating landmarks on the 3D renderings alone can lead to error [12]. Bassam Hassan et al. in 2009 stated that performing cephalometric analysis on 3D-rendered models seems to be the most appropriate approach with regard to accuracy and convenience [6]. However, in research published in 2011, Bassam Hassan et al. concluded that addition of MPR images to the 3D model does have a positive influence on precision—but on average takes twice as much time [9].

The head atlas we created was uniquely designed to provide reference images for image registration. It was

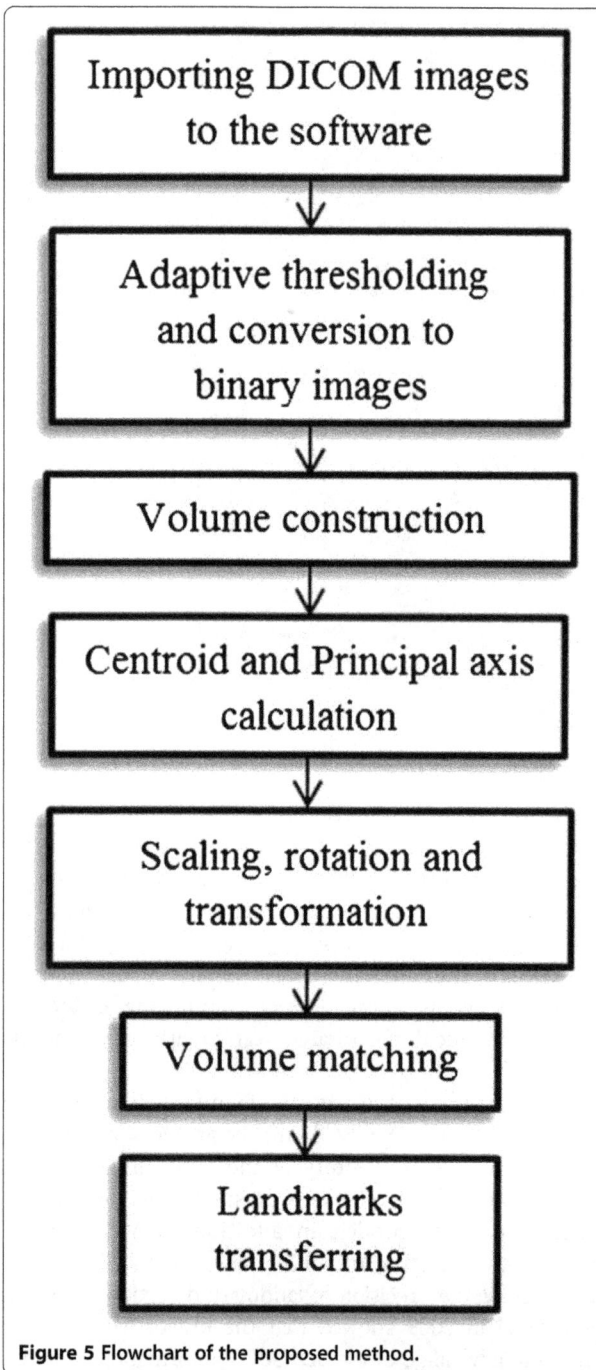

Figure 5 Flowchart of the proposed method.

based on eight CBCT images from subjects at 5-year age intervals. All of the images were evaluated by experts using the 3D + MPR method, which ensures additional precision. Mestiri and Hamrouni stated that they had created a head atlas assisted by medical staff, but they did not explain their exact method [5].

A total of 20 CBCT images were used to evaluate the accuracy of our method. This number was considered suitable by the authors. In a systematic review,

however, the number of images required to appraise the effectiveness of automated landmark detection in 2D images ranged from 5 to 600 [15]. We could not find similar studies on 3D images that reported such a considerable sample size. In a study performed at the University of El-Manar, only one CT image was used to evaluate the accuracy of their method (Reeb graph) for automated localization of the landmarks. Those authors stated that their method needed to be validated on a larger database [5]. Although we used more images in our study, we recommend repetition of similar studies using a larger sample size.

We used a new method for registration, first proposed by Too et al. They combined the advantages of feature-based and voxel similarity-based methods by converting the volumetric data to a binary volume as a feature, followed by use of Principal Axes Registration (PAR) [19]. We believed PAR to be the most effective one among the feature-based methods because it can find the transformation parameters easily and has less computational complexity [16]. Alpert et al. stated that registration by the principal axes transformation can be accomplished with typical errors in the area of ~1 mm. It also has the advantages of simplicity and speed of computation [19]. To the best of our knowledge, our study is the first conducted to implement and evaluate this method for automated landmark localization on maxillofacial CBCT images.

Although the current study presents a valuable method for automated detection of craniofacial landmarks on CBCT images, it has some limitations. First, we did not exclude images of patients with orthodontic braces. These images were responsible for most of our observed error, which reflects the impact of streak artifacts. We concluded that more errors occur with images of patients who have orthodontic appliances and probably surgical rigid fixation as well.

The radiation dosage in CBCT is another limitation that may limit implementation of this technique. The use of large-volume (craniofacial) CBCT imaging—i.e., the entire facial skeleton—is a common procedure for orthodontic-related radiological assessment by some clinicians [20,21]. According to the SEDENTEXTC guideline, however, its radiation dose, particularly in pediatric patients, is a challenging issue. The use of large volume CBCT may be justified when planning a definitive procedure in complex cases of skeletal abnormality, particularly those requiring combined orthodontic/surgical management [22]. However, it is not plausible to expose all orthodontic patients to the radiologic dose of CBCT with the intention of cephalometric analysis per se.

The database used in the present study included only Iranian patients. Therefore, our results may not

Table 1 The Min. error, Max. error, mean error and the standard error of the mean for the 6 manually detected landmarks' coordinates from the mean of those coordinates as the gold standard

Landmark	Min. error (mm)	Max. error (mm)	Mean error (mm)	Standard error of the mean (mm)	Percentage of cases with <3 mm mean error
A	0.89	1.94	1.72	0.62	100%
B	0.95	1.85	1.36	0.52	100%
ANS	1.15	1.90	1.66	0.46	100%
PNS	1.63	2.35	2.10	0.38	100%
Pog	1.05	1.84	1.70	0.36	100%
N	0.96	1.80	1.64	0.48	100%
S	0.75	1.45	1.26	0.39	100%
Gn	1.05	2.60	2.15	0.89	100%
Me	0.86	1.40	1.24	0.26	100%
Go	1.22	2.54	1.96	0.66	100%
U1T	0.65	1.10	0.93	0.28	100%
U1A	0.54	0.89	0.74	0.22	100%
L1T	0.56	0.80	0.68	0.18	100%
L1A	0.45	0.75	0.59	0.19	100%
Total	0.45 for Point L1A	2.60 for Point Gn	1.41 mm	-	100%

be applicable to other populations. We suggest that further research be undertaken using appropriate databases from other ethnic groups. We also suggest that image registration using other approaches be attempted in the future. Intensity-based methods seem to be accurate and suitable for clinical application [23]. We do recommend evaluations of measurement analyses based on automated landmark detection methods.

Conclusion

We contend that this software is the first to use a combined method (feature-based and voxel similarity-based) for image registration during automated localization of craniofacial landmarks on CBCT images. The accuracy of our method was acceptable. Nevertheless we recommend repetition of this study using other techniques, such as intensity-based methods.

Table 2 The Min. error, Max. error, mean error and the standard error of the mean for the automatically identified landmarks in millimeters from the baselines

Landmark	Min. error (mm)	Max. error (mm)	Mean error (mm)	Standard error of the mean (mm)	Percentage of cases with <3 mm mean error
A	1.58	4.77	3.11	0.74	60%
B	2.48	5.92	3.86	1.41	55%
ANS	2.38	4.52	3.12	0.80	70%
PNS	2.35	5.36	3.60	1.35	60%
Pog	2.02	4.78	3.00	1.02	60%
N	1.62	5.97	3.20	1.64	65%
S	1.83	6.12	3.45	1.82	55%
Gn	1.76	7.10	3.77	2.69	65%
Me	2.24	6.78	3.59	1.79	75%
Go	2.15	5.91	3.72	1.67	70%
U1T	2.22	6.70	3.59	1.76	70%
U1A	2.26	4.81	3.15	0.91	60%
L1T	2.31	4.84	3.30	0.92	60%
L1A	1.98	4.98	3.08	1.08	65%
Total	1.58 mm for Point A	7.10 mm for Point Gn	3.40 mm	-	63.57%

Competing interests
The authors declare that they have no competing interests.

Authors' contributions
ShSh devised the study concept, designed the study, supervised the intervention, data collection and analysis, participated in the coordination of the study, and critically revised the manuscript. BE and SE collected data, ran the study intervention, participated in the study concept, performed the analyses, and drafted the manuscript. ZA participated in the intervention, data collection and revision of the manuscript. OM contributed to the design and analysis of the study data, and revised the manuscript. MM participated in the intervention, data collection and revision of the manuscript. MA contributed to the design and intervention of the study, and manuscript revision. All authors read and approved the final manuscript.

Acknowledgements
The authors thank the Vice-chancellory of Shiraz University of Medical Sciences for supporting this research (Grant #EC-P-925479). This manuscript is based on the thesis by Dr. Ehsan Bahrampour. The authors also thank Dr. Vosough of the Center of Research Improvement of the School of Dentistry for the statistical analysis.

Author details
[1]Biomaterial Research Center, Department of Oral and Maxillofacial Radiology, School of Dentistry, Shiraz University of Medical Sciences, Shiraz, Iran. [2]Department of Oral and Maxillofacial Radiology, School of Dentistry, Shiraz University of Medical Sciences, Shiraz, Iran. [3]Department of Pediatric Dentistry, School of Dentistry, Shiraz University of Medical Sciences, Shiraz, Iran. [4]Medical Physics and Medical Engineering Department, School of Medicine, Shiraz University of Medical Sciences, Shiraz, Iran. [5]Private Practice, Tehran, Iran. [6]Faculty of Nursing and Midwifery, Shiraz University of Medical Sciences, Shiraz, Iran.

References

1. Zamora N, Llamas JM, Cibrian R, Gandia JL, Paredes V: **Cephalometric measurements from 3D reconstructed images compared with conventional 2D images.** *Angle Orthod* 2011, **81**:856–864.
2. Miller SBDM: **Computer-aided head film analysis: the University of California San Francisco method.** *Am J Orthod* 1980, **78**:41–65.
3. Forsyth DB, Shaw WC, Richmond S, Roberts CT: **Digital imaging of cephalometric radiographs, Part 2: Image quality.** *Angle Orthod* 1996, **66**:43–50.
4. Ludlow JB, Gubler M, Cevidanes L, Mol A: **Precision of cephalometric landmark identification: cone-beam computed tomography vs conventional cephalometric views.** *Am J Orthod Dentofacial Orthop* 2009, **136**:312 e311-310; discussion 312-313.
5. Makram M, Kamel H: **Reeb Graph for Automatic 3D Cephalometry.** *IJIP* 2014, **8**:17–29.
6. Hassan B, van der Stelt P, Sanderink G: **Accuracy of three-dimensional measurements obtained from cone beam computed tomography surface-rendered images for cephalometric analysis: influence of patient scanning position.** *Eur J Orthod* 2009, **31**:129–134.
7. Chen YJ, Chen SK, Yao JC, Chang HF: **The effects of differences in landmark identification on the cephalometric meaurements in traditional versus digitized cephalometry.** *Angle Orthod* 2004, **74**:155–161.
8. Houston WJB: **The analysis of errors in orthodontic measurements.** *Am J Orthod* 1983, **83**. http://www.ncbi.nlm.nih.gov/pubmed/?term=Houston+WJB%3A+The+analysis+of+errors+in+orthodontic+measurements+Am+J+Orthod+1983%2C+83.
9. Bassam H, Peter N, Hans V, Jamshed T, Christian V, van der Stelt P, Beek H: **Percision of identifying cephalometric landmarks with cone beam computed tomography in vivo.** *Euro J Orthodontics* 2011. doi:10.1093/ejo/cjr050.
10. Gribel BF, Gribel MN, Manzi FR, Brooks SL, McNamara JA Jr: **From 2D to 3D: an algorithm to derive normal values for 3-dimensional computerized assessment.** *Angle Orthod* 2011, **81**:3–10.
11. Couceiro CP, Vilella OV: **2D/3D Cone-Beam CT images or convensional radiography: Which is more reliable?** *Dental Press J Orthod* 2010, **15**:40–41.
12. de Oliveira AE, Cevidanes LH, Phillips C, Motta A, Burke B, Tyndall D: **Observer reliability of three-dimensional cephalometric landmark identification on cone-beam computerized tomography.** *Oral Surg Oral Med Oral Pathol Oral Radiol Endod* 2009, **107**:256–265.
13. Shahidi S, Oshagh M, Gozin F, Salehi P, Danaei S: **Accuracy of computerized automatic identification of cephalometric landmarks by a designed software.** *Dentomaxillofac Radiol* 2013, **42**:20110187.
14. Pan Z, Bahari B, Rozniza Z, Arash I, Rajion ZA: **Computerized 3D Craniofacial Landmark Identification and Analysis.** *eJCSIT* 2009, 1.
15. Rosalia L, Daniela G, Francesco M, Spampinato C: **Automatic Cephalometric Analysis A Systematic Review.** *Angle Orthod* 2008, **78**:145.
16. Naw Chit TJ, Xuenan C, Shengzhe L, Hakil K: **Fast and Accurate Rigid Registration of 3D CT Images by Combining Feature and Intensity.** *J Comp Sci Eng* 2012, **6**:1–11.
17. Yue W, Yin D, Li C, Wang G, Xu T: **Automated 2-D cephalometric analysis on X-ray images by a model-based approach.** *IEEE Trans Biomed Eng* 2006, **53**:1615–1623.
18. El-Feghi IS-AM, Ahmadi M: **Automatic localization of craniofacial landmarks for assisted cephalometry.** *Pattern Recognit* 2004, **37**:609–621.
19. Alpert NM, Bradshaw JF, Kennedy D, Correia JA: **The principal axes transformation–a method for image registration.** *J Nuc Med* 1990, **31**:1717–1722.
20. Kapila S, Conley RS, Harrell WE Jr: **The current status of cone beam computed tomography imaging in orthodontics.** *Dentomaxillofac Radiol* 2011, **40**:24–34.
21. Smith BRPJ, Cederberg RA: **An evaluation of cone-beam computed tomography use in postgraduate orthodontic programs in the United States and Canada.** *J Dent Educ* 2011, **75**:98–106.
22. **Radiation protection: cone beam CT for dental and maxillofacial radiology. Evidence based guidelines.** 2011. SEDENTEXCT Project [http://www.sedentexct.eu/files/guidelines_final.pdf]
23. Hill DL, Studholme C, Hawkes DJ: *"Voxel similarity measures for automated image registration," Visualization in Biomedical Computing.* Bellingham, WA: SPIE; 1994:205.

10

LAA Occluder View for post-implantation Evaluation (LOVE) - standardized imaging proposal evaluating implanted left atrial appendage occlusion devices by cardiac computed tomography

Michael Behnes[1][*][†], Ibrahim Akin[1][†], Benjamin Sartorius[1], Christian Fastner[1], Ibrahim El-Battrawy[1], Martin Borggrefe[1], Holger Haubenreisser[2], Mathias Meyer[2], Stefan O. Schoenberg[2] and Thomas Henzler[2]

Abstract

Background: A standardized imaging proposal evaluating implanted left atrial appendage (LAA) occlusion devices by cardiac computed tomography angiography (cCTA) has never been investigated.

Methods: cCTA datasets were acquired on a 3rd generation dual-source CT system and reconstructed with a slice thickness of 0.5 mm. An interdisciplinary evaluation was performed by two interventional cardiologists and one radiologist on a 3D multi-planar workstation. A standardized multi-planar reconstruction algorithm was developed in order to assess relevant clinical aspects of implanted LAA occlusion devices being outlined within a pictorial essay.

Results: The following clinical aspects of implanted LAA occlusion devices were evaluated within the most appropriate cCTA multi-planar reconstruction: (1) topography to neighboring structures, (2) peri-device leaks, (3) coverage of LAA lobes, (4) indirect signs of neo-endothelialization. These are illustrated within concise CT imaging examples emphasizing the potential value of the proposed cCTA imaging algorithm: Starting from anatomical cCTA planes and stepwise angulation planes perpendicular to the base of the LAA devices generates an optimal **L**AA **O**ccluder **V**iew for post-implantation **E**valuation (LOVE). Aligned true axial, sagittal and coronal LOVE planes offer a standardized and detailed evaluation of LAA occlusion devices after percutaneous implantation.

Conclusions: This pictorial essay presents a standardized imaging proposal by cCTA using multi-planar reconstructions that enables systematical follow-up and comparison of patients after LAA occlusion device implantation.

Keywords: LAA occlusion device, LAA occluder, Cardiac CTA, Peri-device leak, Lobe coverage, Neo-endothelialization, Thrombus

* Correspondence: michael.behnes@umm.de

[†]Equal contributors

[1]First Department of Medicine, University Medical Center Mannheim, Faculty of Medicine Mannheim, University of Heidelberg, Theodor-Kutzer-Ufer 1-3, 68167 Mannheim, Germany

Full list of author information is available at the end of the article

Background

The left atrial appendage (LAA) represents the main origin of thrombus formation in atrial fibrillation, where the principles of Virchow's triad, such as dysfunction and structural changes of the endothelium as well as abnormal blood stasis and homoeostasis are present [1–3]. The implantation of LAA occlusion devices in patients with atrial fibrillation was shown to prevent cardio-embolic stroke as safe and effective as the treatment with the oral anticoagulant warfarin in patients eligible for oral anticoagulation [2–10]. However, the anatomic morphology of the LAA is highly variable and influences independently the incidence of cardio-embolic stroke [11, 12]. The common classification distinguishes four different LAA morphologies, which can be evaluated at best by computed tomography imaging [12–14]: 1. chicken wing, 2. cactus, 3. windsock, 4. cauliflower. All these morphologies differ extremely by the number of different LAA lobes, folds, tortuosities, diameters and global sizes and complicate individually the percutaneous implantation of LAA occlusion devices. Interestingly, the chicken wing was shown to be associated with lowest rates of cardio-embolic stroke compared to all other LAA morphologies [12].

The WATCHMAN (WM) (Boston Scientific, Natick, MA, USA) and Amplatzer Cardiac Plug (ACP) (St. Jude Medical, St Paul, MN, USA) represent the most commonly implanted LAA occlusion devices with valuable scientific evidence being available at present [2, 7, 15, 16]. Until now, trans-esophageal echocardiography (TEE) is most often applied to guide LAA occlusion device implantation, positioning and sealing both during percutaneous intervention and follow-up after device implantation [17–19]. It was shown that healing response after implantation of these devices differs and might result in harmful impact on neighboring structures [20]. However, a standardized imaging proposal for post-implantation evaluation of LAA occlusion devices by cardiac computed tomography (cCTA) has never been developed.

Therefore, this pictorial essay aims to develop this standardized imaging proposal by cCTA in order to analyze relevant clinical aspects of LAA occlusion devices after percutaneous implantation. This cCTA imaging proposal outlines relevant clinical aspects such as device positioning in relation to the varying morphology and topography of the LAA as well as functional device aspects such as peri-device leaks, lobe coverage and neo-endothelialization of the device and demonstrates illustrations of these conditions.

Methods

Ethics, consent and permissions

All participants of the presented patient-related data within this pictorial assays gave written consent to this analysis. The analyses were carried out according to the principles of the declaration of Helsinki and was approved by the medical ethics commission II of the Faculty of Medicine Mannheim, University of Heidelberg, Germany.

Cardiac CTA (cCTA) protocol and image reconstruction advice for post-implantation evaluation of LAA occlusion devices

Based on our experience, cCTA protocols for the evaluation of LAA occlusion devices do not require significant protocol adjustments, when compared to standard cCTA protocols being performed for the evaluation of coronary artery stenosis [21–24]. Optimal hydration of the patient is recommended in order to achieve best measurements. Similar to a standard cCTA acquisition contrast injection should be performed with a flow rate of at least 5 cc/s followed by a saline chaser in order to have a compact contrast bolus that is washed out mainly in the right atrium and right ventricle during the image acquisition. Depending on the patients' heart rate all available cCTA acquisition protocols in principle qualify for the evaluation of LAA occlusion devices including traditional retrospective ECG gating, prospective ECG triggering as well as high pitch or single heart beat acquisitions [25]. However, since there is no dedicated recommendation and clinical requirement for post-implantation evaluation of LAA occlusion devices in all patients, the acquisition technique that provides the lowest radiation dose depending on the available CT system should be applied. Hereby, a slightly lower image quality of the coronary arteries can be accepted since the LAA is not prone particularly to motion artifacts such as for instance the right coronary artery. Prospective ECG triggered cCTA acquisitions or single heart beat acquisitions can be used in patients with high heart rates or arrhythmias. However, different to a standard cCTA in patients with a low and regular heart rate an end-systolic image acquisition was applied for the evaluation of LAA occlusion devices in all patients independently from the heart rate in order to acquire the image data during the maximum distension of the left atrium and LAA.

Reconstruction of cCTA raw data was performed with a slice thickness between 0.5 and 0.6 mm using a sharp convolution kernel that is also used for the reconstruction of cCTA images in patients with coronary artery stent grafts or heavily calcified plaques. If available iterative reconstruction techniques should be used to lower image noise and blooming artifacts originating from metal components of the devices [26–28]. Table 1 summarizes the proposed cCTA protocol of patients after LAA occlusion device implantation.

Table 1 Protocol example for imaging of LAA occlusion devices using a 3rd generation dual source CT system

	Heart rate <70 bpm	Heart rate 71–85 bpm	Heart rate >85	Arrhythmia
cCTA technique	High pitch single heart beat acquisition	Prospective ECG gating (step-and-shot)	Retrospective ECG gating	Retrospective ECG gating
Tube voltage	BMI <28: 70 kVp	BMI <28: 70 kVp	BMI <28: 70 kVp	BMI <28: 70 kVp
	BMI 28.1–30: 80 kVp	BMI 28.1–30: 80 kVp	BMI 28.1–30: 80 kVp	BMI 28.1–30: 80 kVp
	BMI 30.1–33: 90 kVp	BMI 30.1–33: 90 kVp	BMI 30.1–33: 90 kVp	BMI 30.1–33: 90 kVp
	BMI >33: 100–120 kVp	BMI >33: 100–120 kVp	BMI >33: 100–120 kVp	BMI >33: 100–120 kVp
Tube current-time product	Automated tube current modulation (Care Dose 4D, Siemens)	Automated tube current modulation (Care Dose 4D, Siemens)	Automated tube current modulation (Care Dose 4D, Siemens)	Automated tube current modulation (Care Dose 4D, Siemens)
Slice thickness	0.6 mm	0.6 mm	0.6 mm	0.6 mm
Reconstruction increment	0.4	0.4	0.4	0.4
Reconstruction kernel	Bv40 (vascular kernel) (Siemens)	Bv40 (vascular kernel) (Siemens)	Bv40 (vascular kernel) (Siemens)	Bv40 (vascular kernel) (Siemens)
Reconstruction phase	70 % RR	40–70 % RR	20–70 % RR	10–90 % RR
Reconstruction technique	Iterative reconstruction level III (ADMIRE, Siemens)	Iterative reconstruction level III (ADMIRE, Siemens)	Iterative reconstruction level III (ADMIRE, Siemens)	Iterative reconstruction level III (ADMIRE, Siemens)
Contrast medium	80 cc iomeprol 400 (Bracco)[a]	80 cc iomeprol 400 (Bracco)[a]	80 cc iomeprol 400 (Bracco)[a]	80 cc iomeprol 400 (Bracco)[a]

Note: bpm: beats per minute; kVp: kilovoltage peak; ECG: electrocardiogram[a] contrast material is not reduced as it is possible for a standard coronary CT angiography in order to reduce blood stasis artifacts within the left atrial appendage; the scan start is determined using bolus tracking within the descending aorta using a threshold of 120 HU and an additional delay of 7 s in order to have a slightly delayed scan start when compared to standard

Generating a standardized proposal by multi-planar imaging
0.6 mm thick images reconstructed with a medium convolution kernel are uploaded on a simple 3D multi-planar rendering workstation with the 3 planes locked at a 90° angle (Figs. 1 and 2, panels I) (Additional files 1 and 2). The axial slices should be moved to the level of the left atrium, in which the LAA occlusion device is visible (Figs. 1 and 2, panels II). These initial steps are independent of different type of implanted LAA occlusion devices (either WM or ACP).

Amplatzer cardiac plug (ACP) device
Specifically for the ACP device, move the coronal axis within the transverse window perpendicular to the disc of the ACP device (Fig. 1, panel III). Afterwards, align the axes on the two other viewers also perpendicular to the disc of the ACP device (Fig. 1, panels IV and V). Lastly, the center of the axes should be placed to the center of the screw-hub.

WATCHMAN (WM) device
Since the WM device is not equipped with a disc, the alignment might become more challenging. Here, using maximum intensity projection (MIP) images with a slab thickness of approximately 10 mm allows visualization of the whole nitinol frame of the WM device. Afterwards, move the coronal axis within the transverse window perpendicular to the coves of the parachute of the WM device (Fig. 1, panel III). Afterwards, align the axes on the

two other viewers also perpendicular to the coves of the parachute of the ACP device (Fig. 1, panels IV and V). Lastly, the center of the axes should be placed to the center of the screw-hub.

Starting from anatomical cCTA planes while applying all of the described imaging steps above will generate the optimal **LAA O**ccluder **V**iew for post-implantation **E**valuation (LOVE) (Figs. 1 and 2, Additional files 1, 2, 3 and 4). This standardized imaging reconstruction view can be applied for the two most commonly implanted LAA occlusion devices (i.e. ACP and WM). The LOVE view allows optimal evaluation of the most relevant clinical aspects of the post-implantation follow-up of patients with LAA occlusion devices: (1) peri-device leaks, (2) coverage of LAA lobes, (3) indirect signs of neo-endothelialization.

Results
Clinical scenarios reflecting relevant clinical aspects after implantation of LAA occlusion devices
Imaging reports about percutaneously implanted LAA occlusion devices should focus on the following important clinical aspects:

Morphologic and topographic aspects of LAA occlusion device positioning

- Global positioning of the device including rotation around the entry axis to the LAA. This can be best measured on LOVE axial and LOVE sagittal views.

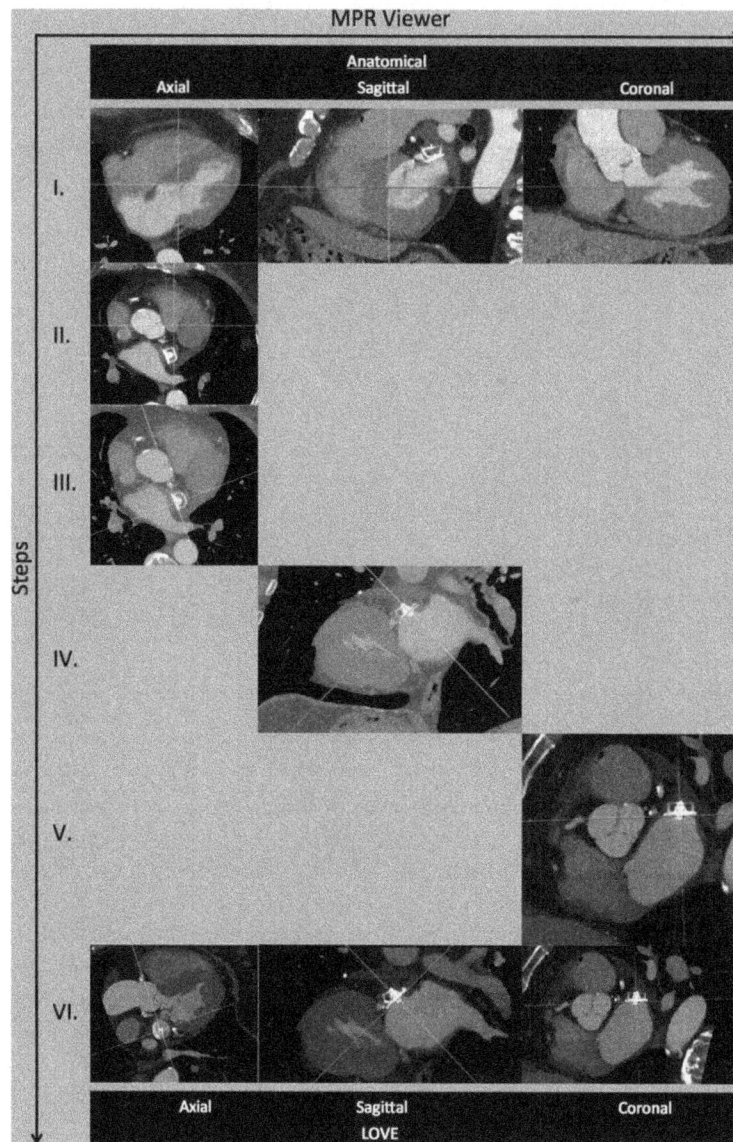

Fig. 1 Illustration of a stepwise standard multimodal imaging to generating optimal LAA Occluder View for post-implantation Evaluation (LOVE) planes from anatomical cCTA planes. Figure shows 5 standardized steps (panels I-V) for the ACP® device

- LOVE axial views allow optimal evaluation of global compression of both devices:
  WM device: compression of 10–20 % referred to the original device size is recommended.
  ACP device: concave disc; device lobe positioned 2/3 distal to the LCX inside and engaged within the LAA; ACP device axis in line with the LAA neck axis.
- LOVE axial views allow optimal evaluation of impairment to neighboring structures by the LAA occlusion device: including positioning in relation to the mitral valve annulus, pulmonary artery, left pulmonary veins as well as LCX that is best visible in LOVE axial views (Fig. 3).

Functional aspects of LAA occlusion devices

- Peri-device leaks:
  These can be seen best on LOVE sagittal views. The presence of a peri-device leak should be measured in all reports (Figs. 4, 5 and 6). Higher resolution measurements of peri-device leak diameters can be performed by cCTA compared to TEE. Accordingly, further studies are needed to evaluate the additional value of cCTA measurements in this context and whether definitions of the PROTECT AF study can accordingly be transferred (i.e. minor (<1 mm width), moderate (1 to 3 mm width) or major

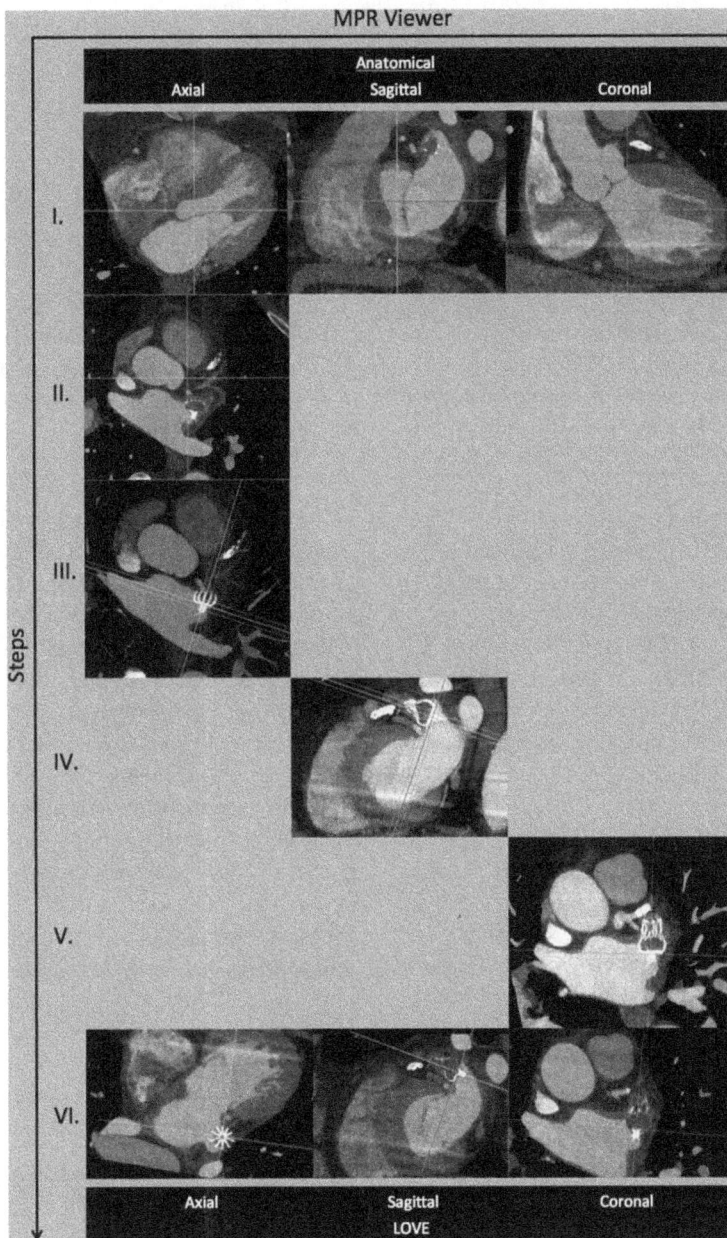

Fig. 2 Illustration of a stepwise standard multimodal imaging to generating optimal LAA Occluder View for post-implantation Evaluation (LOVE) planes from anatomical cCTA planes. Figure shows 5 standardized steps (panels I-V) for the WATCHMAN® device

(3 mm width)). A sole peri-device leak should be reported in case the sealing part of the device (either proximal disk or cap) is parallel to the plane of the LAA ostium. Remaining contrast filling will then be visible around the device on the LOVE views (Fig. 6).

- Coverage of all lobes:
  The LAA often consists of different lobes not corresponding necessarily to the fixed shape of the LAA occlusion device. Therefore, complete coverage of all LAA lobes is not always achievable.

Assessment of lobe coverage should consider the angle between the sealing part of the device (either proximal disk or cap) and the plane of the LAA ostium. This angle corresponds to the incompletely covered LAA lobe. Accordingly, Fig. 7 illustrates a small residual LAA lobe due to over-angulation of the device. Rotation around the entry axis to the LAA should be measured on LOVE axial and LOVE sagittal views. Lobe coverage should be assessed on all LOVE reformations (Figs. 4, 5, 7 and 8).

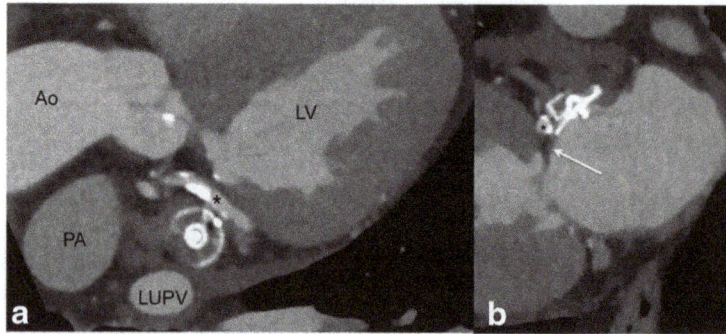

Fig. 3 LOVE coronal (panel **a**) and sagittal (panel **b**) reformations demonstrating the anatomic relationship to relevant neighboring structures that should be reported. Panel **a** shows the close anatomic relationship to the left upper pulmonary vein (LUPV) and the left circumflex coronary artery (LCX) that is adjacent directly to the LAA occlusion device (* in panels **a** and **b**). The pulmonary artery (PA) is the third relatively close neighboring structure that should be inspected carefully on LOVE axial reformations

- Complete neo-endothelialization:
  Absence of contrast enhancement within the LAA without any peri-device leak suggests complete neo-endothelialization. Accordingly, contrast enhancement in the LAA of less than 50 Hounsfield units compared to the left atrium suggests incomplete neo-endothelialization. Equal contrast enhancement in both LAA and left atrium suggests no or very early stages of neo-endothelialization (Figs. 4, 5, 7 and 8).

Discussion

This pictorial essay presents a standardized imaging proposal by cCTA using multi-planar reconstructions that enables systematical follow-up and comparison of patients after LAA occlusion device implantation. As described above and being accompanied by a case series of striking illustrations this imaging proposal intends to cover the most relevant clinical challenges of implanted LAA occlusion devices including morphologic, topographic as well as functional device-related aspects. The presented imaging proposal generates novel hypotheses, which have to be proven by ongoing prospective, randomized imaging studies.

Based on the so far available literature on safety and patient outcome, it is likely that the number of patients undergoing percutaneous LAA occlusion device implantation will raise significantly within the near future similar to the growing number of patients undergoing transcatheter aortic valve replacement (TAVR). However, in order to identify patients with poor outcome and/or post-procedural complications, such as a residual LAA larger than a specific device size that still leads to thrombus formation, accurate, reproducible and reader-independent imaging is crucial. This is of particular importance in order to generate more evidence about optimal placement of LAA occlusion devices.

For instance, the presence of relevant peri-device leaks or incomplete coverage of residual LAA lobes might be

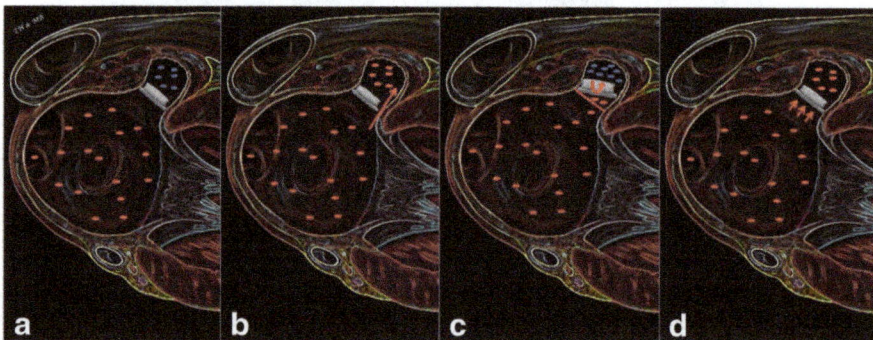

Fig. 4 The figure summarizes schematically the four main follow-up scenarios on cardiac CTA after LAA occlusion device implantation. Panel **a** demonstrates optimal positioning of the LAA occlusion device without any residual lobe, any peri-device leak and without any residual contrast filling (blue dots in LAA) indicating complete neo-endothelialization. Panel **b** demonstrates a peri-device leak with contrast filling of the LAA. Panel **c** shows sub-optimal positioning of the LAA occlusion device with in-complete lobe coverage leaving a residual left atrial appendage. Panel **d** shows optimal positioning of the LAA occlusion device with in-complete neo-endothelialization that is suggested indirectly by the contrast enhancement of the LAA (blue dots in LAA). Please note that all three scenarios can occur in combination. In case of an existing peri-device leak with contrast filling of the LAA assessment of endothelialization is not feasible with cardiac CT

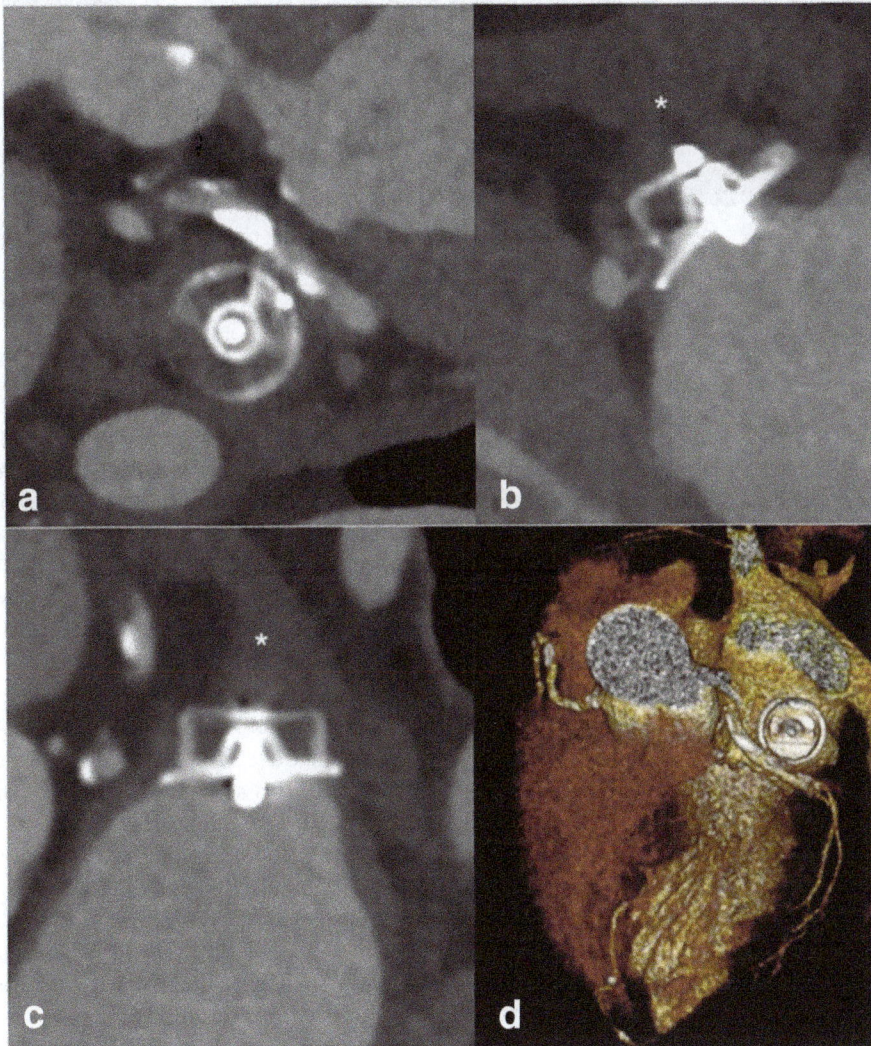

Fig. 5 LOVE - axial (panel **a**), – sagittal (panel **b**), - coronal (panel **c**), and 3D (panel **d**) reformations of a 72 year-old male patient who underwent cardiac CTA 9 months after implantation of a ACP® LAA occlusion device. Panels **a**, **b**, and **c** show optimal positioning of the device with no peri-device leak, complete lobe coverage as well as complete neo-endothelialization of the device suggested by the absence of contrast enhancement < 50 Hounsfield units in the LAA (* in B and C). Volume rendered reconstructions

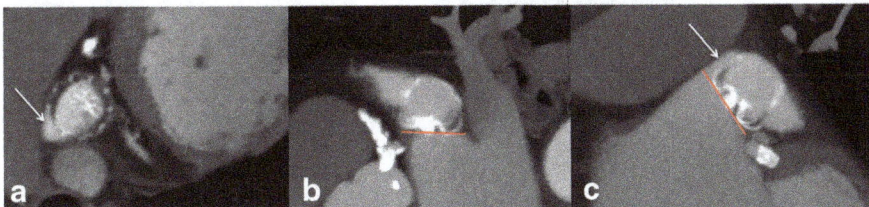

Fig. 6 LOVE - axial (panel **a**), – sagittal (panel **b**), and - coronal (panel **c**) reformations of a 80-year-old male patient who underwent cardiac CTA 8 months after implantation of a WATCHMAN® LAA occlusion device. Panels **a** and **c** show a small peri-device leak <3 mm at the cranial LAA entry causing complete contrast filling of the LAA (*white arrow*). Panel **b** demonstrates the correct positioning of the device with complete lobe coverage, as indicated by the correctly positioned sealing part (proximal cap of the WM device) parallel to the plane of the LAA ostium (*red line*). Due to the presence of the peri-device leak the assessment of endothelialization is not feasible with cardiac CTA

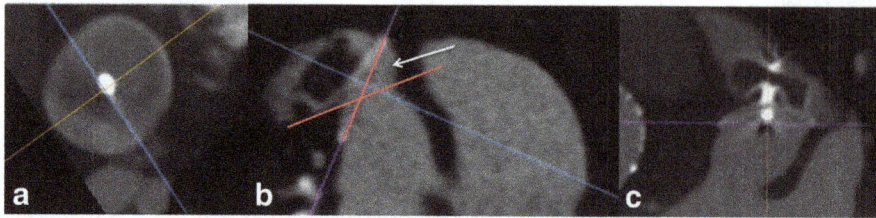

Fig. 7 LOVE - axial (panel **a**), – sagittal (panel **b**), and - coronal (panel **c**) reformations of a 83-year-old female patient who underwent cardiac CTA 9 months after implantation of the ACP® LAA occlusion device. Panels **a**, **b** and, **c** demonstrate no peri-device leak. Panel **b** shows incomplete lobe coverage with a small residual LAA lobe. The uncovered LAA lobe is seen between the angle of the sealing part of the ACP device (proximal disk) and the plane of the LAA ostium (angle in between *red lines*, marked by *white arrow*). The contrast filling of the LAA in combination with the clear absence of a peri-device leak reflects indirectly in-complete endothelialization of the ACP® LAA occlusion device

associated with individually impaired neurologic outcome of the patients. These mal-appositions of LAA occlusion devices have been attributed to clinical overt neurologic disability and silent cerebral ischemia being caused by cerebral micro-embolism and visualized by cerebral magnetic resonance imaging (cMRI) [17]. Importantly, cCTA might also allow the evaluation of complete neo-endothelialization of the LAA occlusion device. From the treating physician's perspective complete neo-endothelialization without any peri-device leak might facilitate future clinical decision-making to stop concomitant anticoagulation or dual antiplatelet therapy (DAPT).

Little is known regarding incidences of device related complications after successful percutaneous implantation of LAA occlusion devices, such as device compression, peri-device leaks, lobe coverage and progress of neo-endothelialization related to study-specific antithrombotic treatments. The latter were evaluated for DAPT (i.e. aspirin and clopidogrel) lasting 6 months, as within the present study, or for warfarin for 45 days, followed by clopidogrel for 4.5 months and lifelong aspirin [2, 7, 10, 16]. There is a lack of data comparing the quality of TEE versus CT follow-up imaging after device implantation and the optimal time period still needs to be investigated. Device compression and shape in relation to surrounding vessels is of importance for

optimal device and hemodynamic stability over time in order to prevent relevant dislodgment or obstruction of neighboring structures as being recommended by the manufacturer [29]. It was shown recently, that compression and shape of LAA occlusion devices are changing temporarily within three months after implantation, however its clinical relevance besides complete LAA closure is still under debate [30, 31].

Furthermore, accurate differentiation between thrombus formation and blood stasis within the LAA is challenging using standard cCTA. An additional delayed cCTA approximately 70 s after the start of the contrast injection is recommended [32]. Imaging the patients in prone position is another theoretical approach in order to minimize the effects of blood stasis in the LAA. However, data is lacking about the usefulness of performing cCTA in a prone position. Dual energy cCTA using calculated iodine maps has been proposed in order to differentiate accurately blood stasis from thrombus formation within the LAA of patients with cardio-embolic stroke [33].

As outlined, post procedural image analysis with cCTA might bear the potential of a standardized imaging using defined multi-planar reformations that best display the complex 3-dimensional shape of the LAA and the device. In our opinion, cCTA has the main advantage that the images can be very standardized analyzed and reconstructed

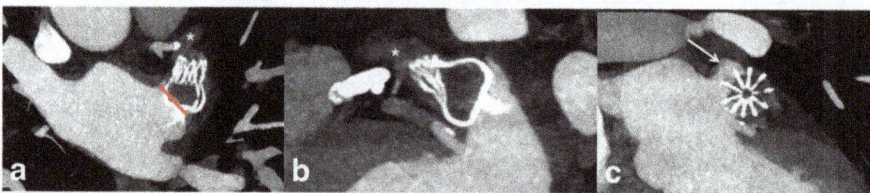

Fig. 8 LOVE - axial (panel **a**), – sagittal (panel **b**), and - coronal (panel **c**) reformations of a 75-year-old male patient who underwent cardiac CTA 4 months after implantation of a WATCHMAN® LAA occlusion device. Panel **a** shows a 20° offset of the device around the entry axis to the LAA (red line in A). The rotation led to an in-complete lobe coverage with a small residual left atrial appendage < 5 mm that is best seen on the LOVE coronal reformation (arrow in panel **c**). The residual slight contrast enhancement (* in panels a and b) of the LAA that is approximately 50 % lower when compared to the contrast enhancement in the left atrium suggests beginning, but still in-complete neo-endothelialization of the device

and make quantitative measurements reliable. This is of particular importance to generate more evidence on relevant clinical questions: (1) What size of a residual LAA is acceptable with different devices? (2) What size of peri-device leaks still leads to a complete occlusion over time? However, the advantages of cCTA for post-implantation LAA occlusion device evaluation have to outscore the patients' individual risk being associated with an additional radiation dose and additional administration of iodinated material.

Potential value and limitations of cardiac CTA in the context of LAA occlusion devices

Cardiac CTA allows the comprehensive non-invasive visualization of the whole heart including coronary arteries as well as all important neighboring structures of the LAA and thus accurate evaluation of post-implantation evaluation of LAA occlusion devices by the described LOVE view. The main arguments for the use of cCTA in this context, besides its non-invasiveness, are firstly, the whole volume coverage with a high spatial resolution and secondly, the high reproducibility of the technique that allows to angulate the isotropic dataset retrospectively after the procedure in all desired projections. Thereby generating an investigator's independency, cCTA becomes particularly attractive for clinical studies that require a high standardization of follow-up examinations. Thirdly, image artifacts do not hamper cCTA image quality because all available LAA occlusion devices do not lead to metal artifacts such as other metal implants. Based on our experience, cCTA allows assessing all relevant clinical questions including indirect visualization of LAA occlusion device neo-endothelialization if no peri-device leak is present. For instance, no contrast enhancement within the LAA suggests complete neo-endothelialization, whereas contrast enhancement in the LAA of less than 50 Hounsfield units compared to the enhancement within the left atrium suggests incomplete neo-endothelialization. Contrast enhancement within the LAA that is equal to the left atrium suggests no or very early stages of neo-endothelialization.

The main concerns with cCTA in the context of LAA occlusion device evaluation are the additional radiation dose that is given to the patient. However, with low radiation dose techniques of state-of-the-art CT systems the radiation dose has been reduced significantly over the past 5 years [25]. Thus, the risk of ionizing radiation in this mainly elderly population should be weighted clinically against potential overseen significant clinical findings potentially being detected by cCTA (such as thrombus formation or indirect signs of incomplete neo-endothelialization), whereas their clinical impact still needs to be proven within prospective clinical studies.

The second relevant concern of cCTA is the need for iodinated contrast material, which is crucial in patients with impairment of renal function. Although the amount of contrast material for the evaluation of LAA occlusion devices can be reduced to a minimum of 30–40 cc of contrast in patients with elevated serum creatinine levels, the indication should be checked strictly in patients with serum creatinine levels above 1.5 mg/dL. Additionally, cCTA is more expensive and not as widely available compared to echocardiography.

Conclusions

This pictorial essay describes a standardized imaging proposal including examples of (ab)normal findings after percutaneous implantation of LAA occlusion devices. Whether the proposed cCTA imaging instructions might facilitate future clinical follow-up, cost effectiveness and therapeutic decisions needs to be evaluated further in larger, prospective and randomized imaging studies evaluating this specific subset of cardiac patients.

Additional files

Additional file 1: Movie demonstrating the generation of the **L**AA **O**ccluder **V**iew for post-implantation **E**valuation (LOVE) for the Amplatzer cardiac plug (ACP) device by cardiac CTA.

Additional file 2: Movie demonstrating the generation of the **L**AA **O**ccluder **V**iew for post-implantation **E**valuation (LOVE) for the WATCHMAN (WM) device by cardiac CTA.

Additional file 3: Movie revealing the potential diagnostic insights of cardiac CTA imaging for an implanted ACP device by optimal alignment of LOVE planes.

Additional file 4: 3D animation illustrating optimal implantation of an ACP device within the LAA after optimal alignment of LOVE planes by cardiac CTA.

Abbreviations
ACP: amplatz cardiac plug; BMBF: German Ministry of Education and Research; cCTA: cardiac computed tomography; cMRT: cerebral magnetic resonance imaging; CT: computed tomography; DAPT: dual antiplatelet therapy; DZHK: Deutsches Zentrum für Herz-Kreislauf-Forschung - German Centre for Cardiovascular Research; LAA: left atrial appendage; LOVE: LAA occluder view for post-implantation evaluation; MIP: maximum intensity projection; TEE: transesophageal echocardiography; WM: Watchman.

Competing interests
The authors declare that they have no competing interests.

Authors' contributions
MBe conceived the study, participated in its design and coordination, performed imaging analysis, participated in data analysis and interpretation and drafted the manuscript. IA conceived the study, participated in its design and coordination, performed imaging analysis, participated in data analysis and interpretation and drafted the manuscript. BS participated in the study design and coordination, data acquisition and analysis, and helped to draft the manuscript. CF participated in the study design and coordination, data acquisition and analysis, and helped to draft the manuscript. IE-B participated in the study design and coordination, data acquisition and analysis, and helped to draft the manuscript. MBo participated in the study design and coordination, data acquisition and analysis, and helped to draft the manuscript. HH participated in the study design and coordination, data acquisition and analysis, and helped to draft the manuscript. MM participated

in the study design and coordination, data acquisition and analysis, and helped to draft the manuscript. SS participated in the study design and coordination, data acquisition and analysis, and helped to draft the manuscript. TH conceived the study, participated in its design and coordination, performed imaging analysis, participated in data analysis and interpretation and drafted the manuscript. All authors read and approved the final manuscript.

Acknowledgements
Supported by the DZHK (Deutsches Zentrum für Herz-Kreislauf-Forschung - German Centre for Cardiovascular Research) and by the BMBF (German Ministry of Education and Research). None of the authors received any funding with respect to study design, collection, analysis, interpretation of data, writing of the manuscript or decision to submit the manuscript for publication.

Author details
[1]First Department of Medicine, University Medical Center Mannheim, Faculty of Medicine Mannheim, University of Heidelberg, Theodor-Kutzer-Ufer 1-3, 68167 Mannheim, Germany. [2]Institute of Clinical Radiology and Nuclear Medicine, University Medical Center Mannheim, Faculty of Medicine Mannheim, University of Heidelberg, Theodor-Kutzer-Ufer 1-3, 68167 Mannheim, Germany.

References
1. Watson T, Shantsila E, Lip GY. Mechanisms of thrombogenesis in atrial fibrillation: Virchow's triad revisited. Lancet. 2009;373(9658):155–66.
2. Bergmann MW, Landmesser U. Left atrial appendage closure for stroke prevention in non-valvular atrial fibrillation: rationale, devices in clinical development and insights into implantation techniques. EuroIntervention. 2014;10(4):497–504.
3. Camm AJ et al. 2012 focused update of the ESC Guidelines for the management of atrial fibrillation: an update of the 2010 ESC Guidelines for the management of atrial fibrillation. Developed with the special contribution of the European Heart Rhythm Association. Eur Heart J. 2012; 33(21):2719–47.
4. Alli O et al. Quality of life assessment in the randomized PROTECT AF (Percutaneous Closure of the Left Atrial Appendage Versus Warfarin Therapy for Prevention of Stroke in Patients With Atrial Fibrillation) trial of patients at risk for stroke with nonvalvular atrial fibrillation. J Am Coll Cardiol. 2013; 61(17):1790–8.
5. Bayard YL et al. PLAATO (Percutaneous Left Atrial Appendage Transcatheter Occlusion) for prevention of cardioembolic stroke in non-anticoagulation eligible atrial fibrillation patients: results from the European PLAATO study. EuroIntervention. 2010;6(2):220–6.
6. Nietlispach F et al. Amplatzer left atrial appendage occlusion: single center 10-year experience. Catheter Cardiovasc Interv. 2013;82(2):283–9.
7. Reddy VY et al. Left atrial appendage closure with the Watchman device in patients with a contraindication for oral anticoagulation: the ASAP study (ASA Plavix Feasibility Study With Watchman Left Atrial Appendage Closure Technology). J Am Coll Cardiol. 2013;61(25):2551–6.
8. Urena M et al. Percutaneous left atrial appendage closure with the AMPLATZER cardiac plug device in patients with nonvalvular atrial fibrillation and contraindications to anticoagulation therapy. J Am Coll Cardiol. 2013;62(2):96–102.
9. Wiebe J, et al. Safety of percutaneous left atrial appendage closure with the amplatzer cardiac plug in patients with atrial fibrillation and contraindications to anticoagulation. Catheter Cardiovasc Interv. 2014;83(5): 796–802.
10. Holmes Jr DR et al. Prospective randomized evaluation of the Watchman Left Atrial Appendage Closure device in patients with atrial fibrillation versus long-term warfarin therapy: the PREVAIL trial. J Am Coll Cardiol. 2014; 64(1):1–12.
11. Anselmino M et al. Left atrial appendage morphology and silent cerebral ischemia in patients with atrial fibrillation. Heart Rhythm. 2014;11(1):2–7.
12. Di Biase L et al. Does the left atrial appendage morphology correlate with the risk of stroke in patients with atrial fibrillation? Results from a multicenter study. J Am Coll Cardiol. 2012;60(6):531–8.
13. Laura DM et al. The role of multimodality imaging in percutaneous left atrial appendage suture ligation with the LARIAT device. J Am Soc Echocardiogr. 2014;27(7):699–708.
14. Lopez-Minguez JR, et al. Anatomical Classification of Left Atrial Appendages in Specimens Applicable to CT Imaging Techniques for Implantation of Amplatzer Cardiac Plug. J Cardiovasc Electrophysiol. 2014;25(9):976–84.
15. Holmes DR et al. Percutaneous closure of the left atrial appendage versus warfarin therapy for prevention of stroke in patients with atrial fibrillation: a randomised non-inferiority trial. Lancet. 2009;374(9689):534–42.
16. Reddy VY et al. Percutaneous left atrial appendage closure for stroke prophylaxis in patients with atrial fibrillation: 2.3-Year Follow-up of the PROTECT AF (Watchman Left Atrial Appendage System for Embolic Protection in Patients with Atrial Fibrillation) Trial. Circulation. 2013; 127(6):720–9.
17. Viles-Gonzalez JF et al. The clinical impact of incomplete left atrial appendage closure with the Watchman Device in patients with atrial fibrillation: a PROTECT AF (Percutaneous Closure of the Left Atrial Appendage Versus Warfarin Therapy for Prevention of Stroke in Patients With Atrial Fibrillation) substudy. J Am Coll Cardiol. 2012;59(10):923–9.
18. Viles-Gonzalez JF et al. Incomplete occlusion of the left atrial appendage with the percutaneous left atrial appendage transcatheter occlusion device is not associated with increased risk of stroke. J Interv Card Electrophysiol. 2012;33(1):69–75.
19. Anter E, et al. Comparison of intracardiac echocardiography and transesophageal echocardiography for imaging of the right and left atrial appendages. Heart Rhythm. 2014.
20. Kar S et al. Impact of Watchman and Amplatzer Devices on Left Atrial Appendage Adjacent Structures and Healing Response in a Canine Model. JACC Cardiovasc Interv. 2014;7(7):801–9.
21. Mahesh M, Cody DD. Physics of cardiac imaging with multiple-row detector CT. Radiographics. 2007;27(5):1495–509.
22. Schoepf UJ et al. CT coronary angiography: indications, image acquisition, and interpretation. Radiologia. 2008;50(2):113–30.
23. Weininger M et al. Cardiothoracic CT angiography: current contrast medium delivery strategies. AJR Am J Roentgenol. 2011;196(3):W260–72.
24. Xu L, Zhang Z. Coronary CT angiography with low radiation dose. Int J Cardiovasc Imaging. 2010;26 Suppl 1:17–25.
25. Henzler T et al. Practical strategies for low radiation dose cardiac computed tomography. J Thorac Imaging. 2010;25(3):213–20.
26. Ebersberger U et al. CT evaluation of coronary artery stents with iterative image reconstruction: improvements in image quality and potential for radiation dose reduction. Eur Radiol. 2013;23(1):125–32.
27. Moscariello A et al. Coronary CT angiography: image quality, diagnostic accuracy, and potential for radiation dose reduction using a novel iterative image reconstruction technique-comparison with traditional filtered back projection. Eur Radiol. 2011;21(10):2130–8.
28. Renker M et al. Evaluation of heavily calcified vessels with coronary CT angiography: comparison of iterative and filtered back projection image reconstruction. Radiology. 2011;260(2):390–9.
29. Corporation, B.S. WATCHMAN™ 12 F Left Atrial Appendage Closure Device with Delivery System. 2014; Instruction for Use]. Available from: http://www.bostonscientific.com/watchman-de/assets/pdf/WATCHMAN_DFU_90893601-01A.pdf.
30. Neuzner J et al. Left atrial appendage closure with the Amplatzer Cardiac Plug: Rationale for a higher degree of device oversizing at implantation. Cardiol J. 2015;22(2):201–5.
31. Sepahpour A et al. Death from pulmonary artery erosion complicating implantation of percutaneous left atrial appendage occlusion device. Heart Rhythm. 2013;10(12):1810–1.
32. Romero J et al. Detection of left atrial appendage thrombus by cardiac computed tomography in patients with atrial fibrillation: a meta-analysis. Circ Cardiovasc Imaging. 2013;6(2):185–94.
33. Hur J et al. Cardioembolic stroke: dual-energy cardiac CT for differentiation of left atrial appendage thrombus and circulatory stasis. Radiology. 2012; 263(3):688–95.

11

Distal radius plate of CFR-PEEK has minimal effect compared to titanium plates on bone parameters in high-resolution peripheral quantitative computed tomography

Joost J. A. de Jong[1,2*], Arno Lataster[3], Bert van Rietbergen[4], Jacobus J. Arts[4,5,6], Piet P. Geusens[2,6,7], Joop P. W. van den Bergh[1,2,7,8] and Paul C. Willems[5,6]

Abstract

Background: Carbon-fiber-reinforced poly-ether-ether-ketone (CFR-PEEK) has superior radiolucency compared to other orthopedic implant materials, e.g. titanium or stainless steel, thus allowing metal-artifact-free postoperative monitoring by computed tomography (CT). Recently, high-resolution peripheral quantitative CT (HRpQCT) proved to be a promising technique to monitor the recovery of volumetric bone mineral density (vBMD), micro-architecture and biomechanical parameters in stable conservatively treated distal radius fractures. When using HRpQCT to monitor unstable distal radius fractures that require volar distal radius plating for fixation, radiolucent CFR-PEEK plates may be a better alternative to currently used titanium plates to allow for reliable assessment. In this pilot study, we assessed the effect of a volar distal radius plate made from CFR-PEEK on bone parameters obtained from HRpQCT in comparison to two titanium plates.

Methods: Plates were instrumented in separate cadaveric human fore-arms (n = 3). After instrumentation and after removal of the plates duplicate HRpQCT scans were made of the region covered by the plate. HRpQCT images were visually checked for artifacts. vBMD, micro-architectural and biomechanical parameters were calculated, and compared between the uninstrumented and instrumented radii.

Results: No visible image artifacts were observed in the CFR-PEEK plate instrumented radius, and errors in bone parameters ranged from −3.2 to 2.6%. In the radii instrumented with the titanium plates, severe image artifacts were observed and errors in bone parameters ranged between −30.2 and 67.0%.

Conclusions: We recommend using CFR-PEEK plates in longitudinal in vivo studies that monitor the healing process of unstable distal radius fractures treated operatively by plating or bone graft ingrowth.

Keywords: Injury/fracture healing, HRpQCT, Implant, Distal radius, CFR-PEEK

* Correspondence: joost.dejong@maastrichtuniversity.nl
[1]NUTRIM School for Nutrition and Translational Research in Metabolism, Maastricht University, Maastricht, The Netherlands
[2]Department of Rheumatology, Maastricht University Medical Center, Maastricht, The Netherlands
Full list of author information is available at the end of the article

Background

Carbon-fiber-reinforced poly-ether-ether-ketone (CFR-PEEK) is increasingly being used as a material for orthopedic implants, e.g. in spinal cages, hip prostheses, or intramedullary nails [1–4]. One of the main advantages of this material is that CFR-PEEK has been found to have superior radiolucency as compared to other materials that are conventionally used for orthopedic implants, such as stainless steel or titanium. Therefore, implants made out of CFR-PEEK allow metal-artifact-free postoperative monitoring by computed tomography (CT), magnetic resonance imaging (MRI) and radiographs [5].

Recently, it has been shown that the repair process of stable distal radius fractures can be monitored longitudinally in vivo using high-resolution peripheral computed tomography (HRpQCT) [6, 7]. For clinical and research purposes, it would be of great interest to monitor the repair process of unstable fractures or the ingrowth of bone graft or bone graft substitutes after corrective osteotomy as well. Whereas stable distal radius fractures are usually treated by immobilization with a fiberglass cast, which only has a limited effect on the bone parameters obtained by HRpQCT [8], volar distal radius plates (VDRPs) as internal fixation are a generally accepted treatment in case of unstable distal radius fractures or after corrective osteotomy [9]. Since VDRPs are usually made from stainless steel or, more common, from titanium, they cause severe artifacts on CT and HRpQCT images [10], including scattering, beam hardening and streak occurrence [11]. Besides reduced sensitivity of CT measurements, this may result in an over- or underestimation of the bone density, micro-architectural and biomechanical parameters that are derived from such images [10].

Besides other implants, VDRPs made of CFR-PEEK were recently developed. Whereas it is known that the polymers alone will not cause major artifacts in clinical CT scans, potentially they could affect the density and morphology measurements in HRpQCT images due to changes in beam hardening or scatter-related noise. Also, such plates typically contain metal fibers or other additions to increase their visibility on radiographs that may cause artifacts. It therefore is unknown whether the quantitatively obtained bone parameters obtained from HRpQCT images remain unaffected. We expect that a CFR-PEEK plate will lead to less artifacts in HRpQCT images as compared to metal plates, and thus might be a suitable alternative to the currently used titanium plates in studies monitoring the healing process of unstable fractures or ingrowth of bone graft or bone graft substitutes after corrective osteotomy.

Therefore, the aim of this study was to compare the effect of VDRPs made of titanium or made of CFR-PEEK on the occurrence of artifacts in HRpQCT images and on the volumetric bone mineral density (vBMD), micro-architectural and biomechanical parameters that are obtained from these images.

Methods

Volar distal radius plates

Three types of commercially available VDRPs from different firms were compared in this study. Plate #1 (Standard 5-hole Volar Distale Radius Plate, Icotec AG, Switzerland) had a thickness of 2.5 mm and consisted of CFR-PEEK to which 0.5% tantalum fibers were added for radiological visibility. Plate #2 (VariAx™ Standard Anatomical Volar Distal Radius Plate, Strycker Corporation, United States of America) was 2 mm thick and made of titanium alloy Ti6Al4V, which contained 89% titanium, 6% aluminum and 4% vanadium. Plate# 3 (2.4 mm Variable Angle LCP Volar Extra-Articular Distal Radius Plate, Synthes AG, Switzerland) was 2.4 mm thick and also made of a titanium alloy, i.e. Ti6Al7Nb containing 86% titanium, 6% aluminum and 7% niobium.

Fresh frozen fore-arms

For this study three intact human fore-arms (right side) were isolated from three cadavers. A handwritten and signed codicil from each donor, posed when still alive and well, is kept at the Department of Anatomy and Embryology, Faculty of Health, Medicine and Life Sciences, Maastricht University, Maastricht, The Netherlands. This is required by Dutch law for the use of cadavers for scientific research and education. The fore-arms were thawed for 8 h at 16 °C before surgery was started.

Surgery

Each plate was instrumented by an experienced orthopedic surgeon (PW) in one fore-arm by means of a standard volar approach and fixed to the distal radius according to the instruction manual provided by the manufacturer. During surgery, employees of the respective firms were present to support the surgeon and to make sure the proper surgical techniques were used. In all plates, five screws were fixed in the metaphysis distally from the region of interest (ROI) and two screws were fixed in the shaft proximally from the ROI (Fig. 1). The screws were made of the same material as the respective plate. The plates were removed after HRpQCT scans had been performed.

HRpQCT scanning

Both after instrumentation and after removal of the plates, the fore-arms were scanned twice, with repositioning between each scan (thus four times in total) by HRpQCT (XtremeCT, Scanco Medical AG, Switzerland) using clinical in vivo settings by the manufacturer (60 kVp effective energy, 900 µA tube current, and 100 ms

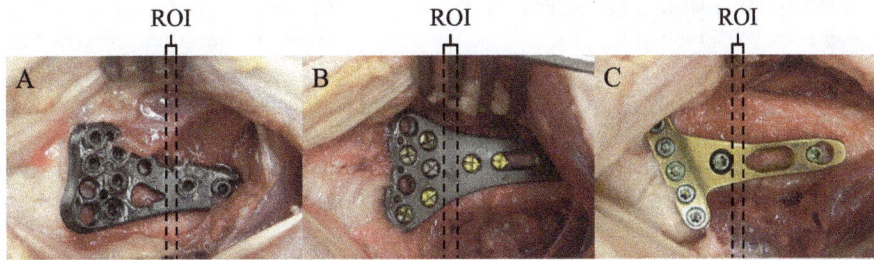

Fig. 1 Each volar distal radius plate was instrumented in one cadaveric forearm by means of a standard volar approach. The CFR-PEEK plate is shown in panel **a** and the two titanium plates in panels **b** and **c**. In each plate, five screws were fixed in the metaphysis and two screws were fixed in the shaft. The region of interest (ROI, *between dotted lines*) was set such that it was fully covered by a part of the plate without screws or holes

integration time). A standard stack of 110 transverse images with an isotropic voxel size of 82 μm was acquired, covering a region of 9 mm in each fore-arm. The ROI was set at the distal end of the radius and which was covered by a part of the plate without screw holes (Fig. 2). Also, the ROI was chosen such that it was located in between the five distal and two proximal screws to eliminate distortion by the screws.

Bone density and micro-architecture

For each forearm, the HRpQCT scans with and without a plate were matched by slice-matching to make sure the same region was analyzed. The HRpQCT images within the ROI were then evaluated using the standard patient evaluation protocol provided by the manufacturer and has been described earlier in detail elsewhere [12]. In short, after contouring of the periosteal boundary of the radius, the total region was separated into a cortical and trabecular region. For each region, the volumetric bone mineral density (Dtot, Dcort and Dtrab, respectively) [mgHA/cm^3] was assessed. The mineralized bone was extracted and a segmented image was created [12] from which the following micro-architectural parameters were assessed: trabecular number (Tb.N) [mm^{-1}], thickness (Tb.Th) [mm] and separation (Tb.Sp) [mm]. For the cortical region, the thickness (Ct.Th) [mm] was calculated [12].

Micro finite element analysis

μFE models were created directly from the segmented HRpQCT images, similar to earlier studies [13, 14]. In short, each voxel representing bone was converted into a brick element of the size, thus creating a representative μFE model of the bone's micro-architecture. Typically, these μFE models consisted of 3 to 4 million elements. Equal material properties were assigned to every element, i.e. a Young's modulus of 10 GPa and a Poisson ratio of 0.3 [14]. By applying a 'high friction' compression test in the axial direction as described by Pistoia et al., the following biomechanical parameters were estimated: stiffness (Scomp) [kN/mm], which can be described as the resistance against displacement; and ultimate failure load (F.Ult) [kN], which is the load at which the fracture criterion is met, e.g. the strain in at least 2% of the volume exceeds 0.7% [13].

Statistics

Reproducibility of the bone density, micro-architectural and biomechanical parameters was expressed using the root mean-square coefficient of variation (RMSCV%) [15]:

$$RMSCV\% = \sqrt{\frac{d^2}{2}} \bigg/ \bar{x} \cdot 100\% \qquad (1)$$

with d the difference between the first and second measurement, and $\bar{x}$ the mean of the two measurements.

Means for the bone parameters in each instrumented and uninstrumented radius were calculated from the duplicate measurements. The errors in the bone parameters introduced by each plate were expressed as percent differences

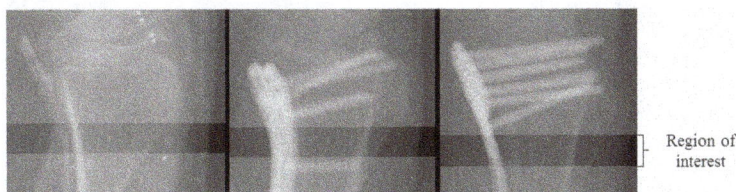

Fig. 2 Lateral scoutviews of each instrumented radius showing the region of interest (ROI) in each radius. The ROI was chosen at a location where the radius was fully covered by a part of the plate without holes and that was not intersected by screws. The tantalum fibers in the CFR-PEEK plate (*left*) allow visualization of the plate

between the instrumented and uninstrumented radius, with the uninstrumented radius as 100% reference.

Results

HRpQCT images

HRpQCT images of each radius with and without plate are shown in Fig. 3. The tantalum fibers that were incorporated into the CFR-PEEK plates were clearly visible, and no visible image artifacts were observed when the CFR-PEEK plate was instrumented (Fig. 3a). In the radii instrumented with the titanium plates, severe image artifacts were seen (Fig. 3b and c). These image artifacts consisted of streaks and a higher intensity of the bone voxels that are closely located to the plate.

Errors in bone parameters

The reproducibility (RMSCV%) of the bone density, micro-architectural and biomechanical parameters ranged from 0.0 to 2.3% (Table 1).

In Table 2, the bone parameters measured per uninstrumented and instrumented distal radius are shown, together with the percent errors that were introduced by each plate. All errors in bone parameters are in comparison to the same but uninstrumented radius. For the radius instrumented with the CFR-PEEK plate, percent errors in bone parameters ranged from −3.2% in Ct.Th to +2.6% in Tb.Sp, and the smallest error was observed in Dtrab, with −0.8%. For the radii instrumented with the titanium plates, in general the percent errors were

larger. For the radius instrumented with plate #2, the percent errors in bone parameters ranged from −43.2% in Tb.Sp to +67.2% in Dtrab, and the smallest error was observed in Scomp, with +7.5%. For the radius instrumented with plate #3, the largest percent errors in bone parameters were also found in Tb.Sp and Dtrab, being −11.2% and +30.2%, respectively. The smallest error was observed in F.Ult, with +0.1%.

Discussion

This study tested the effect of CFR-PEEK and two titanium VDRPs on bone density, micro-architectural and biomechanical parameters at the distal radius obtained by HRpQCT in combination with µFEA. Compared to conventional VDRPs that are made from titanium alloys, the plate made from CFR-PEEK introduced no visible image artifacts and had a minimal effect on the assessment of vBMD, micro-architectural and biomechanical parameters.

As expected, severe image artifacts were introduced by the titanium plates, which in turn led to an overestimation of the BMD, trabecular number and thickness and biomechanical properties, and an underestimation of trabecular separation at the distal radius. The errors in these bone parameters, however, differed between both titanium plates and this difference is probably related to the positioning and geometry of the plates: plate #2 was wider, thicker, and as can be seen in Fig. 3, more closely instrumented onto the radius, whereas plate #3 was smaller and a small gap between the bone and the

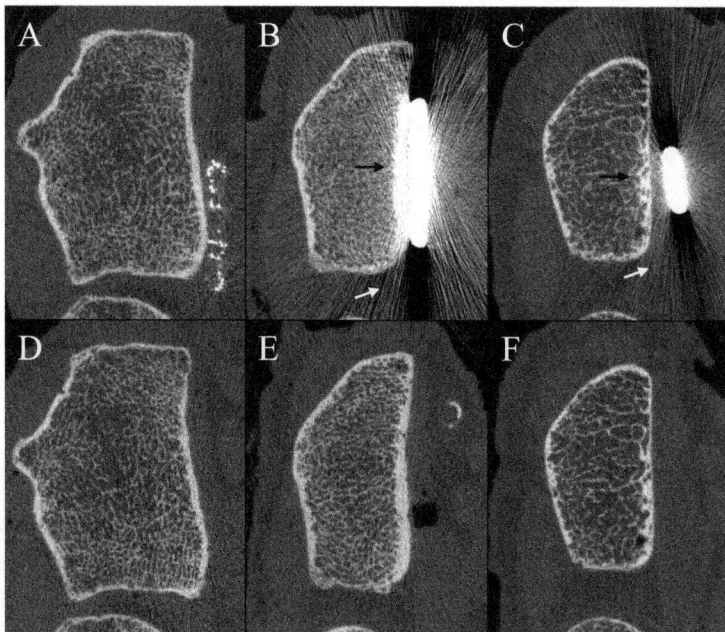

Fig. 3 Representative HRpQCT slices in each radius with (**a**, **b** and **c**) and without instrumented plate (**d**, **e** and **f**). The CFR-PEEK plate with tantalum fibers (panel **a**) caused less visible image artifacts as compared to the titanium plates (panel **b** and **c**), which caused streak artifacts (*white arrows*) and an increased intensity of voxels close to the titanium plates (*black arrows*)

Table 1 Reproducibility (RMSCV%) calculated from duplicate HRpQCT measurements at the uninstrumented and instrumented radii

Bone parameter	RMSCV% Radius #1		RMSCV% Radius #2		RMSCV% Radius #3	
	Un-instrumented	Instrumented (CFR-PEEK)	Un-instrumented	Instrumented (Titanium)	Un-instrumented	Instrumented (Titanium)
vBMD						
Dtot	0.52	2.18	0.02	1.29	0.00	0.20
Dtrab	0.10	1.95	0.34	0.00	0.31	0.62
Dcort	0.31	1.48	0.24	1.13	0.01	0.06
Micro – architecture						
BV/TV	0.00	1.76	0.47	0.00	1.25	0.00
Tb.N	2.24	0.92	0.00	1.19	0.72	0.67
Tb.Th	1.84	0.90	0.00	1.66	0.00	1.11
Tb.Sp	2.16	0.99	0.16	1.13	0.37	0.08
Ct.Th	1.50	1.55	0.00	1.65	0.93	0.00
Biomechanical						
Scomp	0.42	1.38	0.28	1.71	0.02	0.49
F.Ult	0.28	1.30	0.40	2.23	0.06	0.54

Abbreviations: *vBMD* volumetric bone mineral density, *Dtot* total density, *Dtrab* trabecular density, *Dcort* cortical density, *BV/TV* bone to total volume, *Tb.N* trabecular number, *Tb.Th* trabecular thickness, *Tb.Sp* trabecular separation, *Ct.Th* cortical thickness, *Scomp* compression stiffness, *F.Ult* ultimate failure load

plate was left after instrumentation. Nevertheless, the magnitude of the errors introduced by the titanium plates is higher than the reproducibility of the HRpQCT technique. Additionally, due to differences in positioning and size of the implants it seems almost impossible to correct the bone parameters in a systematic way, which makes these titanium plates unsuitable in studies when one wants to monitor bone healing with HRpQCT.

The CFR-PEEK plate, on the other hand, introduced relatively small errors that were of the same order as the reproducibility of the HRpQCT technique [8, 12, 16]. A plate made from CFR-PEEK would therefore be a suitable

Table 2 Bone mineral density, micro-architectural and biomechanical parameters measured with HRpQCT at the uninstrumented and instrumented distal radius and the percent difference between them

Bone parameter	Radius #1			Radius #2			Radius #3		
	Un-instrumented	Instrumented (CFR-PEEK)	Error (Δ%)	Un-instrumented	Instrumented (Titanium)	Error (Δ%)	Un-instrumented	Instrumented (Titanium)	Error (Δ%)
vBMD									
Dtot [mgHA/cm^3]	273	266	(−2.5)	343	520	(+51.8)	229	245	(+6.7)
Dtrab [mgHA/cm^3]	146	145	(−0.8)	181	304	(+67.2)	62	80	(+30.2)
Dcort [mgHA/cm^3]	862	848	(−1.6)	839	1004	(+19.6)	853	850	(−0.3)
Micro – architecture									
BV/TV [–]	0.122	0.121	(−1.2)	0.152	0.253	(+67.0)	0.052	0.067	(+30.1)
Tb.N [mm^{-1}]	1.58	1.54	(−2.2)	1.92	2.98	(+55.0)	0.96	1.06	(+10.5)
Tb.Th [mm]	0.077	0.079	(+1.9)	0.079	0.085	(+7.6)	0.054	0.064	(+17.6)
Tb.Sp [mm]	0.557	0.571	(+2.6)	0.442	0.251	(−43.2)	0.996	0.885	(−11.2)
Ct.Th [mm]	0.94	0.91	(−3.2)	1.01	1.29	(+27.2)	0.76	0.76	(+0.7)
Biomechanical									
Scomp [N/mm]	150	147	(−1.9)	133	143	(+7.5)	70	69	(−1.0)
F.Ult [kN]	7.17	7.06	(−1.5)	6.24	6.85	(+9.8)	3.28	3.28	(+0.1)

Abbreviations: *vBMD* volumetric bone mineral density, *Dtot* total density, *Dtrab* trabecular density, *Dcort* cortical density, *BV/TV* bone to total volume, *Tb.N* trabecular number, *Tb.Th* trabecular thickness, *Tb.Sp* trabecular separation, *Ct.Th* cortical thickness, *Scomp* compression stiffness, *F.Ult* ultimate failure load

alternative to the conventional volar distal radius plates, if one wants to monitor the healing process of unstable distal radius fractures with HRpQCT or any other X-ray technique.

Besides the low number of subjects, a limitation of the present study is that each plate was instrumented on a different radius. However, all results were specified relative to those of the same radius without a plate, and the density and micro-architectural parameters of the radius on which the CFR-PEEK plate was instrumented was in-between those of the radii to which a titanium plate was attached, making it unlikely that this has affected the results in any way. Another important limitation of this pilot study is the difference in geometry between the three plates that were tested. It is likely that a thick, wide plate, such as plate #2, introduces more severe image artifacts and hence larger errors in bone parameters, than a thin, small plate. Furthermore, we did not test VDRPs made from stainless steel. The main reason is that at present in the Netherlands, where the study was conducted, the commonly used plates are made from titanium alloy. However, since stainless steel causes more severe image artifacts in CT than titanium [17], it is expected that stainless steel plates would lead to higher errors in HRpQCT-derived bone parameters as compared to titanium plates.

Conclusions

In conclusion, the results of this pilot study indicate that a volar distal radius plate made from CFR-PEEK has minimal effect on bone parameters obtained at the distal radius with HRpQCT. We therefore recommend the use of CFR-PEEK plates instead of conventional titanium plates in studies that aim to monitor the healing process of distal radius fractures or bone graft ingrowth at the distal radius over time using HRpQCT.

Abbreviations

BMD: Bone mineral density; BV/TV: Bone to total volume; CFR-PEEK: Carbon-fiber-reinforced poly-ether-ether-ketone; Ct.Th: Cortical thickness; Dcort: Cortical density; Dtot: Total density; Dtrab: Trabecular density; F.Ult: Ultimate failure load; HRpQCT: High-resolution peripheral quantitative computed tomography; MRI: Magnetic resonance imaging; RMSCV: Root-mean-square coefficient of variation; ROI: Region of interest; Scomp: Compression stiffness; Tb.N: Trabecular number; Tb.Sp: Trabecular separation; Tb.Th: Trabecular thickness; VDRP: Volar distal radius plate

Acknowledgements

We thank A. Gisep (Icotec AG), H. Gerritsen (Stryker) and D. Mobers (Synthes GmbH) for providing the plates, screws, instrumentation kits and technical assistance. Furthermore, we thank J. Hekking and L. Huiberts from the Anatomy and Embryology department of Maastricht University for their support before and after surgery and preparation of the cadaver materials.

Funding

This study was supported by funding of the Weijerhorst Foundation (WH2).

Authors' contributions

Research design: JdJ, AL, JA and PW. Acquisition, analysis or interpretation of the data: JdJ, AL, BvR, JA, PG, JvdB and PW. Drafting the manuscript: JdJ, AL, BvR and PW. Revising the manuscript: JdJ, AL, BvR, JA, PG, JvdB and PW. All authors have read and approved the final submitted manuscript.

Competing interests

B. van Rietbergen is a consultant for Scanco Medical AG. JJ. Arts is a board member of workgroup Biotechnology of the Dutch Orthopedic Association (NOV) and a board member of the Dutch Society for Biomaterials and Tissue Engineering (NBTE). P.C. Willems is a board member of the Dutch Spine Society (association of spine surgeons).

Consent for publication

Not applicable.

Author details

[1]NUTRIM School for Nutrition and Translational Research in Metabolism, Maastricht University, Maastricht, The Netherlands. [2]Department of Rheumatology, Maastricht University Medical Center, Maastricht, The Netherlands. [3]Department of Anatomy and Embryology, Maastricht University, Maastricht, The Netherlands. [4]Faculty of Biomedical Engineering, Eindhoven University of Technology, Eindhoven, The Netherlands. [5]Department of Orthopedic Surgery, Maastricht University Medical Center, Maastricht, The Netherlands. [6]CAPHRI School for Public Health and Primary Care, Maastricht University, Maastricht, The Netherlands. [7]Faculty of Medicine and Life Sciences, Hasselt University, Hasselt, Belgium. [8]Department of Internal Medicine, VieCuri Medical Center, Venlo, The Netherlands.

References

1. Zimel MN, Hwang S, Riedel ER, Healey JH. Carbon fiber intramedullary nails reduce artifact in postoperative advanced imaging. Skeletal Radiol. 2015;44:1317–25.
2. Heary RF, Kheterpal A, Mammis A, Kumar S. Stackable carbon fiber cages for thoracolumbar interbody fusion after corpectomy: long-term outcome analysis. Neurosurgery. 2011;68:810–8.
3. Pace N, Marinelli M, Spurio S. Technical and histologic analysis of a retrieved carbon fiber-reinforced poly-ether-ether-ketone composite alumina-bearing liner 28 months after implantation. J Arthroplasty. 2008;23:151–5.
4. Nakahara I, Takao M, Bandoh S, Bertollo N, Walsh WR, Sugano N. In vivo implant fixation of carbon fiber-reinforced PEEK hip prostheses in an ovine model. J Orthop Res. 2013;31:485–92.
5. Zimel MN, Farfalli GL, Zindman AM, Riedel ER, Morris CD, Boland PJ, et al. Revision distal femoral arthroplasty with the compress((R)) prosthesis has a low rate of mechanical failure at 10 years. Clin Orthop Relat Res. 2016;474:528–36.
6. de Jong JJ, Heyer FL, Arts JJ, Poeze M, Keszei AP, Willems PC, et al. Fracture repair in the distal radius in post-menopausal women: a follow-up two years post-fracture using HRpQCT. J Bone Miner Res. 2016;31:1114–22.
7. de Jong JJ, Willems PC, Arts JJ, Bours SG, Brink PR, van Geel TA, et al. Assessment of the healing process in distal radius fractures by high resolution peripheral quantitative computed tomography. Bone. 2014;64C:65–74.
8. de Jong JJ, Arts JJ, Meyer U, Willems PC, Geusens PP, van den Bergh JP, et al. Effect of a cast on short-term reproducibility and bone parameters obtained from HR-pQCT measurements at the distal end of the radius. J Bone Joint Surg Am. 2016;98:356–62.
9. Hammert WC, Kramer RC, Graham B, Keith MW. AAOS appropriate use criteria: treatment of distal radius fractures. J Am Acad Orthop Surg. 2013;21:506–9.
10. Mueller TL, Wirth AJ, van Lenthe GH, Goldhahn J, Schense J, Jamieson V, et al. Mechanical stability in a human radius fracture treated with a novel

tissue-engineered bone substitute: a non-invasive, longitudinal assessment using high-resolution pQCT in combination with finite element analysis. J Tissue Eng Regen Med. 2011;5:415–20.

11. Boas FE, Fleischmann D. Evaluation of two iterative techniques for reducing metal artifacts in computed tomography. Radiology. 2011;259:894–902.

12. Boutroy S, Bouxsein ML, Munoz F, Delmas PD. In vivo assessment of trabecular bone microarchitecture by high-resolution peripheral quantitative computed tomography. J Clin Endocrinol Metab. 2005;90:6508–15.

13. Pistoia W, van Rietbergen B, Lochmuller EM, Lill CA, Eckstein F, Ruegsegger P. Estimation of distal radius failure load with micro-finite element analysis models based on three-dimensional peripheral quantitative computed tomography images. Bone. 2002;30:842–8.

14. Pistoia W, van Rietbergen B, Lochmuller EM, Lill CA, Eckstein F, Ruegsegger P. Image-based micro-finite-element modeling for improved distal radius strength diagnosis: moving from bench to bedside. J Clin Densitom. 2004;7:153–60.

15. Gluer CC, Blake G, Lu Y, Blunt BA, Jergas M, Genant HK. Accurate assessment of precision errors: how to measure the reproducibility of bone densitometry techniques. Osteoporos Int. 1995;5:262–70.

16. MacNeil JA, Boyd SK. Improved reproducibility of high-resolution peripheral quantitative computed tomography for measurement of bone quality. Med Eng Phys. 2008;30:792–9.

17. Knott PT, Mardjetko SM, Kim RH, Cotter TM, Dunn MM, Patel ST, et al. A comparison of magnetic and radiographic imaging artifact after using three types of metal rods: stainless steel, titanium, and vitallium. Spine J. 2010;10: 789–94.

12

Atypical findings of perineural cysts on postmyelographic computed tomography: a case report of intermittent intercostal neuralgia caused by thoracic perineural cysts

Hirokazu Iwamuro[1,2*], Taro Yanagawa[1], Sachiko Takamizawa[1] and Makoto Taniguchi[1]

Abstract

Background: Perineural cysts are sometimes found incidentally with magnetic resonance imaging, and clinical symptoms requiring treatment are rare. Perineural cysts typically exhibit delayed filling with contrast medium on myelography, which is one of the criteria used by Tarlov to distinguish perineural cysts from meningeal diverticula. We present a case of multiple thoracolumbar perineural cysts, one of which was considered the cause of intermittent intercostal neuralgia with atypical findings on postmyelographic computed tomography seen as selective filling of contrast medium.

Case presentation: A 61-year-old woman presented with intermittent pain on her left chest wall with distribution of the pain corresponding to the T10 dermatome. Magnetic resonance imaging showed multiple thoracolumbar perineural cysts with the largest located at the left T10 nerve root. On postmyelographic computed tomography immediately after contrast medium injection, the largest cyst and another at left T9 showed selective filling of contrast medium, suggesting that inflow of cerebrospinal fluid to the cyst exceeded outflow. Three hours after the injection, the intensity of the cysts was similar to the intensity of the thecal sac, and by the next day, contrast enhancement was undetectable. The patient was treated with an intercostal nerve block at T10, and the pain subsided. However, after 9 months of observation, the neuralgia recurred, and the nerve block was repeated with good effect. There was no recurrence 22 months after the last nerve block.

Conclusions: We concluded that intermittent elevation of cerebrospinal fluid pressure in the cyst caused the neuralgia because of an imbalance between cerebrospinal fluid inflow and outflow, and repeated intercostal nerve blocks resolved the neuralgia. Our case demonstrates the mechanism of cyst expansion.

Keywords: Perineural cysts, Tarlov cysts, Computed tomography, Myelography, Intercostal nerves, Neuralgia, Thoracic wall, Nerve block

* Correspondence: iwamuroh-tky@umin.ac.jp
[1]Department of Neurosurgery, Tokyo Metropolitan Neurological Hospital, 2-6-1 Musashidai, Fuchu 1830042, Japan
[2]Department of Research and Therapeutics for Movement Disorders, Juntendo University Graduate School of Medicine, 2-1-1 Hongo, Bunkyo-ku, Tokyo 1138421, Japan

Background

Perineural cysts, a subtype of meningeal cysts also called Tarlov cysts [1], are spinal extradural cysts at nerve roots. Most are asymptomatic, found incidentally with magnetic resonance imaging (MRI), and have an estimated prevalence between 1.2% [2] and 9.8% [3]. They commonly occur in the sacrum [4]. The etiology of these cysts is largely unknown; however, several studies have proposed that a ball-valve effect of cerebrospinal fluid (CSF) flow contributes to enlargement of the cysts [5], which is supported by delayed filling with contrast medium on myelography [6]. However, delayed filling implies only that CSF inflow into the cysts is restricted. We present a case of multiple thoracolumbar perineural cysts, some of which showed atypical findings on myelography as selective filling of contrast medium, suggesting restricted CSF outflow from the cysts.

Case presentation

A 61-year-old woman presented with pain in her chest wall for two months, and had no significant medical history, such as trauma, infection, or tumor. The pain was located in the left lower chest in a band-like pattern overlapping the T10 dermatome. The pain was intermittent and occurred several times a day, continuing for 10–20 min each episode and alleviated when lying down. The pain was considered to be intercostal neuralgia.

To identify the cause of the neuralgia, we performed MRI, which revealed multiple cysts at the T9–T11 nerve roots bilaterally (Fig. 1). No other causal abnormality for the chest wall pain was found other than the cysts. The interior of the cysts showed similar intensity to the CSF on imaging. The largest cyst was at the level of the left T10 vertebra and had a linear shadow that suggested the presence of nerve root fibers. Computed tomography

(CT) with myelography was also performed to study CSF communication between the thecal sac and the cysts. After 10 mL of 240 mg I/mL iodinated contrast medium (Omnipaque 240, Daiichi Sankyo, Inc., Japan) was injected into the thecal sac at L4/5 in the lateral recumbent position, the first CT image was taken immediately (left and middle columns of Fig. 2), and revealed multiple cysts from T6–L2, including small cysts. The cysts were enhanced by the contrast medium and most showed the same intensity as that of the thecal sac at the corresponding level; however, the largest cyst at left T10 and another at left T9 showed much higher concentrations of the contrast medium. Three hours after the injection, the intensities of the cysts and the thecal sac were equal on the second CT (right column of Fig. 2). The next day, another CT examination showed no detectable contrast enhancement. Based on these findings, we suggested a diagnosis of multiple perineural cysts.

The patient was treated with an intercostal nerve block at T10 (Fig. 3) with 50 mg of mepivacaine hydrochloride (Carbocain, AstraZeneca, Inc., Japan) and 4 mg of dexamethasone sodium phosphate (DEXART, FujiPharma, Inc., Japan), and the pain subsided. Nine months later, the neuralgia recurred and another nerve block again relieved the pain. There was no recurrence 22 months after the last nerve block.

Discussion

Perineural cysts are defined as CSF-filled saccular lesions in the extradural space of the spinal canal and are formed within the nerve root sheath at the dorsal root ganglion. Diagnosis should be based on histopathological findings because the presence of spinal nerve root fibers in the wall or cavity of the cyst are required for confirmation. However, magnetic resonance neurography has

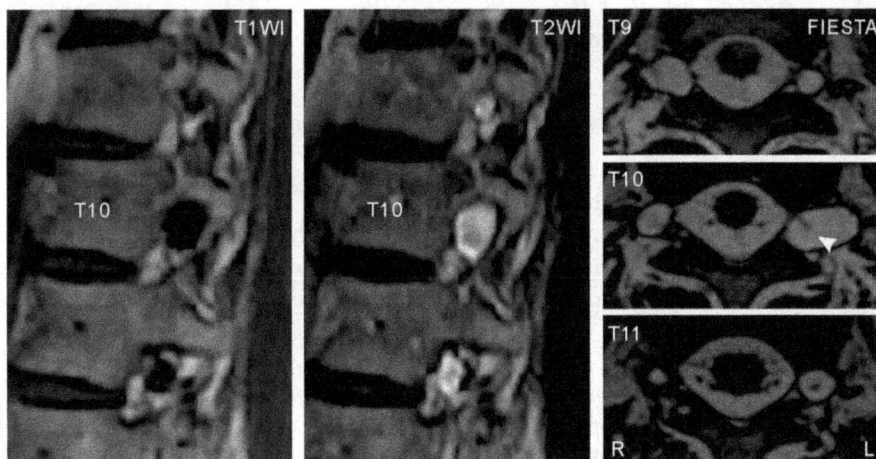

Fig. 1 Magnetic resonance images at T9–T11 showing multiple perineural cysts. Sagittal views at the level of the left intervertebral foramina on T1- (left) and T2-weighted (middle) images show multiple cysts on the left side. In axial views acquired by fast imaging employing steady-state acquisition (FIESTA, right), a linear shadow (arrowhead) is seen in the largest cyst at left T10

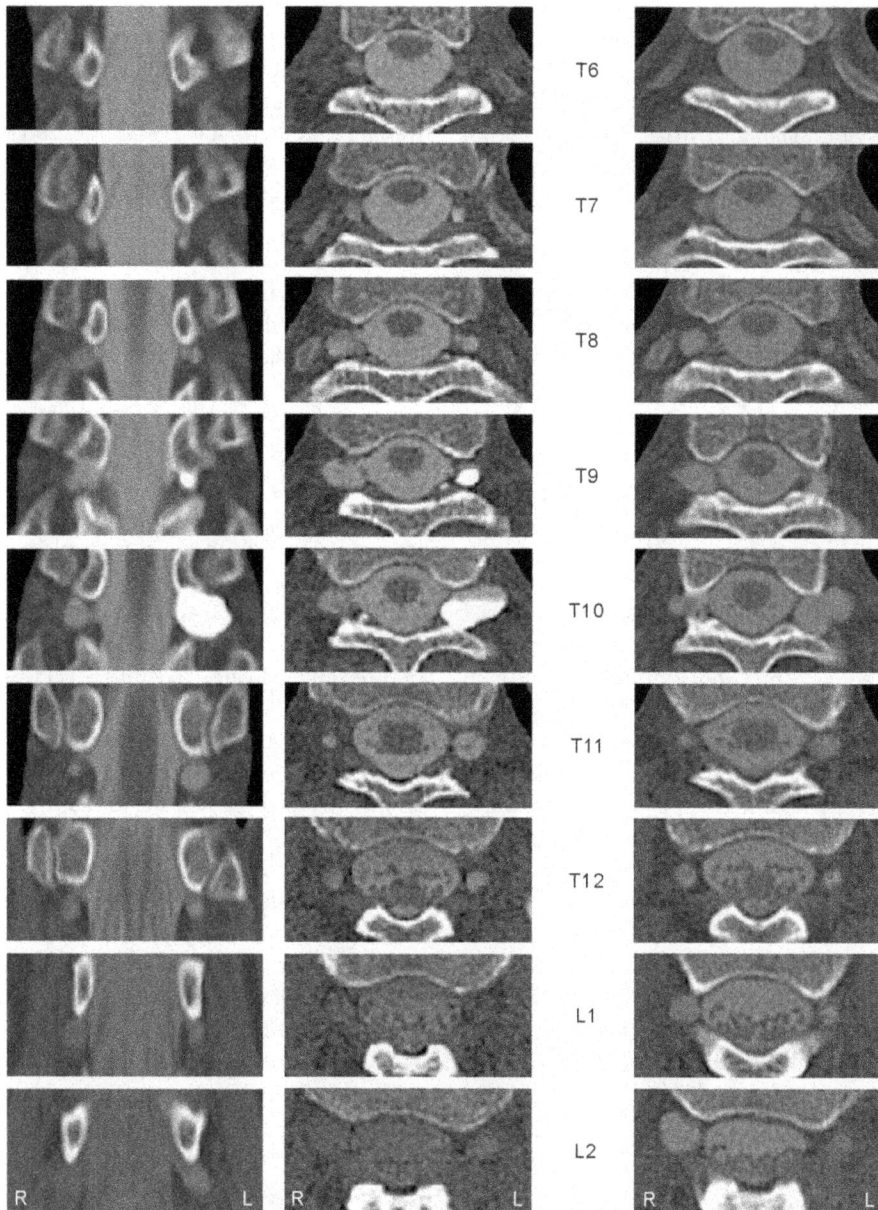

Fig. 2 Computed tomography immediately after contrast medium injection (*left* and *middle* images) and 3 h later (*right* images). Two cysts at left T9 and T10 showed much higher intensity than the other cysts immediately after contrast medium injection

been recently proposed for diagnosis [7]. In our case, histopathology was not performed because non-surgical treatment was effective in relieving the associated neuralgia; but, results of the imaging studies supported our diagnosis.

Delayed filling with contrast medium on CT myelography is a typical finding with perineural cysts [6]. However, in our case, the largest cyst and one other showed immediate selective filling on the first CT, suggesting that the contrast medium flowed selectively into these cysts. We did not have an opportunity to observe the lesions directly, and therefore, do not know the exact mechanism of this inflow. However, considering the anatomical background of the lesions, we presume that the aspiration force was caused by negative pleural pressure. Several reports have stressed that delayed filling on CT myelography is a required finding for diagnosis of perineural cysts [6], but this may not always be true, especially in thoracic cases.

The etiology of perineural cysts remains unclear [8]. However, regarding cyst enlargement, the ball-valve theory has achieved consensus as an underlying mechanism, suggesting that enlargement is caused by restricted CSF outflow from the cyst as a result of CSF pulsatile

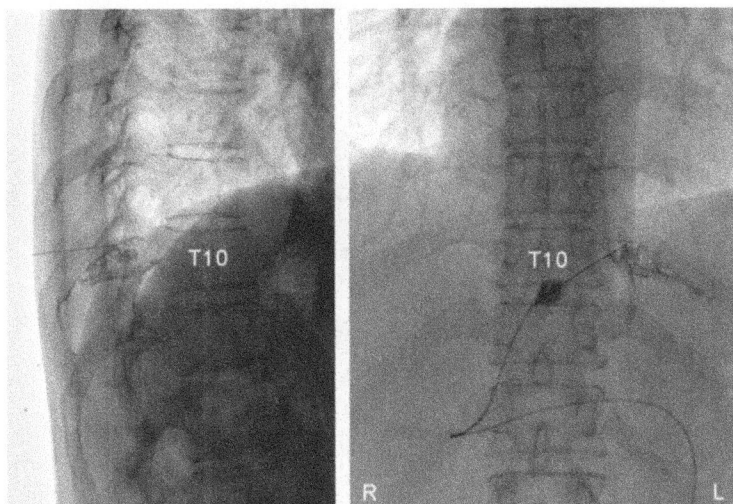

Fig. 3 Thoracic X-ray images (*left*, lateral view; *right*, anterior-posterior view) during the left T10 intercostal nerve block. Contrast medium was injected to indicate the site of the nerve block

and hydrostatic forces [9, 10]. The first CT results in our case suggested that CSF inflow into the two cysts exceeded outflow, which supports this theory.

We considered surgical treatment but ultimately decided to follow the patient conservatively because her symptoms resolved after the nerve block. It was difficult to prove a causal relationship between the perineural cysts and the intercostal neuralgia; however, we concluded that the chest wall pain was caused by the pressure of the largest cyst at left T10 for several reasons: 1) this cyst was considerably larger and involved the nerve root fibers that were causing the symptoms; 2) this cyst showed an imbalance between CSF inflow and outflow; 3) because the pain was intermittent and alleviated when the patient was lying down, the cause of the pain was expected to be easily resolved, considering its relationship to head position; and 4) we found no other causal abnormality to explain the neuralgia other than the cyst. If the patient's symptoms reappear in the future, we would reconsider invasive treatment as the patient would meet the criteria for surgery [9].

Conclusions

We report a rare case of thoracolumbar multiple perineural cysts, one of which was considered the cause of intermittent intercostal neuralgia. The cyst showed immediate selective filling of the contrast medium on CT myelography, which suggested an aspirating force resulting from pleural negative pressure. Because repeat intercostal nerve blocks resolved the neuralgia and we did not perform surgery, our suggested etiology was difficult to prove directly; however, we concluded that intermittent elevation of pressure in the cyst caused the

neuralgia because of an imbalance between CSF inflow and outflow. This case demonstrates the mechanism of perineural cyst expansion.

Abbreviations
CSF: Cerebrospinal fluid; CT: Computed tomography; FIESTA: Fast imaging employing steady-state acquisition; MRI: Magnetic resonance imaging.

Acknowledgements
Not applicable.

Funding
This research was partially supported by JSPS KAKENHI Grant Number JP17K10907 to HI.

Authors' contributions
HI, TY, and ST collected and analyzed the patient data, and drafted part of the case presentation. HI and MT interpreted the data and drafted parts of the Background, Discussion, and Conclusions. HI was involved in overall supervision of the case and manuscript. All authors read and approved the final manuscript.

Competing interests
The authors declare that they have no competing interests.

References

1. Nabors MW, Pait TG, Byrd EB, Karim NO, Davis DO, Kobrine AI, et al.
    Updated assessment and current classification of spinal meningeal cysts.
    J Neurosurg. 1988;68:366–77.
2. Langdown AJ, Grundy JR, Birch NC. The clinical relevance of Tarlov cysts.
    J Spinal Disord Tech. 2005;18:29–33.
3. Tani S, Hata Y, Tochigi S, Ohashi H, Isoshima A, Nagashima H, et al.
    Prevalence of spinal meningeal cyst in the sacrum. Neuro Med Chir (Tokyo).
    2013;53:91–4.
4. Burdan F, Mocarska A, Janczarek M, Klepacz R, Łosicki M, Patyra K, et al.
    Incidence of spinal perineural (Tarlov) cysts among East-European patients.
    PLoS One. 2013;8:e71514.
5. Mummaneni PV, Pitts LH, McCormack BM, Corroo JM, Weinstein PR.
    Microsurgical treatment of symptomatic sacral Tarlov cysts. Neurosurgery.
    2000;47:74–9.
6. Acosta Jr FL, Quinones-Hinojosa A, Schmidt MH, Weinstein PR. Diagnosis
    and management of sacral Tarlov cysts. Case report and review of the
    literature. Neurosurg Focus. 2003;15:E15.
7. Petrasic JR, Chhabra A, Scott KM. Impact of MR neurography in patients
    with chronic cauda equina syndrome presenting as chronic pelvic pain and
    dysfunction. AJNR Am J Neuroradiol. 2017;38:418–22.
8. Neulen A, Kantelhardt SR, Pilgram-Pastor SM, Metz I, Rohde V, Giese A.
    Microsurgical fenestration of perineural cysts to the thecal sac at the level
    of the distal dural sleeve. Acta Neurochir (Wien). 2011;153:1427–34.
9. Burke JF, Thawani JP, Berger I, Nayak NR, Stephen JH, Farkas T, et al.
    Microsurgical treatment of sacral perineural (Tarlov) cysts: case series and
    review of the literature. J Neurosurg Spine. 2016;24:700–7.
10. Lucantoni C, Than KD, Wang AC, Valdivia-Valdivia JM, Maher CO, La Marca F,
    et al. Tarlov cysts: a controversial lesion of the sacral spine. Neurosurg
    Focus. 2011;31:E14.

13

Testing of the assisting software for radiologists analysing head CT images

Petr Martynov[1]* (ID), Nikolai Mitropolskii[1], Katri Kukkola[1], Monika Gretsch[2], Vesa-Matti Koivisto[3], Ilkka Lindgren[2], Jani Saunavaara[4], Jarmo Reponen[5] and Anssi Mäkynen[1]

Abstract

Background: Assessing a plan for user testing and evaluation of the assisting software developed for radiologists.

Methods: Test plan was assessed in experimental testing, where users performed reporting on head computed tomography studies with the aid of the software developed. The user testing included usability tests, questionnaires, and interviews. In addition, search relevance was assessed on the basis of user opinions.

Results: The testing demonstrated weaknesses in the initial plan and enabled improvements. Results showed that the software has acceptable usability level but some minor fixes are needed before larger-scale pilot testing. The research also proved that it is possible even for radiologists with under a year's experience to perform reporting of non-obvious cases when assisted by the software developed. Due to the small number of test users, it was impossible to assess effects on diagnosis quality.

Conclusions: The results of the tests performed showed that the test plan designed is useful, and answers to the key research questions should be forthcoming after testing with more radiologists. The preliminary testing revealed opportunities to improve test plan and flow, thereby illustrating that arranging preliminary test sessions prior to any complex scenarios is beneficial.

Keywords: Computer software, Search engine, Brain imaging, Computed tomography, Research design

Background

Content-based image retrieval (CBIR) in radiology grew to a popular research topic in recent years [1] aimed to make workflow of radiologists more effective in case of increasing numbers of patients and medical images worldwide. The general purpose of CBIR is to help users to find similar items in some set of images, which is especially applicable for automation in radiology. Since the entire field of CBIR technology still faces challenges, evaluation of the usefulness of the CBIR solution applied is also challenging. There are reports addressing implementation and evaluation of applications designed to aid in analysing computed tomography (CT) images [2, 3], mammograms [4, 5], x-ray images [6–8], and other

modalities or complex solutions [9–11]; however, though all those systems are based on CBIR technology, they differ greatly in their workflow and implementation. Therefore, researchers have developed original testing scenarios specific to the case at hand. Such scenarios have typically taken only one aspect of the system into account. The same issue has manifested itself also in other biomedical applications of CBIR [12, 13]. The approach in earlier research has either concentrated on validation of the retrieval system's performance and result quality with users [2, 3, 5, 6, 12] or on usability issues of the solution developed [8, 9, 11, 13]. Notwithstanding significant amount of experience and knowledge that has been accumulated regarding to evaluation of CBIR systems, there is still no comprehensive, unified approach to testing scenarios. This lack is especially evident if one plans to deal with complex

* Correspondence: petr.martynov@oulu.fi; pnmartynov@gmail.com
[1]Optoelectronics and Measurement Techniques Unit, University of Oulu, PO Box 4500, 90014 Oulu, Finland
Full list of author information is available at the end of the article

scenarios or test a novel solution that influences radiologists' existing workflow.

In the CARDS (Computer Assisted Radiology Diagnosis System) project [14], the software application named SeeMIK was developed. The main purpose behind the application was to assist in radiologists' interpretation of CT images of the head by providing tools for image and/or text-based search in hospital's Picture Archiving and Communication System (PACS) and Radiological Information System (RIS) databases. It was designed not to perform diagnosis but as an extension to RIS and PACS for retrieving meaningful textual and image data from them.

In consideration of experiences outlined in the papers mentioned above, a scenario for multifaceted evaluation of the software was designed. The general idea was to find answers to the following questions:

- Are the search results relevant?
- Does the software provide the required level of usability?
- Are the search results useful in decision-making?

The target was to cover the software usability and quality of the search results with a single test process. Due to the complexity of the process, it was decided that preliminary testing of the software should be performed, to verify whether the testing plan was designed well and one could obtain meaningful results and minimise mistakes and systematic bias.

Methods

Two junior radiologists, with six and twelve months of experience, were recruited from Raahe Hospital, Finland, for preliminary testing. Both of the participating radiologists had a separate workroom and computer workstation, and their work was followed by observers during all testing sessions.

The software under test

As a conventional CBIR system the SeeMIK software implements two processing modes: indexing and search. Indexing is needed to determine features (descriptors) for every image in the dataset according to selected algorithm. Features are quantitative characteristics (i.e. color data, textures, shape, size, and location of objects) of visual content, which are necessary for fast image comparison and retrieval. In search mode, conventional CBIR system assesses similarity between image features passed as a query and features stored in the index. Result images returned to the user in a decreasing similarity order.

In the software developed indexing is carried out in two phases: initial indexing (after installation and before normal functioning) and continuous background indexing. In the first phase, a sufficiently large corpus of head CT studies (numbering in the thousands) and associated reports from the hospital's PACS and RIS are used to build a 'bag of visual words' (BoVW) [15] vocabulary for the images and a textual vocabulary. All words in reports are stemmed beforehand so they are indexed in a truncated form. The software does not recognize which terms are significant for diagnosis and consider all the words have the same weight. Then, the software creates an initial 'inverted index' [16], composed of stemmed words and 'visual words', extracted from texts and images of the studies, respectively. In the second phase, it continuously obtains not-yet-indexed studies from PACS and RIS and indexes them using the existing vocabularies.

In search mode, the user interface of the software resembles a typical Web-based DICOM (Digital Imaging and Communications in Medicine) viewer connected to the PACS, which allows radiologists, for example, to browse and manipulate study images, measure tissue density (see Fig. 1). Unlike a conventional viewer, one can also search for similar images or studies (see Fig. 2) and view the search results found from the PACS and RIS of the hospital.

Text, an image, a selected part of an image, or a combination of image and text can be used as the search query. For textual queries, the software determines stemmed forms of words of the provided phrase and then looks for their combinations in the index. For image queries, the search engine developed processes the input image and compares its features, described by the existing vocabulary, with image features in the index database. Those images sharing enough 'visual words' in common with the query image are returned as search results. For combined queries, the search engine shows results matching both text and image on top and those are followed by results matching either image or text queries independently. In addition, it has so called advanced-search mode, which enables limiting search results by additional parameters such as patients' age range, patients' gender and radiological study codes.

The software presents the results as a list of studies/images matching the query. They are shown as blocks, in decreasing-relevance order, and there can be up to 100 radiological reports (studies) for a text-based search and images, grouped by study, for an image search (see Fig. 3). The search engine finds and shows up to five images for each study on results page. The user can open study images for every search result in the DICOM viewer.

During the testing, the software ran on a server in an isolated network created for the CARDS project at the University of Oulu premises. Architecture of the system

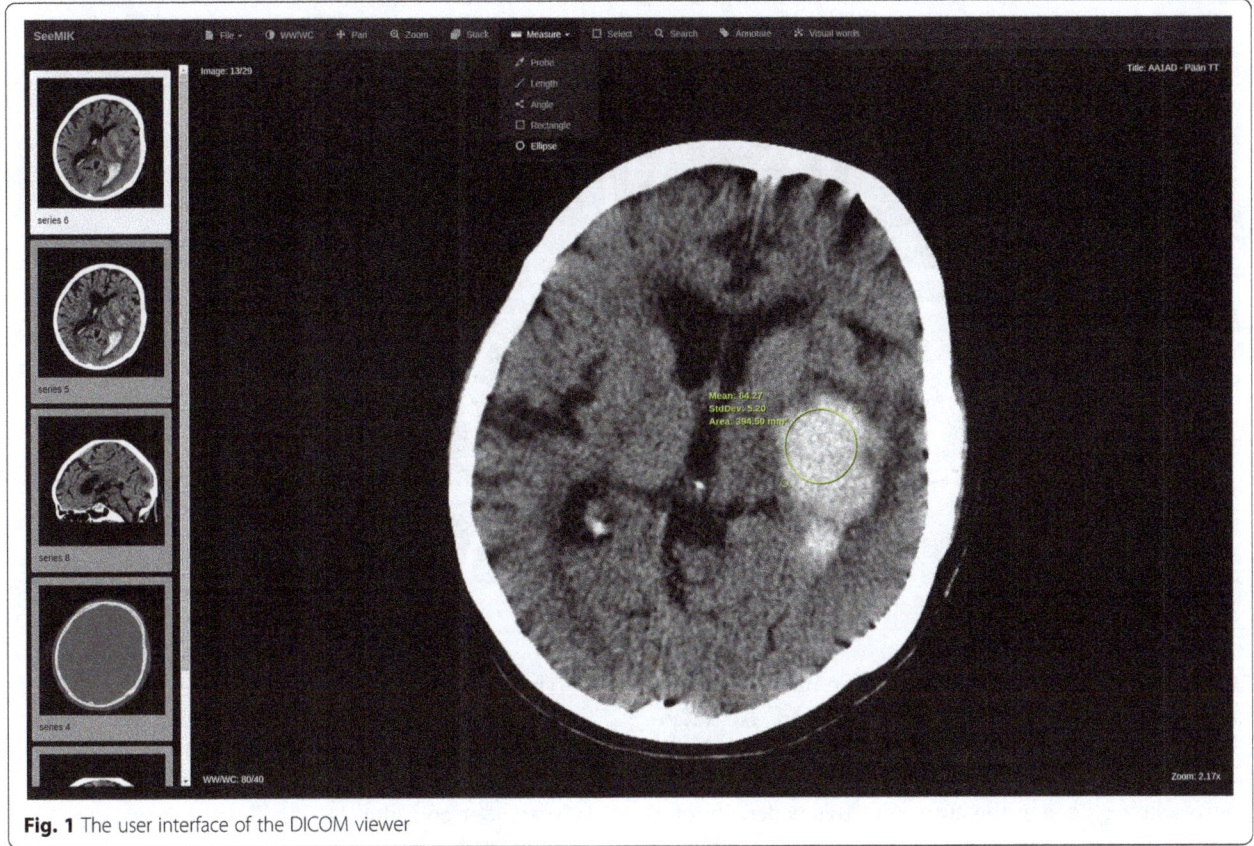

Fig. 1 The user interface of the DICOM viewer

developed represented by several connected modules with separate functions (see Fig. 4).

The testing materials

The Regional Ethics Committee of the Northern Ostrobothnia Hospital District approved this study design and the Northern Ostrobothnia Hospital District gave permission for the registry based data gathering and use for the software development and testing. Only cases which occurrence were high enough were exported to prevent identification after personal data removal. Sample data was exported from the emergency radiology department of Northern Ostrobothnia Hospital District. Radiological studies collected represented all emergency cases processed in the hospital for the last few years. Data exported contained conventional CT studies, enhanced CT studies and mixed studies with both types of CT images made on several different scanners. Text information exported consisted of radiological reports and anamneses linked to image data. For the preliminary testing, a sample of

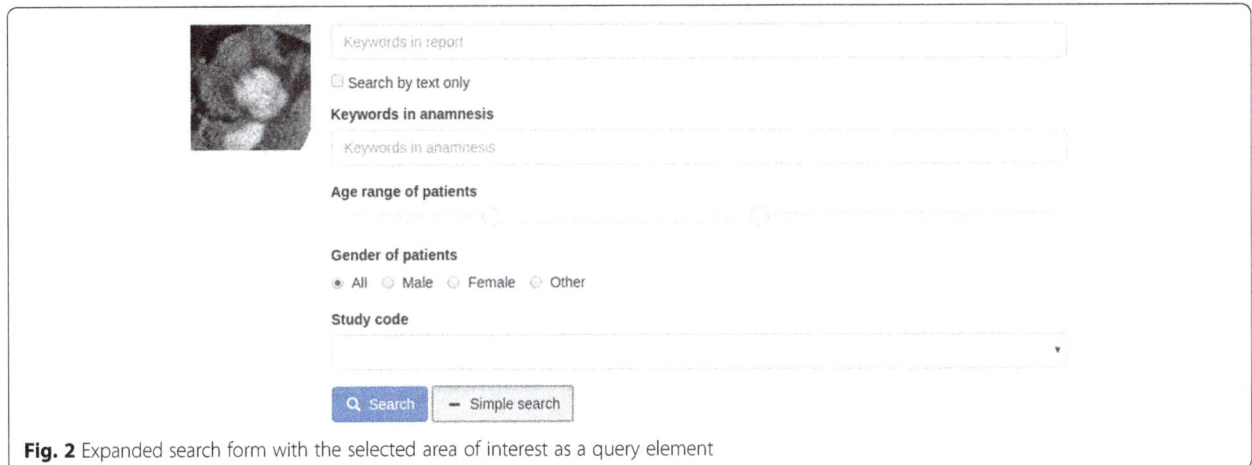

Fig. 2 Expanded search form with the selected area of interest as a query element

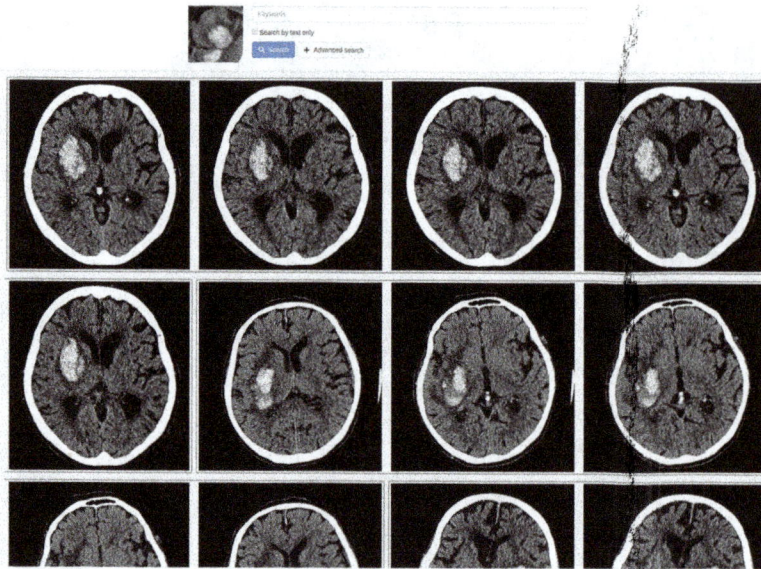

Fig. 3 Concise search form and presentation of image-search results in the software

5975 head CT studies (comprising more than 3.5 million radiological images) was indexed and used. All radiological studies for the test tasks were selected and prepared by an experienced radiologist specializing in neuroradiology, one of the authors of this paper. In total, 16 medical terms and 16 studies, with a wide range of findings, were collected for the relevance testing for the search engine. A study with an obvious finding (intracranial haemorrhage) was chosen for usability testing. For the reporting session, 10 head CT studies were selected in accordance with the following rules:

- The study should not have a conclusion that is obvious to inexperienced radiologists; that is, in a normal work situation, the radiologist would refer to some additional means (literature, an Internet search, or consultation of colleague, for example) to support the decision on the report.
- The CT study should be an appropriate one for observation and decision-making.

Opinions and perceptions of users were collected in several ways: via observation, questionnaires, and

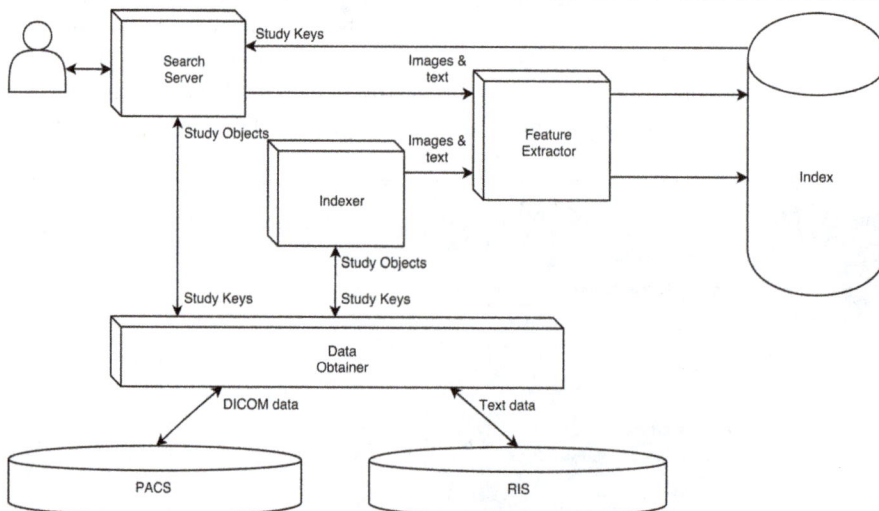

Fig. 4 Functional diagram of the software developed. Search server is a user interface module with which users perform searches and view radiological images. Feature extractor is a central module implementing feature extraction, vocabulary creation and text processing algorithms. Index is a file storage containing extracted image features, text terms and created vocabularies. Indexer is a module for performing initial and/or background processing of available image and textual data. Data obtainer is an integration interface for communicating with PACS and RIS

interviews. The System Usability Scale (SUS) [17] questionnaire was used to collect first impressions after the radiologists had used the search function, and the Usefulness, Satisfaction, and Ease of use (USE) [18] questionnaire was utilised after the software had been used in a situation mimicking normal work. Interviews were conducted immediately after filling in of the forms, so as to collect richer information on users' ideas and perceptions of the test and the software. A structured framework was used for the interview questions. All interviews were carried out in the Finnish language, and the audio was recorded, for later transcription and translation into English.

The SUS questionnaire is a proven and reliable tool for measuring usability of a wide variety of software products and services [19]. While quite brief, consisting of only 10 statements, each with five response options for respondents – from 'strongly agree' to 'strongly disagree' – it highlights the user's general perception of the software. The USE questionnaire contains 30 well-

formulated statements in English, each of which can be assessed with a Likert-type scale from 1 to 7 (representing 'strongly disagree' and 'strongly agree', respectively) or marked as 'not applicable' for the current circumstances. It enables assessing four aspects of software usability: usefulness, ease of use, ease of learning, and satisfaction.

The testing scenario

The preliminary testing addressed three factors: relevance of search results, usability, and usefulness (see Fig. 5). Before testing, the participants were instructed and trained to use the software.

The main aim in the **testing of search results' relevance** was to ascertain a relevance rate for images and studies found by the search engine in the test environment and quantitatively estimate the search results' quality with the aid of the radiologists. The relevance of the search results was assessed by means of three tasks for the participants:

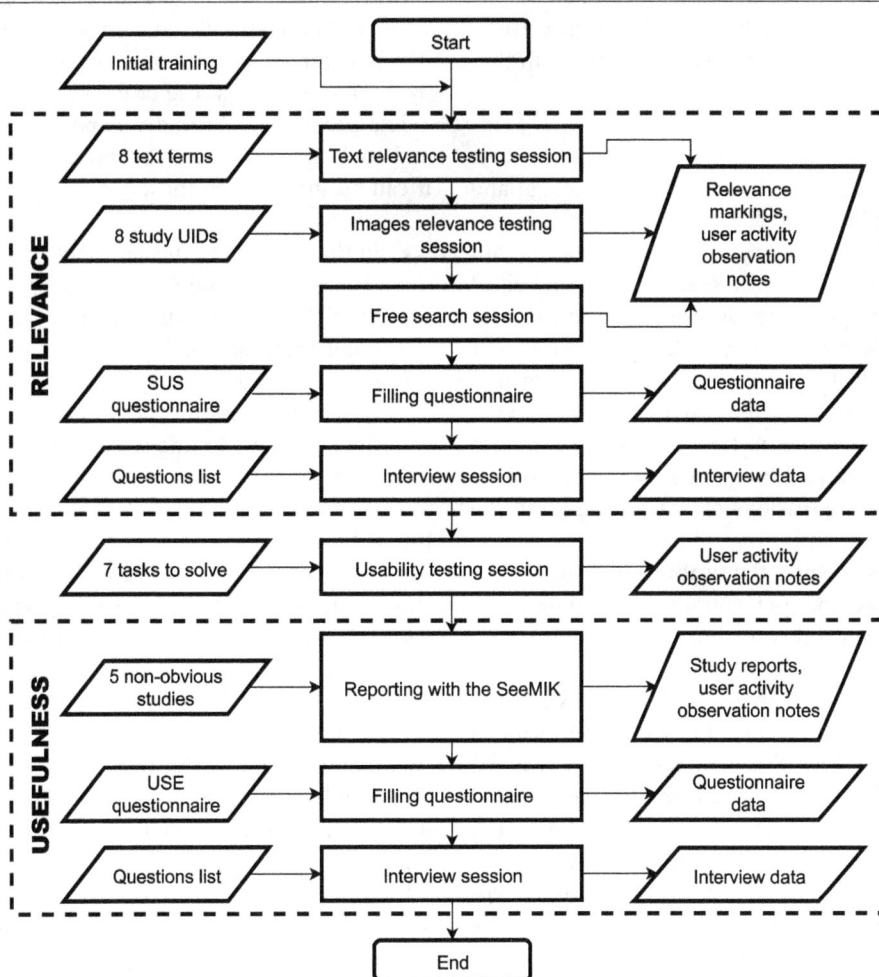

Fig. 5 The flow of the preliminary testing carried out

- Each radiologist was provided with a list of eight medical terms or phrases in Finnish for performing text-based searches. The task for the radiologists was to mark each of the first 10 results for every phrase as a relevant or irrelevant finding with respect to that phrase.
- Each radiologist was provided with a list of eight head CT studies. For each study, the participant's task was to choose a key image, identify an area of interest, and perform a search by that part of the image. The test materials did not inform the radiologists of the main findings in the associated reports, but it was possible to view the reports in the embedded DICOM viewer. The task for the radiologists was to mark the first 10 images returned as relevant or irrelevant for every search query or, if the first 10 results featured no relevant items, identify at least one relevant image from among the results.
- The final task involved free use of the search functionality by the radiologists. They were able to try searches by both image and text (combined-search) or advanced-search mode. Radiologists were asked to mark at least one relevant finding from the result set returned.

For testing purposes, buttons were added to the user interface for marking the relevance of every image and radiological report in the search results. With these buttons, the radiologists could mark the results as relevant or irrelevant with respect to the search query, and all of their markings were permanently stored in the database of the software. For the first two tasks, the 'precision at 10' metric was calculated for each textual or image-based query. The results in the last task were assessed qualitatively. The relevance testing was completed with the SUS questionnaire and interviews with both participants on their first impressions of the software and the test flow.

The main purpose behind the **usability testing** was to ascertain the radiologists' perceptions of the user interface developed, its suitability for image searching, and its applicability in radiologists' workflow. The tasks in the associated testing session were derived from possible use cases and eventual needs of radiologists. These included opening a study, checking the anamnesis (study request) and the details of the study, performing a search and opening its results in the viewer, and refining a search via additional criteria. Activity of users on the screen and facial expressions were recorded in the manner typical in such testing. Because of the number of participants, the assessment was qualitative in nature, no quantitative metrics for user interactions (e.g., task-completion time) were collected. Since observers

followed all testing sessions, the relevance testing and reporting sessions were targeted also for their ability to reveal usability mistakes and bottlenecks in the user interface.

The primary aim with the **usefulness testing** was to determine the real-world utility of the solution for radiologists who need to report on a non-obvious study. In this connection, the target in the preliminary testing was not to compare the time used for reporting with and without the software but solely to determine whether it is possible to report on the study with SeeMIK alone. In this testing, the junior radiologists were asked to open five specially selected head CT studies in the built-in viewer, analyse them, and report on them. The last two studies in each radiologist's list were optional. The information provided on those cases was restricted to the DICOM images and anamnesis. Other background details or previous studies for the same patient were unavailable. When reporting on each case, the radiologists were free to use all tools available in the software, without restriction, and dictate the reports created to a voice recorder. The second questionnaire (USE) and the final interview were completed after all other testing was finished, to gather feedback and cover all experience gained by the radiologists in use of the solution developed.

The preliminary testing was performed in two phases and took approximately five hours for each participant. It can be summarised thus:

- In the first phase, the relevance of the search results was estimated and usability issues were identified via the SUS questionnaire, the interview and observation of radiologists performing tasks.
- In the second phase, usability testing with several typical use cases was performed, with follow-up via the usefulness testing session, the USE questionnaire, and the interview.

Results

The tests showed that it is possible to carry out the desired measurements and collect perceptions of users with the tests used. Although results from actual testing and, especially, questionnaires in preliminary testing with only two participants are, naturally, insufficient for reliable interpretation in the statistical sense, they still yield some insights. Therefore, interviews and observations made during testing are valuable sources of information for evaluation of the successfulness of the test set-up.

Results of relevance tests revealed differences in assumptions as to what was considered relevant between an engineer's and a radiologist's perspective. The engineering view of text search was that a study is relevant if the text searched for appears in text related to that study. At the same time, radiologists in the test conditions assumed a text-search result to be relevant only if the report for the study actually contained the search term in its finding or diagnosis section and sometimes they looked for possible confirmation also in the study images. Differences in interpretations of relevance affected the results, and the average 'precision at 10' was 81% for text search. Most of the results deemed non-relevant contained sought-for terms in the anamnesis part as a question, but without confirmation of such finding in the report part. Though the software attempted to exclude various forms of negative expressions from the results returned, it did not succeed fully in this, especially because there are multiple ways to express both medical terms and their negatives in the Finnish language.

Image search also showed differences in interpretation of what constituted similarity. The engineers and the search engine judged images to be similar on the basis of visually similar features: areas and edges of areas. For the radiologists, however, the images had to be relevant also in a medical sense, since many different findings can look visually similar (for example, acute haemorrhages and some tumours). In some cases, it was difficult for radiologists to evaluate relevance of images from the results page view alone, so confirmation of similarity was sought in report texts and additional images in the studies found. The software showed up to five images for a study on its results page, so in a few cases the first 10 images represented only two studies in all. The precision at 10 calculated for image search was 39%. Nevertheless, SeeMIK offered at least one relevant study in 93% of image-search attempts.

After the tests, it was noted that one radiologist had accidentally skipped a task in the image relevance test, so only 15 results were gathered in total, rather than the expected 16. When checking the relevance markings collected for analysis after the image-search test, it was noticed that the test users had made a few incorrect markings: indicating relevant images to be irrelevant and vice versa. Occasionally, the image part selected for a search was not the targeted main finding of the study, because the exact finding to search for was not specified in the tasks for the participants.

One of the ideas behind the free-search task was that radiologists could 'play with' the search engine and explore it, but it seemed that the participants were very confused and did not know how to start doing so. With a little guidance by the observers, the radiologists tried advanced-search mode and combined-search by using images and text. Both search modes demonstrated good relevance in a few cases tested because the queries were more specific and accurate.

Because the tests began with relevance testing, a few usability issues, such as inadequate visual assistance and unclear behaviour of the user interface controls, were detected at the very outset. All tasks in the usability testing were completed successfully, but during a couple of them, unclear wording in the test guides prompted the radiologists to demand some assistance from the observers. The usability scores from the questionnaires were at a reasonable level: the SUS questionnaire score in both cases was 77.5 out of 100 points, which can be interpreted as showing 'good' usability according to 'SUS: A Retrospective' [19]. In the interviews, both radiologists raised some minor issues with the user interface and also mentioned a few features they would like to see in the DICOM viewer for reporting, such as multiplanar reconstruction (MPR) and support for several layouts of the working area. However, no serious bugs or stability issues were commented. Both radiologists reported a large number of irrelevant images in some cases, but still they thought the software to have good usability. The search process took time, but neither of the participating radiologists found this to be an issue. As most positive aspects of SeeMIK, the users identified ease of use and that the software is 'a good tool also for general learning'.

In the usefulness testing, one radiologist reported on four studies, the other on three. The reports they created were checked by an experienced radiologist and compared to the original ones made at the hospital. The reports created with the assisting software were deemed of good quality in their description of the pathology and in their diagnostic assessment. There were some minor errors such as missing a finding or incorrectly interpreting a finding, but these had only minor effect on the quality of the report overall. One study report created was more correct than the original report, but for another study, the original report was more correct than that created during test.

The opinions of radiologists collected via the USE questionnaire and interviews were assessed. Analysis showed generally positive results from the questionnaire: the median was six on the seven-point Likert-type scale for both radiologists. The statements receiving extreme responses were 'It is useful' (7), 'It makes the things I want to accomplish easier to get done' (7), and 'I can use it successfully every time' (3). Both radiologists considered the example cases to suit the testing purposes well: the studies consisted of single findings with a clear place to focus but were still such that junior radiologists without help of the software would have routinely consulted a more experienced radiologist for aid and going through the study together. The software was perceived as useful. The less experienced of the radiologists stated that the solution developed could be a good aid because it offers a reliable, quick, and easy way to compare and verify images. It was described as very interesting for students because information can be searched for in many ways. Especially with unfamiliar findings, it led the participants on the right track. Image search found at least some images for which the findings were suitable, and then it was possible to continue with word search or combined search.

Discussion

Many aspects of the assisting software were evaluated directly or indirectly during the testing process, and it yielded experience and knowledge that were highly useful for larger-scale testing scenario design. The testing functioned well as a preliminary step, as it revealed weaknesses in the test set-up and the guidance given to the participating radiologists. In addition, it highlighted a few usability issues that should be resolved before larger-scale testing begins. The DICOM viewer used as the user interface had limited functionality in comparison to the software usually used in clinical work, but the participants considered it, for the most part, adequate for the search function.

The relevance test guidance should be extended

The results of relevance testing revealed that judgement of relevance differed slightly between radiologists and the developers of the software. The initial assumption was that conception of relevance would be intuitive for a radiologist, so it was not described in the testing guides. The test results showed, in contrast, that the concept of relevance should be clearly and precisely defined, lest radiologists employ different interpretations, which could bias results related to search relevance. In addition, for image relevance testing, the testing radiologists should

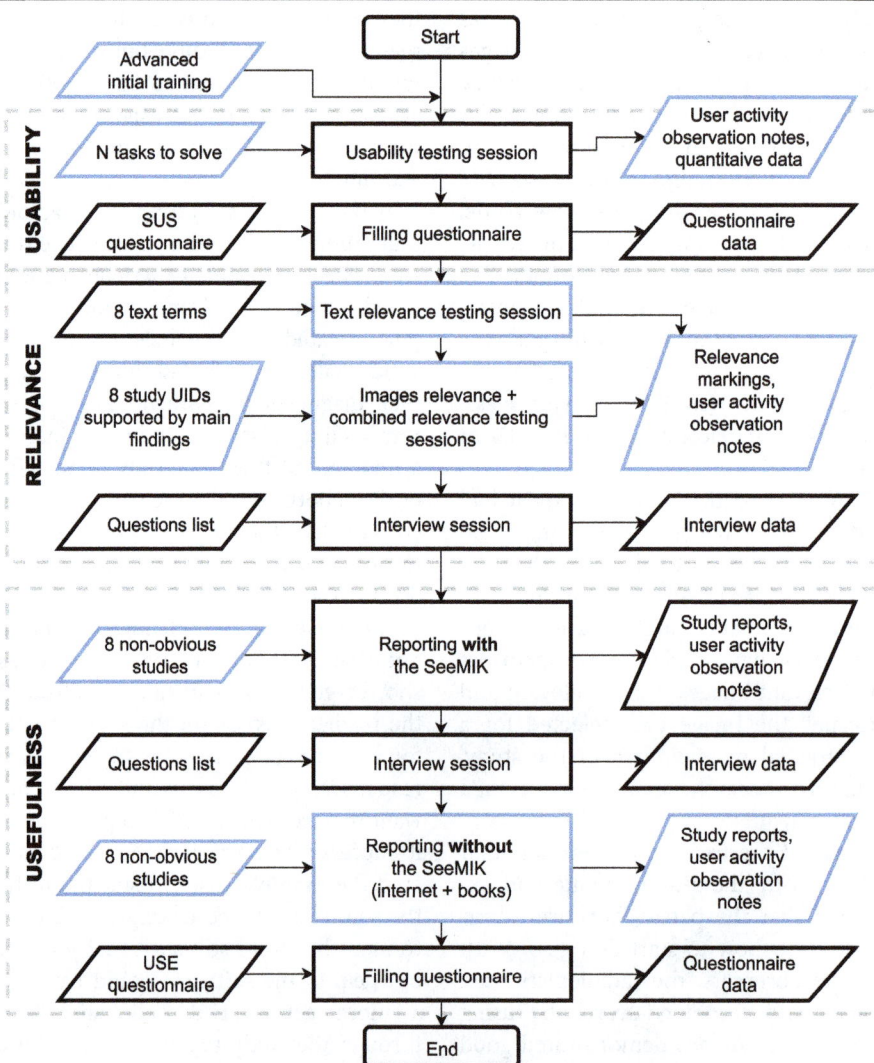

Fig. 6 The improved flow for pilot testing, with the changed steps highlighted

be supplied with the main finding of the study at hand, to make them select the targeted finding.

The relevance test assessment should be modified

The approach for calculating image-search results relevance should be changed. It became clear that, since the search engine grouped image results by study and showed up to five images related to a single study, marking only the first 10 images may result in incomplete assessment, because in some cases these images represent only two studies. Therefore, it was concluded that, while suitable for studies, calculating the 'precision at 10' metric would not be applicable for images in further tests.

The initial training and testing conditions should be rethought

A need was identified by observing user behaviour and issues such as accidental task-skipping in the preliminary testing: better and longer initial training could leave participants more confident in what is expected from them and, hence, both less nervous and more attentive. At the same time, the accuracy of task performance should be managed better by the observers during the tests, with assistance given as needed.

Usability testing should be rearranged

The usability testing should be scheduled as the first test, for capturing the first hands-on experience of users. In this case, it may also serve to shape the attitude of participants better, since the tasks are relatively easy and should not impose an excessive cognitive burden. Additionally, the usability testing tasks should be refined such that they are clearer and more natural for the participating radiologists.

Free-search task should be replaced

The free-search task proved confusing, so it is probably better to use combined-search testing instead. This can be designed as a continuation or further refinement of the image-search task wherein text terms supplement the image-search queries after evaluation of purely image-based results.

Text-search relevance can be improved via changes in software functioning

The software should search only the report text by default. Thereby, the questions in the anamnesis are excluded from the results and more relevant results are provided. Also, filtering out of negation should be improved by defining and adding new filtering rules.

Conclusions

Finally, the results of the tests performed show that the test plan designed is useful and that it should be possible to answer the main research questions after testing of the software with more radiologists. Useful qualitative data and opinions of prospective users were collected. Moreover, the assumption was validated that even junior radiologists can report on non-obvious cases with the aid of the assisting software. The tests performed enabled improvements to the test conditions and materials (see Fig. 6) and preparation of a more mature version of SeeMIK, for testing with a larger user group. It seems clear that when one's test plan cannot be evaluated with all planned conditions (a large enough group of users, the final test materials, sufficient data samples, etc.), simplifying or scaling down the original scenario and performing a test on its basis is still worthwhile. Moreover, with such tests it is possible to provide motivation for further development and gather new ideas and proposals from real users.

Abbreviations

BoVW: Bag of visual words; CBIR: Content-based image retrieval; CT: Computed tomography; DICOM: Digital imaging and communications in medicine; MPR: Multiplanar reconstruction; PACS: Picture archiving and communication system; RIS: Radiological information system; SUS: System usability scale (questionnaire).; USE: Usefulness, satisfaction, and ease of use (questionnaire).

Acknowledgements

Not applicable.

Funding

The entire CARDS project was funded by Tekes – the Finnish Funding Agency for Innovation, decision number 2490/31/2014. The funding body have not influenced in any way the design of the study, collection, analysis, and interpretation of data and the manuscript writing.

Authors' contributions

MP, MN, KK and GM participated in preparation of the testing, collection, analysis and interpretation of the results. All authors participated in the manuscript preparation, read, and approved the final manuscript.

Consent for publication

Not applicable.

Competing interests

The authors declare that they have no competing interests.

Author details
[1]Optoelectronics and Measurement Techniques Unit, University of Oulu, PO Box 4500, 90014 Oulu, Finland. [2]Department of Radiology, Oulu University Hospital, PO Box 50, 90029 Oulu, Finland. [3]Department of Radiology, Lapland Hospital District, PO Box 8041, 96101 Rovaniemi, Finland. [4]Medical Imaging Centre of Southwest Finland, Turku University Hospital, PO Box 52, 20521 Turku, Finland. [5]Finntelemedicum, Research Unit of Medical Imaging, Physics and Technology, University of Oulu; Department of Radiology, Hospital of Raahe, PL 25, 92101 Raahe, Finland.

References

1. Akgül CB, Rubin DL, Napel S, Beaulieu CF, Greenspan H, Acar B. Content-based image retrieval in radiology: current status and future directions. J Digit Imaging. 2011; doi:10.1007/s10278-010-9290-9.

2. Aisen AM, Broderick LS, Winer-Muram H, Brodley CE, Kak AC, Pavlopoulou C, Dy J, Shyu CR, Marchiori A. Automated storage and retrieval of thin-section CT images to assist diagnosis: system description and preliminary assessment. Radiology. 2003; doi:10.1148/radiol.2281020126.

3. Moltz JH, D'Anastasi M, Kiessling A, Pinto dos Santos D, Schülke C, Peitgen HO. Workflow-centred evaluation of an automatic lesion tracking software for chemotherapy monitoring by CT. Eur Radiol. 2012; doi:10.1007/s00330-012-2545-8.

4. de Oliveira JE, Machado AM, Chavez GC, Lopes AP, Deserno TM, Araújo Ade A. MammoSys: a content-based image retrieval system using breast density patterns. Comput Methods Prog Biomed. 2010; doi:10.1016/j.cmpb.2010.01.005.

5. Cho HC, Hadjiiski L, Sahiner B, Chan HP, Helvie M, Paramagul C, Nees AV. Similarity evaluation in a content-based image retrieval (CBIR) CADx system for characterization of breast masses on ultrasound images. Med Phys. 2011; doi:10.1118/1.3560877.

6. Hsu W, Antani S, Long LR, Neve L, Thoma GRSPIRS, Web-based A. Image retrieval system for large biomedical databases. Int J Med Inform. 2009; 78(Suppl. 1):S13–24. doi:10.1016/j.ijmedinf.2008.09.006.

7. Avni U, Greenspan H, Konen E, Sharon M, Goldberger J. X-ray categorization and retrieval on the organ and pathology level, using patch-based visual words. IEEE Trans Med Imaging. 2011; doi:10.1109/TMI.2010.2095026.

8. Geldermann I, Grouls C, Kuhl C, Deserno TM, Spreckelsen C. Black box integration of computer-aided diagnosis into PACS deserves a second chance: results of a usability study concerning bone age assessment. J Digit Imaging. 2013; doi:10.1007/s10278-013-9590-y.

9. Kumar A, Kim J, Bi L, Fulham M, Feng D. Designing user interfaces to enhance human interpretation of medical content-based image retrieval: application to PET-CT images. Int J Comput Assist Radiol Surg. 2013; doi:10.1007/s11548-013-0896-5.

10. Mourão A, Martins F, Magalhães J. Multimodal medical information retrieval with unsupervised rank fusion. Comput Med Imaging Graph. 2014; doi:10.1016/j.compmedimag.2014.05.006.

11. Markonis D, Holzer M, Baroz F, De Castaneda RLR, Boyer C, Langs G, Müller H. User-oriented evaluation of a medical image retrieval system for radiologists. Int J Med Inform. 2015; doi:10.1016/j.ijmedinf.2015.04.003.

12. Ballerini L, Li X, Fisher RB, Rees JA. Query-by-example content-based image retrieval system of non-melanoma skin lesions. Medical content-based retrieval for clinical decision support 2009. Lect Notes Comput Sci. 2010; 5853:31–8.

13. Shyr C, Kushniruk A, Wasserman WW. Usability study of clinical exome analysis software: top lessons learned and recommendations. J Biomed Inform. 2014; doi:10.1016/j.jbi.2014.05.004.

14. Martynov P, Mitropolskii N, Kukkola K, Mutanen L, Reponen J, Mäkynen A. CARDS: The decision support tool for radiologists examining head CT images. ECR 2016 / B-0233. 2016; doi:10.1594/ecr2016/B-0233.

15. Sivic J, Zisserman A. Video Google: a text retrieval approach to object matching in videos. International Conference on Computer Vision. 2003;2:1470–7.

16. Lux M, Marques O. Visual information retrieval using java and LIRE. Synthesis Lectures on Information Concepts, Retrieval, and Services. 2013;5(1) doi:10.2200/S00468ED1V01Y201301ICR025.

17. Brooke JSUS. A 'quick and dirty' usability scale. In: Jordan PW, Thomas B, Weerdmeester BA, McClelland AL, editors. Usability evaluation in industry. London: Taylor & Francis; 1996. p. 189–94.

18. Lund AM. Measuring usability with the USE questionnaire. STC SIG newsletter, usability. Interface. 2001;8(2):3–6.

19. Brooke JSUS. A retrospective. J Usability Stud. 2013;8(2):29–40.

14

Development of an algorithm to automatically compress a CT image to visually lossless threshold

Chang-Mo Nam[1], Kyong Joon Lee[1], Yousun Ko[1], Kil Joong Kim[1], Bohyoung Kim[2] and Kyoung Ho Lee[1*]

Abstract

Background: To develop an algorithm to predict the visually lossless thresholds (VLTs) of CT images solely using the original images by exploiting the image features and DICOM header information for JPEG2000 compression and to evaluate the algorithm in comparison with pre-existing image fidelity metrics.

Methods: Five radiologists independently determined the VLT for 206 body CT images for JPEG2000 compression using QUEST procedure. The images were divided into training ($n = 103$) and testing ($n = 103$) sets. Using the training set, a multiple linear regression (MLR) model was constructed regarding the image features and DICOM header information as independent variables and regarding the VLTs determined with median value of the radiologists' responses (VLT_{rad}) as dependent variable, after determining an optimal subset of independent variables by backward stepwise selection in a cross-validation scheme.

The performance was evaluated on the testing set by measuring absolute differences and intra-class correlation (ICC) coefficient between the VLT_{rad} and the VLTs predicted by the model (VLT_{model}). The performance of the model was also compared two metrics, peak signal-to-noise ratio (PSNR) and high-dynamic range visual difference predictor (HDRVDP). The time for computing VLTs between MLR model, PSNR, and HDRVDP were compared using the repeated ANOVA with a post-hoc analysis. $P < 0.05$ was considered to indicate a statistically significant difference.

Results: The means of absolute differences with the VLT_{rad} were 0.58 (95% CI, 0.48, 0.67), 0.73 (0.61, 0.85), and 0.68 (0.58, 0.79), for the MLR model, PSNR, and HDRVDP, respectively, showing significant difference between them ($p < 0.01$). The ICC coefficients of MLR model, PSNR, and HDRVDP were 0.88 (95% CI, 0.81, 0.95), 0.85 (0.79, 0.91), and 0.84 (0.77, 0.91). The computing times for calculating VLT per image were 1.5 ± 0.1 s, 3.9 ± 0.3 s, and 68.2 ± 1.4 s, for MLR metric, PSNR, and HDRVDP, respectively.

Conclusions: The proposed MLR model directly predicting the VLT of a given CT image showed competitive performance to those of image fidelity metrics with less computational expenses. The model would be promising to be used for adaptive compression of CT images.

Keywords: Visually lossless threshold, CT compression, DICOM header

* Correspondence: kholeemail@gmail.com
[1]Department of Radiology, Seoul National University Bundang Hospital, Seoul National University College of Medicine, 82 Gumi-ro 173 Beon-gil, Bundang-gu, Seongnam-si, Gyeonggi-do 13620, Korea
Full list of author information is available at the end of the article

Background

Although the cost of storage and network resources have continued to drop, there is still a demand for irreversible compression of computed tomography (CT) images for long-term preservation and efficient transmission of data, especially between institutions at the regional or national level [1–4]. However, the irreversible compression is not always accepted by radiologists due to concern about compression artifacts that might hinder diagnosis. Therefore, the importance of achieving an optimal compression level for a CT image, which provides the maximum data reduction while preserving the diagnostic accuracy, has gained the attention of radiologists [5].

Regarding the estimation of such optimal compression level, many researchers have advocated that visually lossless threshold (VLT) is robust and conservative sufficiently to be adopted for the compression of medical images [6–11]. This approach focuses on image fidelity (i.e. the visual equivalence between the original and compressed images). The underlying idea of this approach is that if a compressed image is visually indistinguishable from its original, the artifacts should not affect the diagnosis.

However, because the compressibility of an image is affected by various factors including body parts, scanning protocols, and image contents itself, the establishment of a robust VLT for various images would require a very large study [12, 13]. Instead, if a computerized algorithm can accurately predict visual perception of radiologists, it can be used for compressing a CT image adaptively and automatically to its own VLT. For that purpose, several researchers have experimented with using image fidelity metrics, which measure the fidelity of a distorted image, in predicting the VLT, and some of the metrics showed promising results [5, 14–18]. However, to achieve the VLT of a given CT image, it is necessary to iteratively compress the image to multiple compression levels and to measure the image fidelity at each compression level until the measured fidelity reaches a cutoff value predefined by the metric.

It has been advocated that some of the factors influencing the compressibility of CT images can be derived directly from the Digital Imaging and Communications in Medicine (DICOM) header information [19, 20], especially related to the image noise which is known as an important factor affecting the compressibility of CT images as well as from image contents themselves [21–25]. Thereby, it is plausible to hypothesize that the VLTs of CT images can be predicted by using those DICOM header information and image features derived from the original images.

This study aimed to develop a computerized algorithm to predict the VLTs of CT images solely using the original images by exploiting the image features and DICOM header information for Joint Photographic Experts Group 2000 (JPEG2000) compression and to evaluate the performance of the algorithm in comparison with pre-existing image fidelity metrics.

Methods

Our institutional review board approved this study and waived informed patient consent. The study design was described in Fig. 1.

A. Image acquisition and selection

A body radiologist with 13 years of clinical experience, who did not participate in the human visual analysis, retrospectively reviewed CT scans of adults which were obtained from 256-channel or 64-channel multi-detector row CT scanners (Brilliance; Philips Medical Systems, Cleveland, OH) in Seoul National University Bundang Hospital in early 2012. He compiled 206 studies (84 abdomen scans, 82 chest scans obtained by using our standard radiation dose, and 40 low-dose chest scans; 79 scans from 256-channel scanners and 127 scans from 64-channel scanners) containing common abnormalities.

Of the 84 abdomen scans, 42 scans were randomly selected and then reconstructed into 4-mm-thick transverse sections and the remaining 42 scans were reconstructed into 2-mm-thick sections. Likewise, 41 of the 82 standard-dose chest scans were reconstructed into 3-mm-thick sections and the remaining 41 scans were reconstructed into 2-mm-thick sections. The 40 low-dose chest scans were reconstructed into 3-mm-thick sections. From each reconstructed image dataset, the same radiologist selected a single section that most clearly represented pathology. Therefore, the final study sample was a set of 206 images, which was composed of five subsets of different body regions (i.e., abdomen or chest) and image noise levels (i.e., different section thicknesses and radiation doses): 4-mm-thick abdomen images (abdomen thick), 2-mm-thick abdomen images (abdomen thin), 3-mm-thick lung images (chest thick), 2-mm-thick chest images (chest thin), and 3-mm-thick low-dose chest CT images (low-dose chest).

Among various clinical CT protocols, we focused on these five CT protocols because they are performed very frequently in daily practice of our hospital and thus cover a large portion of the image archive. The scan parameters and patient demographics for each subset are tabulated in Table 1. All scan parameters followed the clinical scan protocols of our hospital. Also, using the five different subsets was to introduce heterogeneity in the test dataset to some extent in terms of structural content and image noise. The heterogeneity was considered important in measuring the robustness of the prediction model in predicting the VLTs of CT images, as it is well known that the image compressibility is

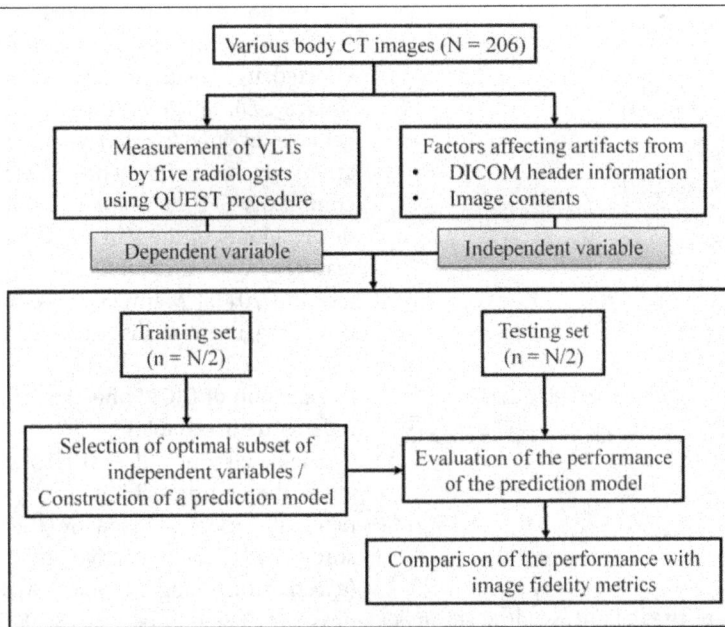

Fig. 1 Study design. *Independent variables include five image features (image standard deviation, image entropy, relative percentage of low frequency energy, variation in high frequency, and visual complexity) and DICOM header information (effective mAs, field of view, section thickness, and reconstruction filter). DICOM: digital imaging and communications in medicine; VLT: visually lossless threshold

significantly affected by structural content [17, 26] and image noise level [12, 13].

B. VLT measurement by radiologists using QUEST procedure

Five radiologists with 10, 9, 7, 6, and 4 years of clinical experience, respectively, participated in the VLT measurement. The 206 images were randomly assigned to five reading sessions. The order of the reading sessions was changed for each reader. Sessions were separated by a minimum of 24 h to minimize reader fatigue.

Images were displayed in a monochrome monitor calibrated according to the Digital Imaging and Communications in Medicine part 14 grayscale standard display function [26]. Detailed specifications of the display system and viewing condition were described in Table 2. The window level and width were set as 20 and 400 HU for abdomen CT images and as –600 and 1500 HU for

Table 1 CT imaging parameters and patient demographics

	Subsets				
	Abdomen thick	Abdomen thin	Chest thick	Chest thin	Low-dose chest
Common scan parameters	Detector collimation, 64 × 0.625 mm for 64-channel MDCT and 2 × 128 × 0.625 mm for 256-channel MDCT; gantry rotation time, 0.42 s for 64-channel MDCT and 0.27 s for 256-channel MDCT; tube potential, 120 kVp; pitch, 1.077 to 1.172; matrix, 512 × 512				
Body part	Abdomen	Abdomen	Chest	Chest	Chest
Field of view[ab]	277.2 ± 20.7 (245–323)	281.0 ± 23.5 (249–321)	319.0 ± 27.1 (262–383)	317.9 ± 26.5 (271–375)	291.5 ± 22.9 (248–329)
Section thickness (mm)	4	2	3	2	3
Effective mAs[ac]	121.5 ± 38.0 (69–222)	127.5 ± 34.2 (62–191)	152.3 ± 45.1 (58–249)	151.1 ± 30.5 (72–181)	25.6 ± 2.3 (22–31)
Effective radiation Dose (mSv)[ad]	7.5 ± 1.0 (4.5–9.8)	7.5 ± 1.5 (4.1–10.2)	7.2 ± 1.1 (4.3–9.5)	7.3 ± 0.9 (4.1–9.3)	1.6 ± 0.1 (1.4–1.7)
Reconstruction filter	Soft-tissue	Soft-tissue	Medium-sharp	Medium-sharp	Medium-sharp
Age[a]	57.2 ± 27.2 (15–88)	55.3 ± 24.8 (15:82)	50.6 ± 26.4 (18–88)	53.1 ± 24.4 (22–91)	45.4 ± 22.4 (19–84)
Sex (Male:Female)	22:20	23:19	22:19	20:21	23:17

Note: [a]Data are means ± standard deviations, with ranges in parentheses. [b]The field of view was set for each patient to match the maximum transverse diameter of the body to the image size. [c]Automatic tube-current modulation was used. [d]Estimated by multiplying the dose-length product measured on the CT console by a conversion factor (0.017 and 0.019 mSv•mGy-1•cm-1 for abdomen and chest, respectively) [39]

Table 2 Display system and viewing conditions in human visual analysis

Display system	
Display resolution	1536 × 2048 pixels
Display size	31.8 × 42.3 cm
Image resolution	1483 × 1483 pixels (stretched using bilinear interpolation)
Luminance	1.5–408.2 cd/m²
Viewing conditions	
Ambient room light	30 lux
Reading distance	42–77 cm
Window setting	level, 20 HU; width, 400 HU for abdomen CT,
	level, −600 HU; width, 1500 HU for chest CT, not adjustable
Magnification	not allowed
Reading time	not constrained

lung CT images, which were the default window settings in our clinical practice.

The five readers independently measured the VLT of each image by visually comparing the image with its distorted versions compressed to various compression ratios (CRs) using the JPEG2000 algorithm (Accusoft-Pegasus Imaging, Tampa, Fla) [27–30]. The VLT of each image was determined through 25 comparison trials. In each trial, the image pair of the original and compressed version was alternately displayed on a single monitor. The reader selectively toggled between the two images (returning to the first image as desired) and was forced to answer if they are distinguishable or not. Based on the reader's response, the QUEST algorithm [31] calculated the CR for the next trial. The CR for the initial trial was 5:1. Details of the QUEST were described in elsewhere [31].

Prior to the formal visual analysis, the readers were instructed on how to perform the visual analysis with five example images which were not included in the test dataset. The readers also had a chance to perform the analysis with another three example image pairs by themselves so that they could become familiar with the visual analysis.

Although we selected images containing abnormalities, the readers were asked not to confine their visual analysis to the pathologies. Instead, the readers were asked to examine an entire image to find any image differences. When analyzing the abdomen CT images, the readers were asked to focus particularly on the small vessels and edges of the organs and the texture of solid organs and soft tissues. For the chest CT images, the readers were asked to focus on the small airways, pulmonary vessels, interlobular septa, interlobar fissures, and the texture of the pulmonary parenchyma.

C. Selection of image features as independent variables

As inspired from the literature and our observations, we selected five image features of image standard deviation (*Image_SD*), image entropy (*Image_entropy*), relative percentage of low frequency energy (*Percentage_LF*), variation in high frequency (*Variation_HF*), and visual complexity (*Visual_complexity*) as the candidates for the determinants of the VLTs of CT images. Those five image features were measured for each image using Matlab (version 2011a, Mathworks, Nattick, Mass). The detail of those image features is described elsewhere [25].

D. Selection of DICOM header information as independent variables

We selected four DICOM tags which were considered to affect the compressibility as the candidates for the independent variables based on the results of the previous study: [19] the effective tube current-time product (*effective mAs*; tag number: 0018, 9332); section thickness (*ST*; tag number: 0018, 0050); field of view (*FOV*; tag number: 0018, 0090), and reconstruction filter type (tag number: 0018, 9320).

E. Construction of the VLT prediction model

To construct and validate a prediction model, we applied an analysis scheme widely used in the machine learning field [32]. The 206 images were divided randomly into two groups: 103 images for the training set and 103 images for the testing set. With the training set, an optimal subset of independent variables was determined using multiple linear regression (MLR) by performing backward stepwise selection using the likelihood-ratio statistic ($p = 0.05$ for entry and $p = 0.10$ for removal) as a selection criterion [32]. At each step in the backward stepwise selection, four-fold cross-validation scheme was used.

With the determined subset of independent variables, a final model was constructed by fitting the MLR on the entire training set while regarding the VLTs determined with median value of the radiologists' responses (VLT_{rad}) as dependent variable. The constructed MLR model was then validated using the testing set. The detail of the validation is described in the subsequent statistical analysis section.

The time for computing the VLTs predicted by the model (VLT_{model}) was measured for each image. In this calculation, we included the time to load input files to the memory and to save output files to the storage. We used a PC platform running 64-bits Windows 7 (Microsoft Co., Redmond, WA) with a 3.2 GHz quad-core processor (i7-3930 k; Intel Co., Santa Clara, CA) and 32 GB main memory.

F. Image fidelity metrics

To compare the performance of the prediction model with those of the pre-existing image fidelity metrics, we tested two metrics, peak signal-to-noise ratio (PSNR) [15] and high-dynamic range visual difference predictor (HDRVDP) [33]. These metrics have been widely tested in predicting radiologists' perception of compression artifacts in CT images [5, 14–17, 34]. The detail of the metrics is described in Appendix.

Each of the two metrics takes two images (original and distorted images) as input and calculates the degree of the fidelity of the distorted image. Thereby, to calculate the VLT of a CT image using the metrics, it is necessary to iteratively compress and measure the image fidelity for multiple CRs until the measured fidelity reaches a cutoff value predefined by the metric.

The cutoff value of each of the metrics was determined using the training set as follows. First, each image on the training set was compressed to its VLT_{rad}. Second, the metric value was calculated for each pair of the original image and compressed image to VLT_{rad}. Note that if a metric is completely accurate in predicting the VLT_{rad}, then the metric outputs for the VLT_{rad}-compressed images should be a constant value. The cutoff value was defined as the mean of the metric values for the entire training set ($N = 103$) to minimize the deviation between the cutoff value and metric values.

The VLTs of each image using PSNR or HRDVDP ($VLT_{(PSNR\ or\ HDRVDP)}$) on the testing set was calculated with the metrics' own cutoff values using the iteration scheme. The times for computing the $VLT_{(PSNR\ or\ HDRVDP)}$ were measured for each image.

G. Statistical analysis

The sample size of 206 images (103 images for training set and 103 images for testing set) was determined to provide narrow two-sided 95% confidence intervals (CIs) for the absolute difference between VLT_{rad} and VLT_{MLR} ($|VLT_{rad-MLR}|$) as follows. First, to measure the standard deviation (SD) of $|VLT_{rad-MLR}|$, we conducted a preliminary test with 100 images. The 100 images were repeatedly divided (200 times) randomly into two sets, a training (50 images) and testing (50 images) data sets. For each division, an MLR model was constructed on the training and $|VLT_{rad-MLR}|$ was measured on the testing set. The mean of SD of the 200 $|VLT_{rad-MLR}|$ was 0.51. With this SD, the sample size of a testing set was estimated to be 103 to construct a 95% CI of $|VLT_{rad-MLR}|$ with the width of no greater than 0.10. In addition to the testing set, a separate sample of the same size was required for the training set ($n = 103$).

Interobserver agreement between the five readers was evaluated by measuring the ICC coefficient. Using the testing set, the performance of each of the MLR model and the two metrics was evaluated by measuring ICC coefficient, and bland-Altman plot between $VLT_{radiologist}$, and $VLT_{(MLR\ model,\ PSNR,\ or\ HDRVDP)}$. The difference between $|VLT_{rad-model}|$, $|VLT_{rad-PSNR}|$, and $|VLT_{rad-HDRVDP}|$ were compared using the repeated measures analysis of variance (ANOVA) with a post-hoc analysis. The time for computing VLTs between MLR model, PSNR, and HDRVDP were compared using the repeated ANOVA with a post-hoc analysis. $P < 0.05$ was considered to indicate a statistically significant difference.

Results
A. VLT measured by radiologists
The ICC coefficient between the five readers was 0.56 (95% CI, 0.53, 0.57; $p < 0.01$). The VLTs varied with different subsets, especially different section thicknesses (Fig. 2). The VLT_{rad} of thick sections were significantly higher than those of thin sections for both of abdomen (thick vs. thin, 7.3 ± 0.5 vs. 6.3 ± 0.4; $p < 0.01$) and chest (9.2 ± 1.1 vs. 7.1 ± 1.3; $p < 0.01$). The VLTs of chest thick sections were significantly higher than those of low-dose chest images (9.2 ± 1.1 vs. 7.5 ± 1.4; $p < 0.01$).

B. Optimal variable selection
According to the results of backward stepwise selection, the ST, effective mAs, and reconstruction filter among the DICOM tags and Visual_complexity, and Variation_HF among the image features were determined as the optimal subset of independent variables while the remaining variables were excluded.

C. Performance of MLR model, PSNR, and HDR-VDP (Figs. 3 and 4)
The means of $|VLT_{rad-MLR}|$, $|VLT_{rad-PSNR}|$, and $|VLT_{rad-HDRVDP}|$ were 0.58 (95% CI, 0.48, 0.67), 0.73 (0.61, 0.85), and 0.68 (0.58, 0.79), respectively, showing significant difference between them ($p < 0.01$). According to the

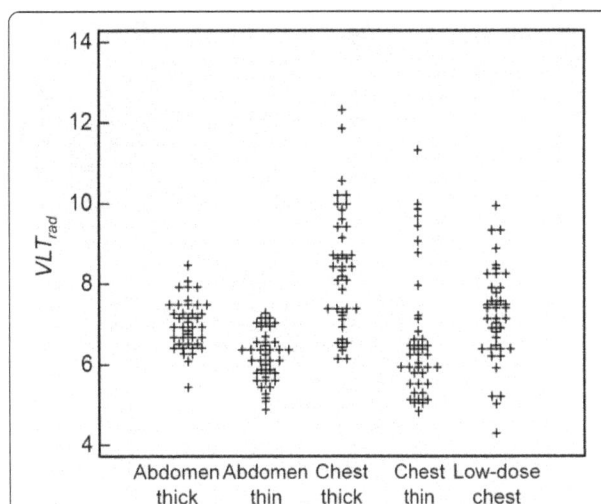

Fig. 2 Scatter plot of the radiologists' pooled responses. The VLT_{rad} represents the visually lossless thresholds determined with median value of the five radiologists' responses for each image

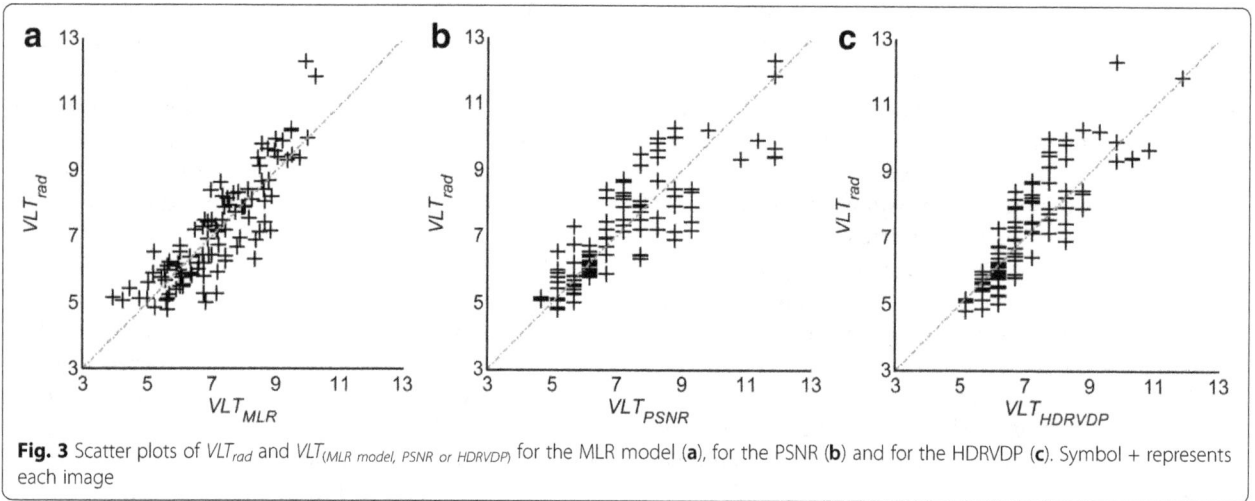

Fig. 3 Scatter plots of VLT_{rad} and $VLT_{(MLR\ model,\ PSNR\ or\ HDRVDP)}$ for the MLR model (**a**), for the PSNR (**b**) and for the HDRVDP (**c**). Symbol + represents each image

post-hoc analysis, the significant difference was shown between $|VLT_{rad\text{-}MLR}|$ and $|VLT_{rad\text{-}PSNR}|$. The ICC coefficients of MLR model, PSNR, and HDRVDP were 0.88 (95% CI, 0.81, 0.95), 0.84 (0.77, 0.91), and 0.85 (0.79, 0.91). The Bland-Altman plot demonstrates the discrepancy between VLT_{rad} and $VLT_{(MLR\ model,\ PSNR,\ or\ HDRVDP)}$ with a mean difference (bias) and a 95% confidence limit of agreement (Fig. 5).

D. Computing time of image features

The mean computing times for calculating VLT per image were 1.5 ± 0.1 s, 3.9 ± 0.3 s, and 68.2 ± 1.4 s, for MLR metric, PSNR, and HDRVDP, respectively. The differences between them were significant ($p < 0.01$).

Discussion

In this study, we proposed a MLR model which predicts the VLT of JPEG2000 compressed CT images using the image features and DICOM header information. The mean of absolute difference between the VLTs measured by radiologists and the VLTs calculated by the MLR model was 0.58. The ICC coefficient of the VLTs measured by radiologists and the VLTs calculated by the MLR model was 0.88. The proposed model showed superior or comparable performance to those of the PSNR and HDRVDP while requiring less computational expenses. Our model utilized "*visually lossless*" compression, and does not interfere with a doctor's diagnosis. Human visual system cannot find the difference between the original image and the compressed image resulting from the model. In clinical applications, it is crucial to compute the optimal VLT value to keep the quality of the compressed image that does not degrade the diagnostic value in any case. Therefore, the proposed model would be promising to be used for adaptive compression of CT images.

According to our results, among the DICOM header tags, the *ST, effective mAs*, and *reconstruction filter*

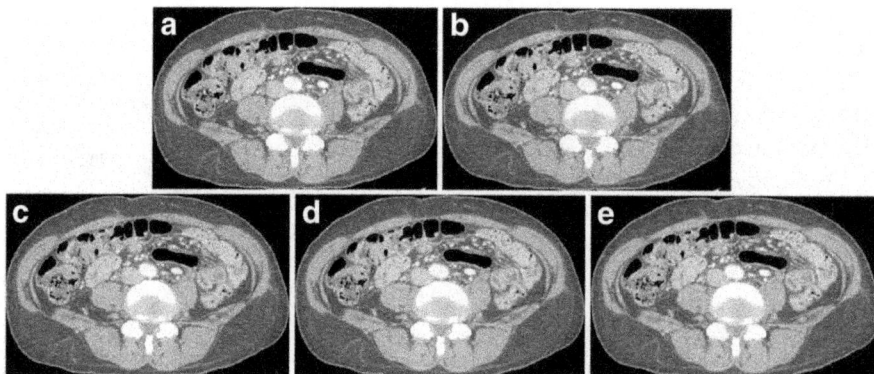

Fig. 4 JPEG 2000 compressed CT images in transverse abdominal view of a 78-year-old female. (**a**) the original image. (**b**) the compressed image by a radiologist. (compression ratio 8.6:1.) The compressed images using (**c**) the MLR model (8.8,1), (**d**) the PSNR (9.5,1), and (**e**) the HDRVDP (9.3,1) respectively. Window width and level are set to 400 and 20 HU. Since the images are generated by visually lossless compression methods, all the images are indistinguishable from the original image

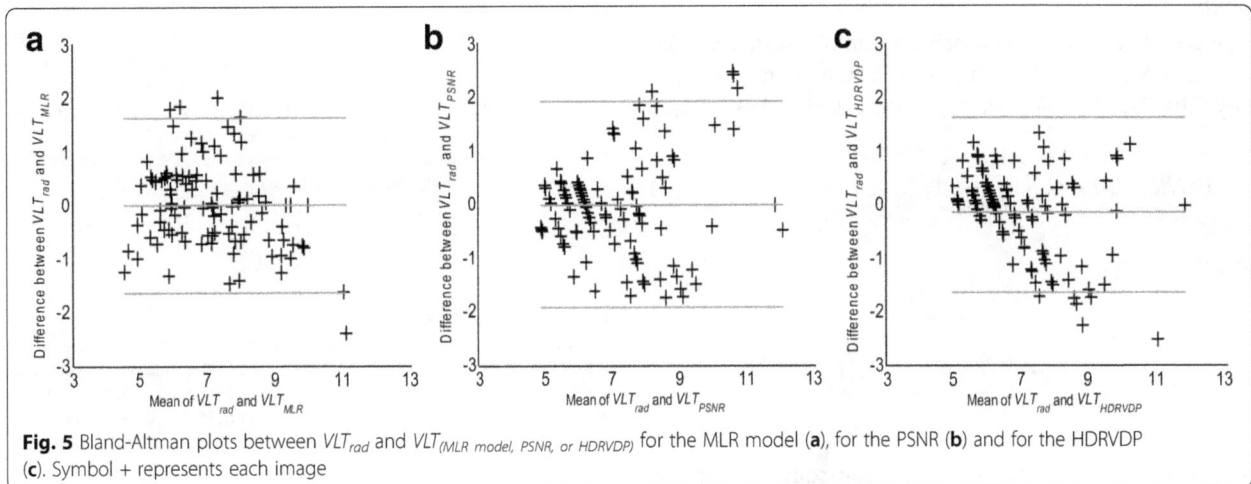

Fig. 5 Bland-Altman plots between VLT_{rad} and $VLT_{(MLR\ model,\ PSNR,\ or\ HDRVDP)}$ for the MLR model (**a**), for the PSNR (**b**) and for the HDRVDP (**c**). Symbol + represents each image

played an important role in predicting the VLT of CT images. These results were expected since those DICOM tags are theoretically related to image noise and thus to the degree of compression artifacts. In addition, the image features of *Variation_HF* and *Visual_complexity* are also shown as factors predicting the VLT of CT images, which are devised by being inspired from the previous research on the modeling of human visual system (HVS) [25]. Note that there might exist other HVS-related image features which outperform those two image features.

Previous studies [5, 14–18] evaluated several image fidelity metrics, such as PSNR and HDRVDP in measuring the fidelity of compressed CT images. The principal goal of these studies was to introduce the image fidelity metrics into an adaptive compression. However, those metrics have a couple of limitations from a practical viewpoint. First, they analyze the image characteristics of a compressed image in comparison to its original, requiring a substantial computational expense. Second, to achieve an optimal compression level for an image, it is necessary to iteratively compress the image to multiple compression levels and to measure the image fidelity at each compression level until the measured fidelity reaches a predefined threshold. In contrast, the prediction model proposed in this study can directly predict VLTs of CT images without the iterative compression and fidelity measurement at multiple CRs, thereby computationally efficient. In an academic medical center with 900-bed tertiary care, where this study is conducted, the total number of CT examinations from August 2011 to January 2012 is 43,854. The required time and computational power for compressing all the CT examinations in such a great scale is not trivial. Using inefficient compression models may increase the waiting time of patients, particularly for the model like HDRVDP which requires about 46 times more

computational cost comparing to our method. Furthermore, the models can probably induce unnecessary load on picture archiving and communication system (PACS) and gradually degenerate durability of the system.

Our model cannot be directly applied to clinical practice due to the following reasons: first, this study used a small number of test images; second, we did not test all available DICOM header information and image features. Furthermore, more sophisticated classification methods exist as an alternative to MLR, such as artificial neural network, support vector machine, and AdaBoost [32]. However, it should be noted that our study did not intend to suggest a prediction model which can serve as a global compression guideline for all CT images. Instead, the purpose of our study is rather to propose a new scheme of adaptive compression which directly predicts the VLT of a given CT image solely using the original image without compression.

Conclusion

In conclusion, we proposed a MLR model which directly predicts the VLT of a given CT image solely using the original image without compression. The proposed model showed superior or comparable performance to those of image fidelity metrics while requiring less computational expenses. The model would be promising to be used for adaptive compression of CT images.

Appendix
Description of image fidelity metrics

The PSNR and HDRVDP were performed after converting the 12-bit images to 8-bit images by applying the same window settings used in the human visual analysis. This conversion was to reproduce the clinical practice, in which images are displayed with an appropriate window setting.

PSNR

The PSNR [15] has been widely used in measuring the degree of image distortion due to its computational simplicity. The PSNR (in decibels [dB]) was calculated as follows:

$$PSNR = 20 \log_{10}\left(\frac{255}{RMSE}\right), \qquad (1)$$

Where

$$RMSE = \sqrt{\frac{\sum_{x=1}^{512}\sum_{y=1}^{512}(f(x,y)-g(x,y))^2}{512^2}}, \qquad (2)$$

and where RMSE stands for root-mean-square error and $f(x, y)$ and $g(x, y)$ are the pixel values in the original and compressed images, respectively.

HDRVDP

The HDRVDP, which is publicly available [33, 35], is an extension of Visual Difference Predictor [36], one of the most widely used perceptual metrics simulating individual components of the HVS. Because modern medical display systems are significantly brighter than general-purpose displays, the HDRVDP, which covers a wide range of luminance, is likely suitable for medical applications. The HDRVDP has been reported to accurately reproduce radiologists' perception of compression artifacts in CT images [5, 14–17, 37].

The HDRVDP takes two images as input and then outputs a probability-of-detection map in which the pixel value indicates the probability, ranging from 0 to 1, that an observer viewing the two images will detect the difference at that pixel location. The map was summarized into a single value representing the overall perceptual image fidelity using the Minkowski metric [38] as follows:

$$HDR\text{--}VDP = \left(\sum_u \sum_v \left\{p(u,v)^\beta\right\}\right)^{\frac{1}{\beta}}, \qquad (3)$$

where $p(u, v)$ is the probability-of-detection map. β was set to 2.4 according to the results of previous studies [18].

Abbreviations

ANOVA: Analysis of variance; CI: Confidence interval; CR: Compression ratio; CT: Computed tomography; DICOM: Digital imaging and communications in medicine; FOV: Field of view; HDRVDP: High-dynamic range visual difference predictor; HVS: Human visual system; ICC: Intra-class correlation; JPEG2000: Joint photographic experts group 2000; MLR: Multiple linear regression; PACS: Picture archiving and communication system; PSNR: Peak signal-to-noise ratio; SD: Standard deviation; ST: Section thickness; VLT: Visually lossless threshold

Acknowledgements
Not applicable.

Funding
This research was supported by grants of the Korean Health Technology R&D Project through the Korea Health Industry Development Institute (KHIDI), funded by the Ministry of Health & Welfare, Republic of Korea (No. HI13C0004 and HI15C1052), and Seoul National University Bundang Hospital Research Fund (No. 02-2012-056), and the Interdisciplinary Research Initiatives Program from College of Engineering and College of Medicine, Seoul National University (No. 800-20170169).

Authors' contributions
C-MN participated in the study design, data collection, statistical analysis, and drafted the manuscript. KJL and YK participated in the statistical analysis and drafted the manuscript. KJK and BK participated in the study design and were major contributors in writing the manuscript. KHL conceived and designed the study, supervised the project. All authors read and approved the final manuscript.

Consent for publication
Not applicable.

Competing interests
Kyoung Ho Lee received grants from the Korea Health Industry Development Institute (KHIDI), funded by the Ministry of Health & Welfare, Republic of Korea, and Seoul National University Bundang Hospital. Kyong Joon Lee received grants from Seoul National University. All other authors declare no competing interests.

Author details
[1]Department of Radiology, Seoul National University Bundang Hospital, Seoul National University College of Medicine, 82 Gumi-ro 173 Beon-gil, Bundang-gu, Seongnam-si, Gyeonggi-do 13620, Korea. [2]Division of Biomedical Engineering, Hankuk University of Foreign Studies, Oedae-ro 81, Mohyeon-myeon, Cheoin-gu, Yongin-si, Gyeonggi-do 17035, Korea.

References
1. Koff D, Bak P, Brownrigg P, Hosseinzadeh D, Khademi A, Kiss A, Lepanto L, Michalak T, Shulman H, Volkening A. Pan-Canadian evaluation of irreversible compression ratios ("Lossy" compression) for development of national guidelines. J Digit Imaging. 2009;22:569–78.
2. Lee KH, Kim YH, Kim BH, Kim KJ, Kim TJ, Kim HJ, Hahn S. Irreversible JPEG 2000 compression of abdominal CT for primary interpretation: assessment of visually lossless threshold. Eur Radiol. 2007;17:1529–34.
3. Lee KH, Lee HJ, Kim JH, Kang HS, Lee KW, Hong H, Chin HJ, Ha KS. Managing the CT data explosion: initial experiences of archiving volumetric datasets in a mini-PACS. J Digit Imaging. 2005;18:188–95.
4. Rubin GD. Data explosion: the challenge of multidetector-row CT. Eur J Radiol. 2000;36:74–80.
5. Kim KJ, Kim B, Lee KH, Mantiuk R, Kang HS, Seo J, Kim SY, Kim YH. Objective index of image fidelity for JPEG2000 compressed body CT images. Med Phys. 2009;36:3218–26.
6. Cosman PC, Davidson HC, Bergin CJ, Tseng CW, Moses LE, Riskin EA, Olshen RA, Gray RM. Thoracic CT Images: effect of lossy image compression on diagnostic accuracy. Radiology. 1994;190:517–24.

7. Goldberg MA, Gazelle GS, Boland GW, Hahn PF, Mayo-Smith WW, Pivovarov M, Halpern EF, Wittenberg J. Focal hepatic lesions: effect of three-dimensional wavelet compression on detection at CT. Radiology. 1997;202:159–65.

8. Ko JP, Chang J, Bomsztyk E, Babb JS, Naidich DP, Rusinek H. Effect of CT image compression on computer-assisted lung nodule volume measurement. Radiology. 2005;237:83–8.

9. Ko JP, Rusinek H, Naidich DP, McGuinness G, Rubinowitz AN, Leitman BS, Martino JM. Wavelet compression of low-dose chest CT data: effect on lung nodule detection. Radiology. 2003;228:70–5.

10. Ohgiya Y, Gokan T, Nobusawa H, Hirose M, Seino N, Fujisawa H, Baba M, Nagai K, Tanno K, Takeyama K, Munechika H. Acute cerebral infarction: effect of JPEG compression on detection at CT. Radiology. 2003;227:124–7.

11. Zalis ME, Hahn PF, Arellano RS, Gazelle GS, Mueller PR. CT colonography with teleradiology: effect of lossy wavelet compression on polyp detection-initial observations. Radiology. 2001;220:387–92.

12. Bajpai V, Lee KH, Kim B, Kim KJ, Kim TJ, Kim YH, Kang HS. The difference of compression artifacts between thin- and thick-section lung CT Images. Am J Roentgenol. 2008;191:38–43.

13. Woo HS, Kim KJ, Kim TJ, Hahn S, Kim BH, Kim YH, Yoon CJ, Lee KH. JPEG 2000 compression of abdominal CT: difference in compression tolerance between thin- and thick-section images. Am J Roentgenol. 2007;189:535–41.

14. Kim B, Lee KH, Kim KJ, Mantiuk R, Bajpai V, Kim TJ, Kim YH, Yoon CJ, Hahn S. Prediction of perceptible artifacts in JPEG2000 compressed abdomen CT images using a perceptual image quality metric. Acad Radiol. 2008;15:314–25.

15. Kim B, Lee KH, Kim KJ, Mantiuk R, Hahn S, Kim TJ, Kim YH. Prediction of perceptible artifacts in JPEG2000 compressed chest CT images using mathematical and perceptual quality metrics. Am J Roentgenol. 2008;190: 328–34.

16. Kim B, Lee KH, Kim KJ, Mantiuk R, Kim HR, Kim YH. Artifacts in slab average-intensity-projection images reformatted from JPEG 2000 compressed thin-section abdominal CT data sets. Am J Roentgenol. 2008;190:342–50.

17. Kim KJ, Kim B, Lee KH, Kim TJ, Mantiuk R, Kang HS, Kim YH. Regional difference in compression artifacts in low-dose chest CT images: effects of mathematical and perceptual factors. Am J Roentgenol. 2008;191:30–7.

18. Kim KJ, Kim B, Mantiuk R, Richter T, Lee H, Kang HS, Seo J, Lee KH. A comparison of three image fidelity metrics of different computational principles for JPEG2000 compressed abdomen CT images. IEEE Trans Med Imaging. 2010;29:1496–503.

19. Kim KJ, Kim B, Lee H, Choi H, Jeon JJ, Ahn JH, Lee KH. Predicting the fidelity of JPEG2000 compressed CT images using DICOM header information. Med Phys. 2011;38:6449.

20. Digital Imaging and Communications in Medicine (DICOM). Part 14: gray scale standard display function. medical.nema.org/dicom/2004/04_14pu.pdf. Accessed 1 June 2012.

21. Clunie DA, Mitchell PJ, Howieson J, Roman-Goldstein S, Szumowski J. Detection of discrete white matter lesions after irreversible compression of MR images. AJNR Am J Neuroradiol. 1995;16:1435–40.

22. Erickson BJ, Manduca A, Palisson P, Persons KR, Earnest FT, Savcenko V, Hangiandreou NJ. Wavelet compression of medical images. Radiology. 1998; 206:599–607.

23. Fidler A, Skaleric U, Likar B. The impact of image information on compressibility and degradation in medical image compression. Med Phys. 2006;33:2832–8.

24. Janhom A, van der Stelt P, van Ginkel F. Interaction between noise and file compression and its effect on the recognition of caries in digital imaging. Dentomaxillofac Radiol. 2000;29:20–7.

25. Kim KJ, Kim B, Lee KH, Mantiuk R, Richter T, Kang HS. Use of image features in predicting visually lossless thresholds of JPEG2000 compressed body CT images: initial trial. Radiology. 2013; in press

26. Kim TJ, Lee KW, Kim B, Kim KJ, Chun EJ, Bajpai V, Kim YH, Hahn S, Lee KH. Regional variance of visually lossless threshold in compressed chest CT images: lung versus mediastinum and chest wall. Eur J Radiol. 2008;69:483–8.

27. Antonini M, Barlaud M, Mathieu P, Daubechies I. Image coding using wavelet transform. IEEE Trans Image Processing. 1992;1:205–20.

28. Zeng W, Daly S. An overview of the visual optimization tools in JPEG 2000. Signal Process: Image Comm. 2002;17:85–104.

29. Liu Z, Karam LJ, Watson AB. JPEG2000 encoding with perceptual distortion control. IEEE Trans Image Processing. 2006;15:1763–78.

30. Tan D, Tan C, Wu H. Perceptual color image coding with JPEG2000. IEEE Trans Image Processing. 2010;19:374–83.

31. Macmillan NA. Threshold estimation: the state of the art. Attention, Perception, Psychophysics. 2001;63:1277–8.

32. Friedman J, Hastie T, Tibshirani R. The elements of statistical learning. New York: Springer series in statistics; 2001.

33. R. Mantiuk, HDR visual difference predictor. http://sourceforge.net/projects/hdrvdp. Accessed 4 July 2006.

34. Shannon CE. A mathematical theory of communication. Bell Syst Tech J. 1948;27(379–424):623–56.

35. R. Mantiuk, S. Daly, K. Myszkowski and H.-P. Seidel, Presented at the proc human vision and electronic imaging X, IS&T/SPIE's 17th annual symposium on electronic imaging, 2005.

36. Daly S. The visible differences predictor: an algorithm for the assessment of image fidelity. In: Watson AB, editor. Digital images and human vision. Cambridge: MIT Press; 1993. p. 179–206.

37. Kim B, Lee H, Kim KJ, Seo J, Park S, Shin YG, Kim SH, Lee KH. Comparison of three image comparison methods for the visual assessment of the image fidelity of compressed computed tomography images. Med Phys. 2011;38:836–44.

38. Quick RF. A vector-magnitude model of contrast detection. Biol Cybern. 1974;16:65–7.

39. G. Bongartz, S. J. Golding, A. G. Jurik, M. Leonardi, E. van Persijn van Meerten, R. Rodríguez, K. Schneider, A. Calzado, J. Geleijns, K. A. Jessen, W. Panzer, P. C. Shrimpton and G. Tosi, Bongartz G, Golding SJ, Jurik AG, et al. European guidelines for multislice computed tomography. http://www.drs.dk/guidelines/ct/quality/index.htm. Accessed 1 June 2012.

15

Performance of a feature-based algorithm for 3D-3D registration of CT angiography to cone-beam CT for endovascular repair of complex abdominal aortic aneurysms

Giasemi Koutouzi[1]* ⓘ, Behrooz Nasihatkton[2], Monika Danielak-Nowak[1], Henrik Leonhardt[1], Mårten Falkenberg[1] and Fredrik Kahl[3,4]

Abstract

Background: A crucial step in image fusion for intraoperative guidance during endovascular procedures is the registration of preoperative computed tomography angiography (CTA) with intraoperative Cone Beam CT (CBCT). Automatic tools for image registration facilitate the 3D image guidance workflow. However their performance is not always satisfactory. The aim of this study is to assess the accuracy of a new fully automatic, feature-based algorithm for 3D3D registration of CTA to CBCT.

Methods: The feature-based algorithm was tested on clinical image datasets from 14 patients undergoing complex endovascular aortic repair. Deviations in Euclidian distances between vascular as well as bony landmarks were measured and compared to an intensity-based, normalized mutual information algorithm.

Results: The results for the feature-based algorithm showed that the median 3D registration error between the anatomical landmarks of CBCT and CT images was less than 3 mm. The feature-based algorithm showed significantly better accuracy compared to the intensity-based algorithm ($p < 0.001$).

Conclusion: A feature-based algorithm for 3D image registration is presented.

Keywords: Cone-beam CT, Aortic aneurysm, Image registration, Feature-based registration, Intensity-based registration

Background

Since endovascular aortic repair (EVAR) for abdominal aortic aneurysm (AAA) was first described by Volodos and Parodi [1, 2] there has been a shift away from traditional open surgery towards the less invasive option of endovascular treatment. This has been facilitated by a fast evolution in stent graft design and imaging technology.

Development of fenestrated and branched stent grafts allows treatment of complex juxta-renal and supra-renal AAA [3, 4]. These devices have openings or side-branches, preserving perfusion of vital organs while excluding the aneurysm. Accurate placement of such stent grafts is crucial, not only in the proximal/distal dimension but also in the rotational dimension, matching the fenestrations and branches with the origins of the target vessels. Even after optimal placement of the main aortic device, subsequent catheterization of target vessels to deliver mating stents can be difficult. Treatment of complex AAA with fenestrated or branched EVAR is therefore challenging, and image information on the patient's anatomy is particularly important during these procedures [5–10].

The introduction of cone-beam computer tomography (CBCT) in the interventional suite allows intraoperative acquisition of 3D images. CBCT can be done with or without contrast enhancement. When used for image fusion, CBCT is usually done without contrast, to spare the patient's renal function. Multimodality 3D fusion and projection of selected details on the live fluoroscopy screen enables visualization of the patient's anatomy,

* Correspondence: giasemi.koutouzi@vgregion.se
[1]Department of Radiology, Institute of Clinical Sciences, Sahlgrenska Academy, Gothenburg, Sweden
Full list of author information is available at the end of the article

captured in the preoperative images, to facilitate intraoperative navigation [11, 12].

A crucial step in image fusion for intraoperative guidance is the registration of preoperative computer tomography angiography (CTA) with intraoperative CBCT [13, 14]. Registration can be done by manual alignment in multi-planar reconstruction (MPR) projections or using automatic algorithms. Manual registration is time consuming and requires a high degree of anatomical and procedural insight. In fact, the need for manual registration during the procedure may explain the still limited dissemination of image fusion to vascular centers. Automatic registration algorithms in commercially available systems are often intensity-based. However, fully automatic registration presents several difficulties. First, the fields of view (FOVs) of a CTA and a CBCT differ markedly, the CTA often being approximately three times the size of the CBCT. Secondly, the exact posture of the patient often varies between the preoperative and intraoperative image acquisitions. For example, during CT the patient lies with the knees slightly bent, whereas during the procedure the patient usually lies on the operating table with the legs straight. Thirdly, the contrast-enhanced aorta in the CTA has no image counterpart in the non-enhanced CBCT. Fourthly, the preoperative images may not be perfect with sub-millimeter slices; sometimes only thicker reconstructed slices are available. For all the reasons above, standard intensity-based algorithms for automatic 3D-3D image registration are less than perfect in the clinical situation [14].

Most of the existing CT-CBCT registration algorithms are intensity-based. Many of these techniques are different variants of the well-known Demons algorithm [15] in which a deformable grid models the non-rigid image transformation. For example, Nithiananthan et al. [16] propose a variant of the Demons algorithm in which an intensity correction step is performed on the CBCT image at every iteration of the registration algorithm. A more flexible intensity correction scheme has been proposed in by Lou et al. in 2013 [17].

The registration proposed by Yu et al. [18], is done on 3D gradient fields to deal with the intensity inaccuracies of CBCT in deformable intensity-based registration.

Perhaps the most relevant work to our application of interest is presented by Miao et al. [19], where a multi-stage CBCT to CT registration technique has been proposed for aortic stenting. First, a 2D global search technique is applied to the maximum intensity projection images to estimate an initial translation parameter. Then, the spine in two images are segmented out and rigidly registered. Finally, a deformable registration is applied to fine-tune the alignment around the aorta.

Feature-based methods have also been employed for CT-CBCT image registration. Xie et al. [20] use 3D SIFT features to map the rectal contours from the CT to the CBCT image. The mapping is done by finding a set of SIFT matches between the two volumes and computing a thin-plate spline transformation between them. Xie et al. [21] in 2011 used the same method in a two stage manner for the registration of the liver. In the first stage, the relative position of the liver volumes is found in two images. In the second stage, using manually segmented liver in the first image, a more accurate registration is performed y only exploiting the feature points inside the liver volume in both images. Paganenelli et al. [22] investigated the performance of 3D SIFT features in adaptive radiation therapy. However, the SIFT features are used to evaluate the performance of other non-rigid registration techniques, and not as a means of registration.

Here, we have developed a novel feature-based algorithm for affine 3D-3D image registration. It was first presented at the International Symposium on Biomedical Imaging, 2015 [23], where it was shown to perform well for inter-subject registration, and where both the source and target images were of the same modality (CT or MRI). In the current work, we have developed the method further by allowing more general transformations parametrized by splines in order to improve the registration accuracy in regions of soft tissue. The aim of this study was to evaluate the performance of this feature-based algorithm for 3D-3D registration of CTA to CBCT, and to compare its accuracy with that of a commercially available intensity-based algorithm that optimizes normalized mutual information.

Methods

The algorithm proposed was evaluated offline using data from 14 clinical cases. The study has been approved by the regional research ethics committee. No formal consent was required.

One patient had a common iliac artery aneurysm and was treated with a branched iliac stent graft, and all other patients had a juxta-renal or thoraco-abdominal aneurysm and were treated with fenestrated, branched, or chimney EVAR at the hybrid operating room of Sahlgrenska University Hospital between June 2012 and March 2015 (12 men and two women with a mean age of 73.6 years (standard deviation (SD) ± 5.4)). Characteristics of the patients and procedures are given in Table 1.

All the patients had a pre-procedural multi-detector CTA and an intraoperative CBCT.

CT

Throughout the study, a variety of 64-slice multi-detector spiral CT scanners from different manufacturers were used at our hospital and the referral hospitals of the

Table 1 Characteristics of patients and procedures

Patient	Age (years)	Gender	BMI (kg/m²)	Aneurysm type	Aneurysm size (mm)[1]	Procedure
1	69	M	30	Common iliac artery aneurysm	40	Iliac Branched
2	82	F	34.4	Juxta-renal	62	FEVAR
3	81	M	23.2	Thoraco-abdominal	90	BEVAR
4	71	M	23.8	Juxta-renal	72	FEVAR
5	72	M	27.5	Juxta-renal	58	FEVAR
6	75	M	23.8	Juxta-renal	65	Chimney EVAR
7	76	M	24.3	Juxta-renal	65	FEVAR
8	67	M	24.7	Juxta-renal	70	FEVAR
9	67	M	25.8	Supra-renal	83	BEVAR
10	83	M	33.3	Juxta-renal	62	FEVAR
11	76	M	23.3	Juxta-renal	60	EVAR
12	69	M	24.5	Thoraco-abdominal	90	BEVAR
13	70	F	27.3	Thoraco-abdominal	100	BEVAR
14	73	M	19.6	Thoraco-abdominal	62	BEVAR

F, female; M, male; FEVAR, fenestrated endovascular aneurysm repair; BEVAR, fenestrated endovascular aneurysm repair
[1]Aneurysm size was defined as the maximal aortic diameter perpendicular to the line of flow

region. The preoperative CTA was performed within 6 months (median 3 months, range 2 days to 6 months) before the EVAR procedure.

The CT scans were performed according to routine protocols designed for aortic imaging. The tube voltage varied between 80 and 120 kV. The contrast medium used was of non-ionic low-osmolar type with a concentration of 350 mg I/mL and an injection rate of 4–5 mL/s. The datasets available at the time of the procedures had a median slice thickness of 1.25 mm (0.7–3.0 mm).

CBCT

All procedures were performed in the same hybrid room, which was equipped with a multi-axis robotic C-arm system and a dedicated post-processing workstation (Artis Zeego and Syngo; Siemens Healthcare GmbH, Forchheim, Germany).

A low-dose CBCT without contrast was performed at the start of the each procedure, just before vascular access. During image acquisition, the C-arm (equipped with a 30 × 40-cm flat-panel detector in either landscape or portrait orientation) rotates around the patient in a 200° trajectory. The CBCT protocol used at our institution (5 s DCT Body Care) acquires 248 projection images (0.8°/image) at a configured detector dose of 0.36 μGy. The projection images are transferred automatically to the workstation, where they are reconstructed to.

CT-like images with an isotropic voxel size of 0.5 mm. The cylindrical volume captured by a CBCT has a diameter of 25 cm and a height of 19 cm with the detector in landscape mode.

(19 cm and 25 cm, respectively, in portrait mode).

To provide the best conditions for the 3D fusion process that followed, the patient was centered on the table so that the spine was in the center and the iliac spines were visible at the.

caudal end of a frontal view, and the lumbar vertebrae were visible in the lower aspect of a lateral view.

Feature-based registration

Our approach for registration is based on detecting and matching features. Three-dimensional scale-invariant feature transform (SIFT) features are detected in both CT and CBCT images, and 3D SIFT descriptors are computed for each feature [24]. Each feature point in the CT images is matched to its closest feature point in the CBCT image in terms of the Euclidean distance between the feature descriptors. Similarly, each CBCT feature is matched to a CT feature. Only the feature pairs that are matched in both directions are kept and rest of the feature points are discarded. Then we run a geometry-aware RANSAC test, assuming that the correct feature locations are related by an affine transformation [25] to remove the matches that are not consistent geometrically. Due to nonlinear deformation the body undergoes, the transformation between the two image volumes is not exactly affine. The this reason we use a high threshold of 10 mm to determine the inliers in the RANSAC algorithm.

In all cases we examined on, this gave a very robust affine transformation between the CBCT and CT images. However, one major problem is that most of the matched features are located around the vertebral column. The reason is that there are a large number of features (in the order of few thousands) in both images. In the boundaries of vertebrae, there are clear structures that can be distinguished—even among thousands of features. However, in the soft tissue area, a correct match cannot easily be found among this large number of features. Still, this initial affine estimate of the registration, which aligns vertebrae, gives an accuracy of less than a centimeter even in the soft tissue area. Thus, to find more matches in the soft tissue area, given the initial affine estimate, the algorithm first transforms the CBCT into the CT image space and removes all the CT feature points located outside the boundaries of the transformed CBCT volume (plus a small margin). Then it repeats the feature-matching procedure, but this time, to find the nearest feature descriptors, it performs a local search in which each feature is only searched against the features in a 10 mm radius of its transformed location in the other image. Then the RANSAC algorithm is repeated, but this time with a 5 mm threshold. As a result, we can obtain more matches in the soft tissue area. The feature matches obtained for one CBCT-CT pair are illustrated in Fig. 1. The procedure yields a better affine transformation, as it also tries to align the soft tissue area.

As a final step, the algorithm computes a thin-plate spline transformation between the two images using the feature matches. The thin-plate spline transformation is suitable for when we have an affine transformation plus a rather small nonlinear deformation. Using N three-dimensional point correspondences it gives $3 N + 12$ parameters out of which 12 parameters account for a global affine transformation and $3 N$ parameters model the nonlinearity. This improves the registration accuracy compared to when using a global affine transformation. Fig. 2 illustrates a fused CBCT-CT pair after fully automatic feature based registration.

Registration using the intensity-based algorithm

In order to evaluate the accuracy of the new algorithm, a comparison was made with a commercially available intensity-based, normalized mutual information algorithm (Syngo 3D3D image fusion, Siemens Healthcare),

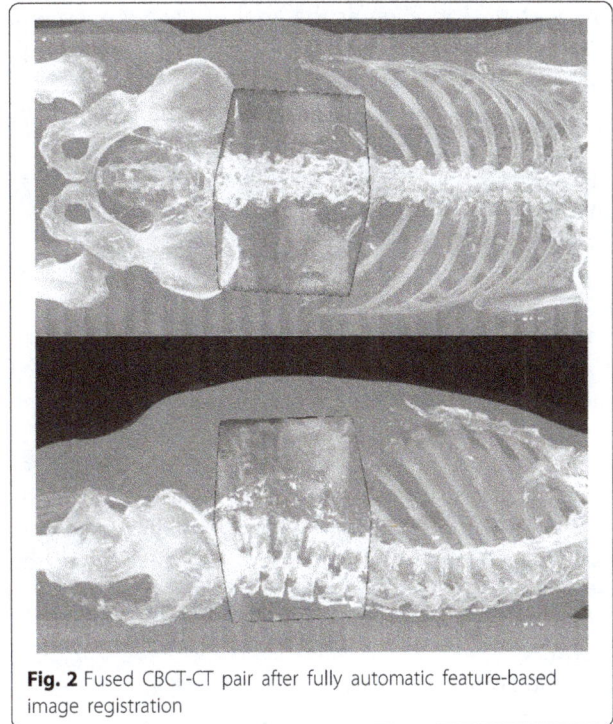

Fig. 2 Fused CBCT-CT pair after fully automatic feature-based image registration

which is a standard algorithm used for 3D3D fusion of CT with CBCT.

Measurements

Registration error was defined as the 3D distance between landmarks on CBCT and corresponding landmarks on CTA.

Six anatomical landmarks on each dataset were used for registration validation. The landmarks were vascular calcifications and bony structures that could be clearly identified in both modalities. Since the benefit of image fusion in complex EVAR procedures lies in position information concerning the ostia of the renal and the visceral arteries, the landmarks chosen were: one aortic calcification at the level of the left renal ostium, one aortic calcification at the level of the right renal ostium, and

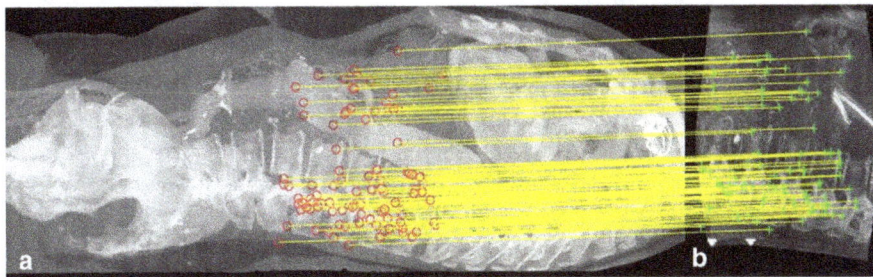

Fig. 1 a CT-Angiography, **b** Cone-Beam CT: feature matching with local correspondence search. Features are obtained from the soft tissue area and from bony structures. For the sake of illustration, only 100 (randomly selected) matches are shown. Lateral views of the 3D volumes are shown using max projection

one aortic calcification at the level of the SMA ostium. The three remaining landmarks were distinct points on each of the nearby vertebrae Th12, L1, and L2.

The landmarks were first identified in the preoperative CT and then in the intraoperative CBCT. After automatic image registration, the 3D alignment error between the corresponding landmarks from the two modalities was calculated.

Measurements were performed using MATLAB for evaluation of the feature-based algorithm and a post-processing workstation (Syngo Workplace; Siemens Healthcare) connected to our angio suite for the intensity-based algorithm. For this purpose, the same landmarks had to be identified twice for each dataset.

Furthermore, for estimation of inter-observer agreement the landmarks were identified in each modality by two independent radiologists who were blind regarding each other's landmarks and regarding the result of the registrations.

Statistics

Continuous data are presented as median with range and as mean with SD. The Wilcoxon signed-rank test was used to test whether there was a statistically significant difference in accuracy between the feature-based algorithm and the intensity-based algorithm. The Wilcoxon signed-rank test was also used to test whether there was a significant difference in accuracy between aortic and bony landmarks for each algorithm. Inter-class correlation coefficient (ICC) (2,1) was used to estimate inter-rater reliability. Statistical analyses were conducted with SPSS for Windows version 24.0 (IBM Corp., Armonk, NY, USA). Any p-value < 0.05 was considered statistically significant.

Spearman's rank correlation coefficient was used to investigate whether the slice thickness of the preoperative CT influenced the accuracy of the algorithms.

Results

The feature-based algorithm was more robust and accurate than the intensity-based algorithm ($p < 0.001$). The median 3D target error for the feature-based algorithm was 2.3 mm (range 0.4–7.9 mm) and the median error for the intensity-based algorithm was 31.6 mm (range 0.5–112.2 mm). A 3D error of < 3 mm was found for 73% of the landmarks using the feature-based registration and for 20% of the landmarks using the intensity-based algorithm. A 3D error of < 5 mm was observed for 94% of the landmarks using the feature-based algorithm and for 28% of the landmarks using the intensity-based algorithm. The feature-based algorithm had a 3D error of < 10 mm in all cases whereas the 3D error for the intensity-based algorithm was < 10 mm for 29% of the landmarks.

The distribution of the 3D errors for the 84 points evaluated for each algorithm was plotted on a cumulative percentage graph (Fig. 3). Figure 4 illustrates the average 3D error for each patient.

There was no significant difference in alignment accuracy between bony landmarks and aortic calcifications in any of the two algorithms.

Correlation analysis revealed that the slice thickness of the preoperative CT had no significant influence on image fusion accuracy (intensity-based algorithm, $P = 0.52$; feature-based algorithm, $p = 0.77$).

Reproducibility

The inter-observer agreement was almost perfect, with an ICC of > 0.8 for both algorithms.

Discussion

In this article we present a robust, fully automatic feature-based algorithm for 3D-3D registration of CTA to CBCT. To our knowledge, this is the first study to validate a feature-based algorithm for image fusion of these modalities using clinical cases.

Image fusion has an expanding role for intraoperative guidance during endovascular repair of complex aortic aneurysms. Fenestrated EVAR (FEVAR) and branched EVAR (BEVAR) are complex and technically challenging operations, demanding precise stent graft positioning, and precise visceral and renal artery cannulation and stenting. These procedures are time consuming and involve risks of embolization and thrombosis.

In the last decade, the introduction of CBCT in radiology suites has revolutionized intraoperative image guidance. Image fusion can facilitate intraoperative guidance by overlaying important anatomical information from pre-procedural CT on the live fluoroscopic image—thus reducing procedure time, radiation dose, and the amount of contrast medium used [5–8].

However, a key determinant of widespread clinical application of the fusion technique is the ease of use and the accuracy of image registration. Manual 3D3D registration of preoperative CTA with intraoperative un-enhanced CBCT is a challenging procedure, requiring the operator to be skilled in using advanced fusion software.

Commercially available systems for automatic registration may be helpful, if they are accurate. However, these systems are still not sufficiently robust and often result in large misalignments, thus requiring inconvenient manual interaction during the procedure.

In 2016, a study on 19 EVAR cases assessed the accuracy of fully automatic registration between CT and CBCT using a feature-based mutual information algorithm. The fully automatic registration alone was not sufficient for EVAR guidance (defined as < 3 mm deviation at the lower renal artery ostium), and in 42% of

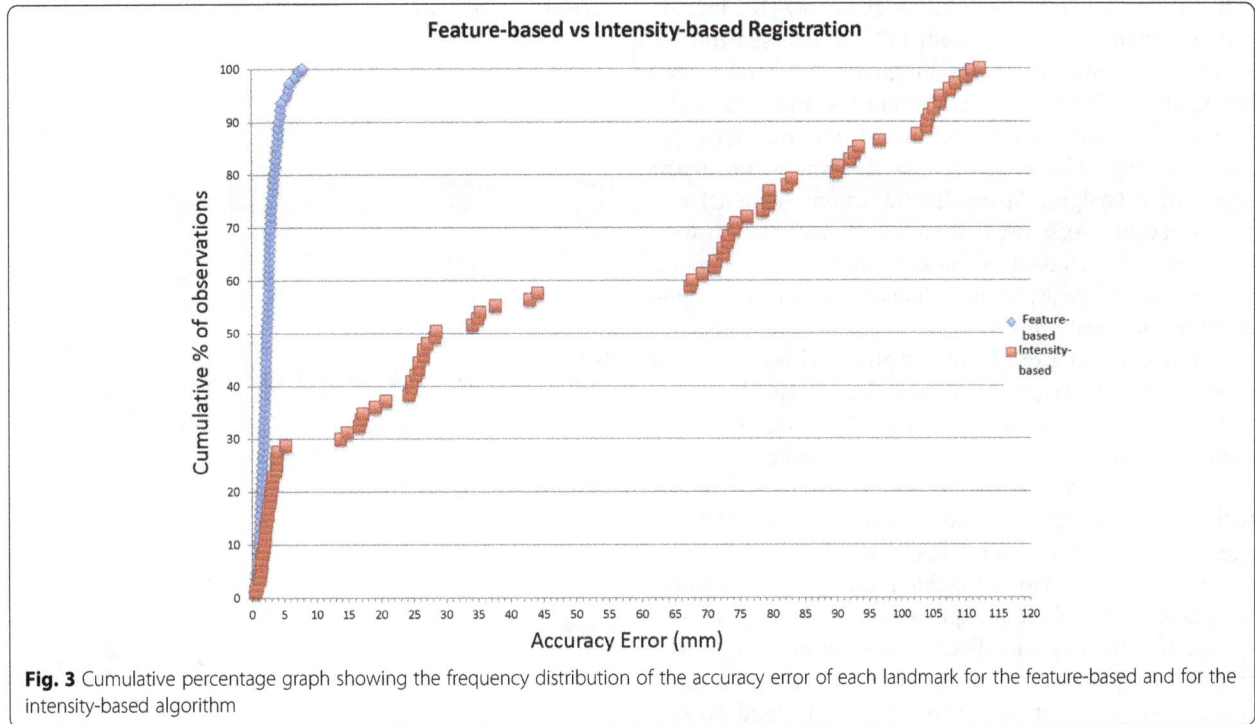

Fig. 3 Cumulative percentage graph showing the frequency distribution of the accuracy error of each landmark for the feature-based and for the intensity-based algorithm

the cases the deviation in registration at the lower renal artery was greater than 20 mm [14].

Schulz et al. (2016) [26] reported their experience with image fusion in a larger cohort of 101 consecutive EVARs using a two-step algorithm designed to automatically align the 3D datasets [19]. First, bony structures were aligned using normalized mutual information and then alignment of vessels and vessel calcifications of the aorta was performed in a second step. This software was included in a prototype workplace with AAA guidance software (Siemens Healthcare). The fully automatic registration was found to be satisfactory without further adjustments in 39% of the cases. In the rest of the cases, the registration error was larger than one renal artery diameter or completely manual registration was required.

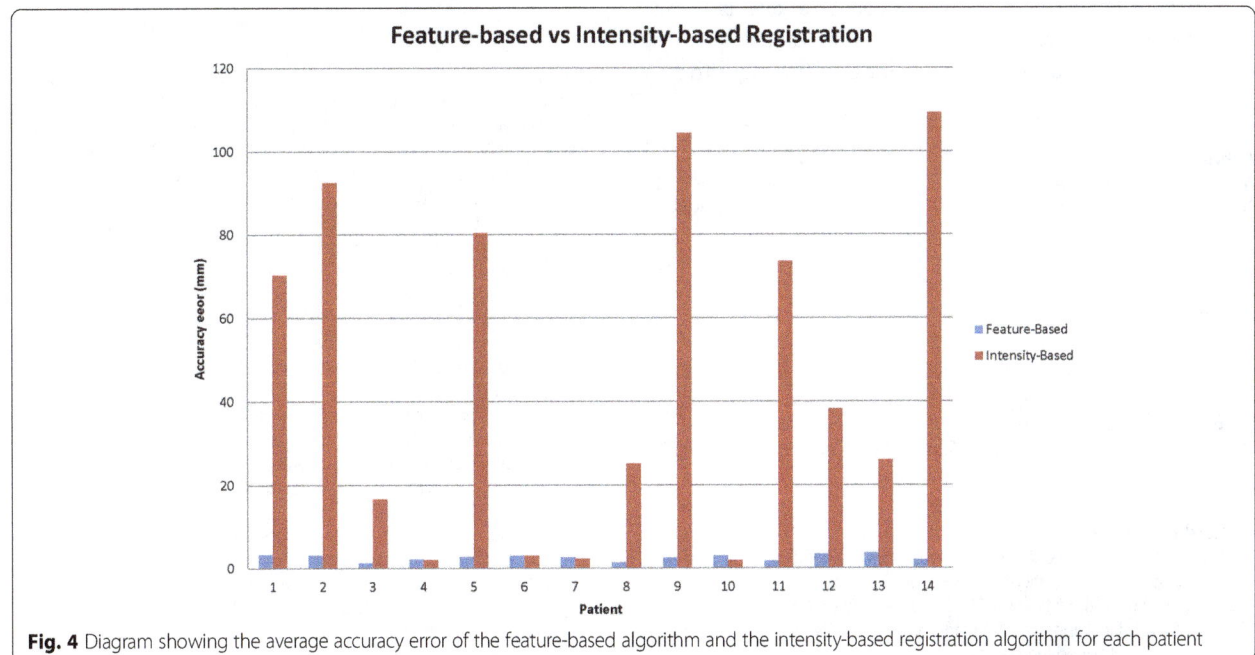

Fig. 4 Diagram showing the average accuracy error of the feature-based algorithm and the intensity-based registration algorithm for each patient

A recent study from Schwein et al. (2018) [10] including 26 patients who underwent FEVAR assessed the accuracy of fusion technique in guiding visceral vessel cannulation. The results were promising and 83% of the target vessels were cannulated based only on image fusion guidance. However, even in this study the image registration (syngo InSpace 3D/3D fusion; Siemens) was performed in two steps; first automatic registration with focus on the alignment of the bone anatomy, and then a semiautomatic registration emphasizing on the alignment of the calcifications.

The experimental results of our proposed feature-based approach for 3D registration showed acceptable registration error in the majority of cases. The algorithm was evaluated using 14 clinical cases. A limitation of the study was that not all of the preoperative CTs were performed with the same equipment, and the reconstructed MPR images available had a slice thickness that varied from 0.7 mm to 3 mm. However, this represents a real-world clinical situation where preoperative examinations are not always of optimal quality. Even so, the performance of the feature-based algorithm was consistently fair with a maximum average registration error of 3.69 mm and no significant difference in the alignment error of aortic calcifications and bony structures.

Conclusions

A new and efficient algorithm for 3D3D registration of CTA with CBCT is proposed. The novelty of this work lies in the fact that the algorithm is feature-based whereas commercially available algorithms are intensity-based. Furthermore, the algorithm was validated in a group of clinical cases where image fusion is highly beneficial and is being increasingly used. Our encouraging results require further studies to confirm the clinical usefulness of this algorithm.

Abbreviations
AAA: Abdominal Aortic Aneurysm; CBCT: Cone Beam Computed Tomography; CTA: Computed Tomography Angiography; EVAR: Endovascular Aortic Repair

Acknowledgements
Not applicable

Funding
The study was funded by research grant from VG region (ALFGBG-218331 to MF).

Authors' contributions
Conception and design: GK, BN, MF, FK. Feature-based algorithm development: BN, FK. Analysis and interpretation: GK, BN, MDN, HL. Data collection: GK, BN, MDN, HL,MF. Writing the article: GK, BN. Critical revision of the article: GK, BN, MDN, HL, MF, FK. Final approval of the article: GK, BN, MDN, HL, MF, FK. Statistical analysis: GK. Obtained funding: MF.

Consent for publication
Not applicable.

Competing interests
The authors declare that they have no competing interests.

Author details
[1]Department of Radiology, Institute of Clinical Sciences, Sahlgrenska Academy, Gothenburg, Sweden. [2]K. N. Toosi University of Technology, Tehran, Iran. [3]Department of Electrical Engineering, Chalmers University of Technology, Gothenburg, Sweden. [4]Center for Mathematical Sciences, Lund University, Lund, Sweden.

References
1. Parodi JC, Palmaz JC, Barone HD. Transfemoral intraluminal graft implantation for abdominal aortic aneurysms. Ann Vasc Surg. 1991;5:491–9.
2. Volodos NL, Karpovich IP, Troyan VI, YuV K, Shekhanin VE, Ternyuk NE, et al. Clinical experience of the use of self-fixing synthetic prostheses for remote endoprosthetics of the thoracic and the abdominal aorta and iliac arteries through the femoral artery and as intraoperative endoprosthesis for aorta reconstruction. VASA Suppl. 1991;33:93–5.
3. ELG V, Katsargyris A, Bekkema F, Oikonomou K, CJAM Z, Ritter W, et al. Editor's choice - ten-year experience with endovascular repair of Thoracoabdominal aortic aneurysms: results from 166 consecutive patients. Eur J Vasc Endovasc Surg. 2015;49:524–31.
4. Guillou M, Bianchini A, Sobocinski J, Maurel B, D'elia P, Tyrrell M, et al. Endovascular treatment of thoracoabdominal aortic aneurysms. J Vasc Surg. 2012;56:65–73.
5. Dijkstra ML, Eagleton MJ, Greenberg RK, Mastracci T, Hernandez A. Intraoperative C-arm cone-beam computed tomography in fenestrated/branched aortic endografting. J Vasc Surg. 2011;53:583–90. https://doi.org/10.1016/j.jvs.2010.09.039.
6. Sailer AM, De Haan MW, Peppelenbosch AG, Jacobs MJ, Wildberger JE, Schurink GWH. CTA with fluoroscopy image fusion guidance in endovascular complex aortic aneurysm repair. Eur J Vasc Endovasc Surg. 2014;47:349–56. https://doi.org/10.1016/j.ejvs.2013.12.022.
7. McNally MM, Scali ST, Feezor RJ, Neal D, Huber TS, Beck AW. Three-dimensional fusion computed tomography decreases radiation exposure, procedure time, and contrast use during fenestrated endovascular aortic repair. J Vasc Surg. 2015;61:309–16. https://doi.org/10.1016/j.jvs.2014.07.097.
8. Dias NV, Billberg H, Sonesson B, Törnqvist P, Resch T, Kristmundsson T. The effects of combining fusion imaging, low-frequency pulsed fluoroscopy, and low-concentration contrast agent during endovascular aneurysm repair. J Vasc Surg. 2016;63:1147–55. https://doi.org/10.1016/j.jvs.2015.11.033.
9. Ahmad W, Gawenda M, Brunkwall S, Shahverdyan R, Brunkwall JS. Endovascular Aortoiliac aneurysm repair with fenestrated stent graft and iliac side branch using image fusion without iodinated contrast medium. Ann Vasc Surg. 2016;33:231.
10. Schwein A, Chinnadurai P, Behler G, Lumsden AB, Bismuth J, Bechara CF. Computed tomography angiography-fluoroscopy image fusion allows visceral vessel cannulation without angiography during fenestrated endovascular aneurysm repair. J Vasc Surg. 2018;68(1):2–11. https://doi.org/10.1016/j.jvs.2017.11.062.
11. Abi-Jaoudeh N, Kruecker J, Kadoury S, Kobeiter H, Venkatesan AM, Levy E, et al. Multimodality image fusion-guided procedures: technique, accuracy, and applications. Cardiovasc Intervent Radiol. 2012;35:986–98.
12. Kaladji A, Daoudal A, Clochard E, Gindre J, Cardon A, Castro M, et al. Interest of fusion imaging and modern navigation tools with hybrid rooms in endovascular aortic procedures. J Cardiovasc Surg. 2017;58:458–66.

13. Tacher V, Lin M, Desgranges P, Deux JF, Grünhagen T, Becquemin JP, et al. Image guidance for endovascular repair of complex aortic aneurysms: comparison of two-dimensional and three-dimensional angiography and image fusion. J Vasc Interv Radiol. 2013;24:1698–706. https://doi.org/10.1016/j.jvir.2013.07.016.

14. Koutouzi G, Sandström C, Roos H, Henrikson O, Leonhardt H, Falkenberg M. Orthogonal rings, fiducial markers, and overlay accuracy when image fusion is used for EVAR guidance. Eur J Vasc Endovasc Surg. 2016;52:604–11. https://doi.org/10.1016/j.ejvs.2016.07.024.

15. Thirion JP. Image matching as a diffusion process: an analogy with Maxwell's demons. Med Image Anal. 1998;2(3):243–60.

16. Nithiananthan S, Schafer S, Uneri A, Mirota DJ, Stayman W, Zbijewski W, Brock KK, et al. Demons deformable registration of CT and cone-beam CT using an iterative intensity matching approach. Med Phys. 2011;38:1785–98.

17. Lou Y, Niu T, Jia X, Vela PA, Zhu L, Tannenbaum AR. Joint CT/CBCT deformable registration and CBCT enhancement for cancerradiotherapy. Med Image Anal. 2013;3:387–400.

18. Yu G, Liang Y, Yang G, Shu H, Li B, Yin Y, Li D, et al. Accelerated gradient-based free form deformable registration for online adaptive radiotherapy. Physics in medicine & Biology. 2015;60:2765.

19. Miao S, Liao R, Pfister M, Zhang L, Ordy V. System and method for 3-D/3-D registration between non-contrast-enhanced CBCT and contrast-enhanced CT for abdominal aortic aneurysm stenting. Lect notes Comput Sci (including Subser Lect notes Artif Intell Lect notes Bioinformatics). 2013; 8149 LNCS PART(1):380–7.

20. Xie Y, Chao M, Lee P, Xing L. Feature-based rectal contour propagation from planning CT to cone beam CT. Med Phys. 2008;35:4450–9.

21. Xie Y, Chao M, Xiong G. Deformable image registration of liver with consideration of lung sliding motion. Med Phys. 2011;38:5351–61.

22. Paganelli C, Peroni M, Riboldi M, Sharp GC, Ciardo D, Alterio D, et al. Scale invariant feature transform in adaptive radiation therapy: a tool for deformable image registration assessment and re-planning indication. Phys Med Biol. 2012;58:287.

23. Svärm L, Enqvist O, Kahl F, Oskarsson M. Improving Robustness for Inter-Subject Medical Image Registration Using a Feature-Based Approach. In Conf. 2015 IEEE 12th International Symposium on Biomedical Imaging (ISBI). https://doi.org/10.1109/ISBI.2015.7163998.

24. Allaire S, Kim JJ, Breen SL, Jaffray DA, Pekar V. Full orientation invariance and improved feature selectivity of 3D SIFT with application to medical image analysis, vol. 2008. Anchorage, AK: 2008 IEEE computer society conference on computer vision and pattern recognition workshops; 2008. p. 1–8. https://doi.org/10.1109/CVPRW.2008.4563023.

25. Sotiras C, Davatzikos NP. Deformable medical image registration: a survey. IEEE Trans Med Imaging. 2013;32(7):1153–90.

26. Schulz CJ, Schmitt M, Boeckler D, Geisbusch P. Fusion imaging to support endovascular aneurysm repair using 3D-3D registration. J Endovasc Ther. 2016;23:791–9. https://doi.org/10.1177/1526602816660327.

16

Evaluation of the diagnostic performance of the simple method of computed tomography in the assessment of patients with shoulder instability

Tingting Liu[1†], Jianpeng Ma[2†], Hetao Cao[1], Dongmei Hou[1] and Lin Xu[3*] (iD)

Abstract

Background: Physical examinations may reveal the instability of a *glenohumeral* joint but cannot diagnose the bony Bankart lesions. Soft tissue Bankart lesion cannot be visualized on traditional radiogram. Magnetic resonance images have high cost and availability issues. The purpose of the study was to access the diagnostic performance of the Computed Tomography (CT) in the assessment of patients with shoulder instability and to diagnose the Bankart and bony Bankart lesions.

Methods: A total of 145 patients with shoulder instability were included in the study. Patients were subjected to clinical examination tests, traditional radiography, and CT. Two orthopedic surgeons, two engineers (trained in musculoskeletal imaging), and two physiotherapists have analyzed the radiological images, CT scans, and the clinical examination tests respectively. The *Chi-square* test or one-way ANOVA/ Dunnett Multiple comparisons test was performed at 99% of confidence level.

Results: Sensitivity (0.972 ± 0.18 vs. 1, $p = 0.11$) and accuracy (0.942 ± 0.17 vs. 1, $p < 0.0001$, $q = 3.88$) for the clinical examination tests combining the traditional radiological images were same to CT. However, the clinical examination tests combining the traditional radiological images had more inconclusive results (5 vs. 1), false-positive results (6 vs. 5), and false negative results (4 vs. 1) than CT. The area that detects the Bankart and bony Bankart lesions at least one time for CT was higher than that of the clinical examination tests combining the traditional radiological images.

Conclusion: CT should be considered for evaluation in patients with shoulder instability and suspected Bankart and bony Bankart lesions.

Keywords: Bankart lesions, Clinical examination tests, Computed tomography, Traditional radiological images, Twin trial

* Correspondence: LivelyLenopalin@yahoo.com
†Tingting Liu and Jianpeng Ma contributed equally to this work.
3Department of Radiology, PLA general hospital, No.28 Fuxing Road, Haidian District, Beijing 100000, China
Full list of author information is available at the end of the article

Background

A *glenohumeral* joint is most frequently dislocated [1]. The recurrent shoulder instability affected patients can develop significant functional deficiencies and symptoms of chronic instability [2]. The reason behind recurrent instability is a glenoid bone loss or the Bankart lesion. Anterior shoulder dislocation due to structural damage to the anterior-inferior labrum with tearing of the anterior capsule is called the Bankart lesion. When it includes osseous fragments, it is called the bony Bankart lesion. The treatment involved in the reattachment of the lesion is arthroscopy with surgical suture [3]. The reason behind the Bankart lesion is a loss of 25% and/or more of the width of the inferior glenoid, which leads to a loss of bony support [4]. The glenoid bone loss is frequent in shoulders with the Bankart lesion [5].

The complexity of the combined motions of the degree of the scapulothoracic and the *glenohumeral* joints creates difficulties in preoperative quantification and identification of the Bankart and bony Bankart lesions for decision making of arthroscopy or open procedures [6]. Surgeons may fail in the surgical repair of the Bankart and bony Bankart lesions if not follow protocol for workup and have addressed a bony problem without being aware of it by the differential diagnosis. Moreover, the management of the Bankart and bony Bankart lesions after a failed surgery could be challenging. Therefore, an adaptation of proper diagnostic modality is crucial in the detection of the Bankart and bony Bankart lesions [7]. The optimal treatment for the Bankart and bony Bankart lesions remains controversial [8]. The accepted diagnostic method of quantifying the Bankart and bony Bankart lesions is not available [9] because physical examinations may reveal instability of the *glenohumeral* joints but cannot diagnose the Bankart or bony Bankart lesions. Generally, orthopedic surgeons have preferred radiography, the Computed Tomography (CT), and magnetic resonance imaging (MRI) in the decision making of surgeries [6].

Soft tissue Bankart lesion cannot be visualized on traditional radiogram. With a Grashey view, an external and internal rotation view, an axillary lateral view, a scapular-Y view, a West Point view, a Stryker notch view, and an apical oblique (Garth) view, the sensitivity of traditional radiography for detection of significant glenoid bone loss is not more than 50% [2]. Moreover, an acute fracture of the glenoid rim is often inaccurately quantified by traditional radiography [10]. Therefore, traditional radiography is underestimated bone defects. MRI has high cost and availability issues [3]. MR images are suggested only if the traditional radiography will fail to provide the necessary information for decision making of surgeries [11]. Therefore, there is a strong need for a consensus on the universally accepted diagnostic method of quantifying the Bankart and bony Bankart lesions.

The goal of the study was to access the diagnostic performance of the simple method of CT in the assessment of patients with shoulder instability and to diagnose the Bankart and bony Bankart lesions. The secondary endpoint of the study was to compare sensitivity and accuracy of the clinical examination tests combining the traditional radiological images with CT for decision making of arthroscopy or open procedures for repair of the bony problem of shoulder(s) at level 2 of evidence (Table 1) without conflict of interest.

Methods

The study had adhered 2013 Declarations of Helsinki, standards for reporting of diagnostic accuracy studies (STARD) guidelines, and the law of China. The work has been reported in line with the strengthening the reporting of cohort studies in surgery (STROCSS) criteria [12].

Inclusion criteria

Patients age 18 years and above, with a complaint of progressively reduced shoulder function, pain located at the front and lateral side of the shoulder, load-dependent pain, or/and delocalization of the shoulder available with outpatient setting of the PLA general hospital, China, Affiliated Hospital of Nantong University, China, and Dingbian County People's Hospital, China from 18 December 2014 to 1 February 2018 were included in the study. Patients who had a bony problem of shoulder(s) and signed an informed consent form were subjected to a pre-index test (the pre-index tests were performed for eligible participants screening purposes).

Pre-index tests

Functional outcomes were measured in pre-index tests as follows to confirm glenoid bone loss:

Oxford instability shoulder score

It contains 12 items questionnaires with four responses (0–3). The total score (the sum of 12 items) ranged from 0 (excellent) to 48 (the worst) [13].

Table 1 Level of Evidence

Level	Diagnostic study
1	Testing previously developed diagnostic criteria
2	Testing diagnostic criteria with gold standard
3	Review article/Meta-analysis on STARD studies
4	Case study
5	Expert opinion

STARD Standards for reporting of diagnostic accuracy studies

Western Ontario shoulder instability index

It has 21 items questionnaires on a visual analog scale score. The total score (the sum of 21 items) ranged from 0 (the excellent) to 100 (the worst) [13].

Simple shoulder test score

It consists of 12 questions with dichotomous response options, which are scored 0 or 1. The total score (the sum of 12 items) ranged from 0 (the worst) to 12 (the excellent) [13].

Disability of the arm, shoulder, and hand score

It is a measurement of physical function and symptoms in patients with musculoskeletal disorders from any condition in any joint in the upper extremity. It has 30-questions (grading 0–3). The average of item scores, subtracting one, and multiplying the result by 25 is the resulting score. It has the range from 0 (no disability) to 100 (extreme disability) [14].

Exclusion criteria

Patients age younger than 18 years and not signed informed consent form were excluded from the study. Patients who had frozen shoulder and arthritis were excluded from the study. Patients who had oxford instability shoulder score, four and less than four were excluded from the study.

A total of 145 patients with the proved shoulder instability were enrolled in a prospective cohort study. The demographic parameters of the enrolled patients are presented in Table 2. STARD flow diagram of the study is presented in Fig. 1.

Diagnosis of the Bankart and bony Bankart lesions
Clinical examination tests

Physical examinations of shoulders were performed as follows:

Apprehension test

The enrolled patients had kept in supine position with the arm in 90^0 abductions, the elbow in 90^0 flexions, and maximum external rotation. The evaluator had applied an anterior, external, rotatory force [15].

The relocation test

In apprehension test position, the force was applied to the humeral head in the posterior direction [16].

The anterior release/ the surprise test

The patient's affected arm was maintained in the position of apprehension and the pressure on the humeral head was suddenly released by the evaluator [17].

The anterior drawer test

Patients were kept in supine positions and affected hand was on the examiner's axilla, the arm was held in 80–120^0 of abduction, 0–20^0 of forwarding flexion, and 0–30^0 of external rotation. With one hand, the evaluator had stabilized the scapula by applying force on the coracoid process. The other hand was grasped the humeral and drew it out anteriorly [18].

The load and shift test/ the push-pull test

Patients were kept in set positions. With the dominant hand, the evaluator was grasped the patient's elbow and the non-dominant hand (of the evaluator) was grasped the patient's upper arm. The evaluator was positioned the patient's arm in 90^0 of abduction in the scapular plane with no rotation and centered the humeral head of subject on the glenoid by applying a force along the axis of the humeral with the dominant hand to shift the humeral head in the anterior direction [19].

The Hyperabduction test

Patients were kept in standing positions, the elbow was flexed at 90^0, the forearm was horizontal, and the evaluator was standing behind the patients. With the evaluator's forearm of the dominant hand, the shoulder girdle was pushed down firmly, while the evaluator's non-dominant hand was lifted the patient's upper limb, which was relaxed in the abduction [13].

All tests were performed by two physiotherapists (evaluators; three years of experience) who were blinded regarding radiological images and in order of those have written. The interpretation of observations of all the tests for considering them positive or negative are presented in Table 3.

Traditional radiographs

All enrolled patients were subjected to axillary traditional radiographs (GE Healthcare, Chicago, IL, USA) at an axial position and at 90^0. Conventional axillary lateral, anteroposterior (in exo-rotation or in endo-rotation) radiographs and the Grashey view of the affected shoulder were performed (Fig. 2).

CT scans

Spiral CT (CATIA, France) was performed at 1.25 mm thickness and 0.625 mm interval of affected shoulder to confirm or exclude the Bankart and Bony Bankart lesions (Fig. 3).

Image analysis

Radiological images were checked by a radiologist (three years of experience) under the lightbox (Efftronics Systems Pvt. Ltd., China). A small bone spur in traditional radiological images of the shoulder was considered as the Bankart or bony Bankart lesions present (Fig. 4). The

Table 2 The demographic parameters of the enrolled patients

Characters		Populations
Patients enrolled in the study (sample size)		145
Gender	Male	66 (46)
	Female	79 (54)
Age (years)		28.52 ± 7.56
Reduced shoulder function	DS	114 (79)
	NDS	29 (20)
	Both	2 (1)
Pain located at the front side of the shoulder	DS	117 (81)
	NDS	24 (17)
	Both	4 (2)
Pain located at the lateral side of the shoulder	DS	113 (78)
	NDS	30 (21)
	Both	2 (1)
Load-dependent pain	DS	125 (86)
	NDS	22 (18)
	Both	8 (6)
Delocalization of the shoulder	DS	112 (77)
	NDS	33 (23)
	Both	0 (0)
Incidence of event	The first time	133 (92)
	The second or third time	12 (8)
Functional outcome measures	Oxford Instability Shoulder Score (48–0) [a]	20.15 ± 1.89
	Western Ontario Shoulder Instability Index (0–100) [a]	44.57 ± 5.28
	Simple Shoulder Test score (0–12) [a]	8.52 ± 1.13
	Disability of the Arm, Shoulder, and Hand score (100–0) [a]	25.47 ± 2.58

Constant data are considered as number (percentage) and continuous data are presented as mean ± SD
[a]The range is reflected as most impaired to the least impaired condition
DS: The dominant side
NDS: The non-dominant side
Oxford Instability Shoulder Score: 0: excellent, 48: The worst
Western Ontario Shoulder Instability Index: 0: excellent, 100: The worst
Simple Shoulder Test score: 0: excellent, 12: The worst
Disability of the Arm, Shoulder, and Hand score: 100: No disability, 0: extreme disability
Enrolled patients had more than one type of demographic characters regarding the bony problem in the shoulder(s)
All patients have China PR origin

surgeons had decided the Bankart or bony Bankart lesions and taken the decision of arthroscopy or open procedures. CT scans were evaluated using CATIA (CATIA V5R21; Dassault Systemes, France). The percentage missing area was calculated by surface area missing and the inferior glenoid circle (Fig. 5) as per Eq. 1 (surface area method) [20]. The Bankart and/or bony Bankart lesions was confirmed if the percentage missing area was minimum 20% [3].

$$\text{The percentage missing area} = \frac{\text{The eroded missing area}}{\text{The inferior glenoid circle}} \times 100 \quad (1)$$

Surgery curative was considered as 'gold standard' in all the operative case. If any kind of bony problem (e.g. inflammation, rupture, ligament straitening, Hill–Sachs lesion) had found in diagnosis, which was lead to arthroscopy or opens surgical procedure and actually it was the Bankart and/or bony Bankart lesions considered as a 'false negative'. If the Bankart and/or bony Bankart lesions had found in diagnosis, which was lead to surgery and actually it was the other than the bony problem (frozen shoulder, arthritis, Hill–Sachs lesion) considered as a 'false positive'. The accurate Bankart and bony Bankart lesions absent category were also found in all diagnosis because all patients who had

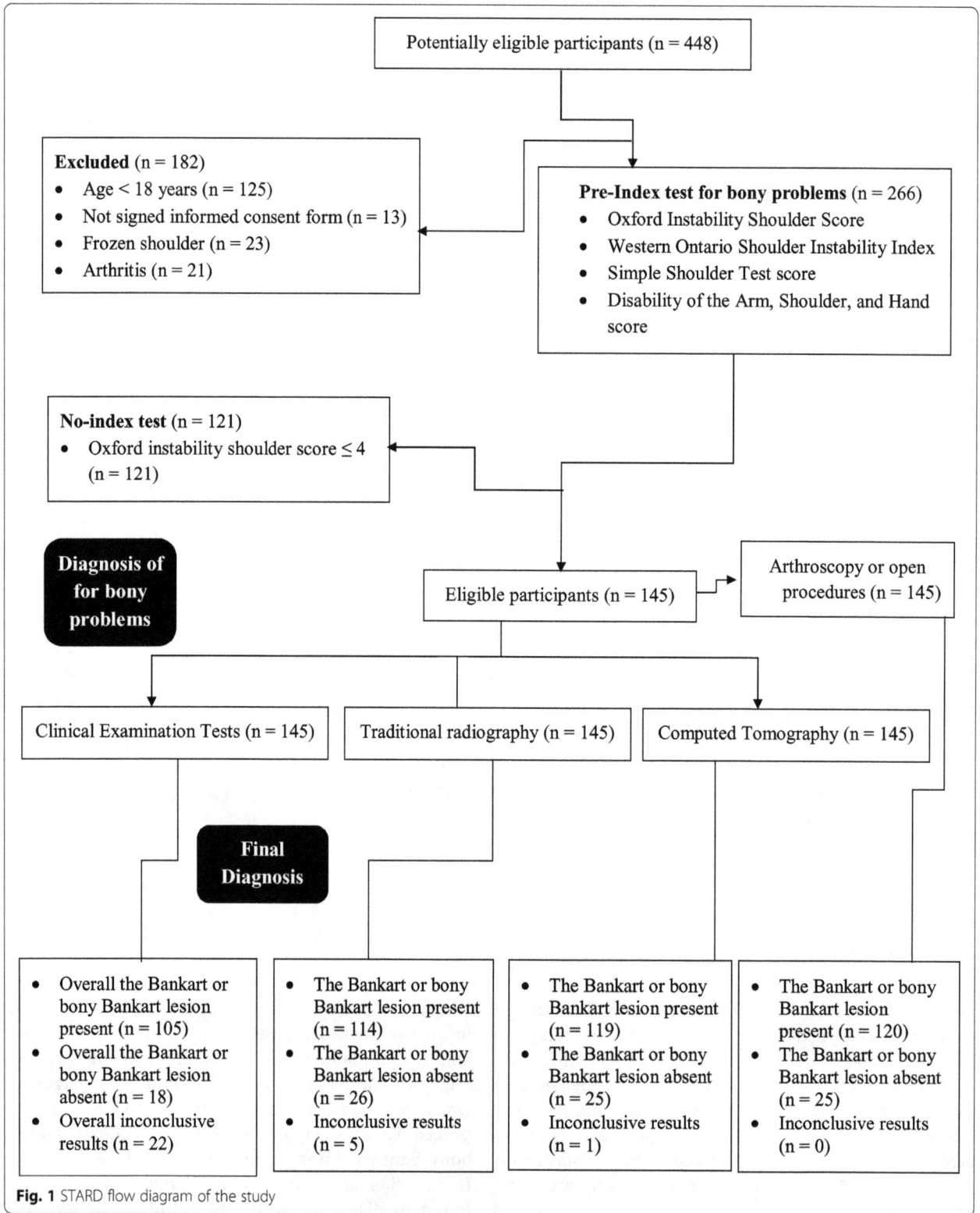

Fig. 1 STARD flow diagram of the study

to complain of the shoulder(s) instability were included and there is no any accurate clinical test until the time to confirm the Bankart and bony Bankart lesions.

Beneficial analysis of diagnostic methods

Decision-making curve for detection of the Bankart and bony Bankart lesions was drawn by decision curve analysis as per Eqs. 2 and 3 [21]:

Table 3 Interpretation of clinical examination tests

Clinical Examination Tests	Observations regarding patients feeling after the test	
	Considered positive	Considered negative
Apprehension Test	An apprehensive feeling	Only pain noticed
The Relocation Test	Apprehensive feeling or pain is reduced	Apprehensive feeling or pain is not reduced
The Anterior Release/ the Surprise Test	An apprehensive experience	Only pain noticed
The Anterior Drawer Test	Humeral head increased translation than the other shoulder	Only pain noticed
The Load and Shift Test/ the Push-Pull Test	displayed apprehension	No apprehension
The hyperabduction Test	Arm hyper-abducted $\geq 105^{\circ}$	Arm hyper-abducted $< 105^{\circ}$

Each patient underwent physical examinations total four times by two physiotherapists (blinded regarding radiological images)

Decision making of the Bankart and bony Bankart lesions

= True Positive ratio of the Bankart and bony Bankart lesions

−(False positive ratio of the Bankart and bony Bankart lesions

×Weighting factor)

$$(2)$$

Weighting factor =

$$\frac{\text{A level of diagnostic confidence above it had performed arthroscopy or opens surgical procedure}}{1 - \text{A level of diagnostic confidence above it arthroscopy or opens surgical procedure had performed}}$$

$$(3)$$

Weighting factor: The risk of overdiagnosis.

Inter-and intra-observer reliability

For purposes of the reliability of assessments, two orthopedic surgeons were analyzed twice times the traditional radiological images, two engineers trained in musculoskeletal imaging assessments (this is diploma course for musculoskeletal imaging assessments in PR. China after MD radiology; three years of experience in image analysis) were evaluated the CT scans twice, and two physiotherapists were evaluated clinical examination tests twice (each patient underwent physical examinations four times). All were blinded to the others' conclusions.

Cost of diagnosis

Cost of diagnosis was included hospitalization, charges of experts, and radiographers.

Statistical analysis

Kappa statistics (considering kappa value (k) ≤ 0.4 low, 0.41–0.6 moderate, 0.61–0.8 substantial, and ≥ 0.81 perfect inter-and intra-observer reliabilities) were used to determine reliability [22]. One-way analysis of variance (ANOVA) following Dunnett Multiple comparisons tests (considering critical value $(q) > 4.148$ as significant) was performed to compare constant diagnostic parameters [23] and the *Chi-square* test was performed for categorical data. All results were considered significant at 99% of confidence level. InStat (vWindow, GraphPad, IL, USA) was used for statistical analysis.

Results

Functional outcome measures were strongly correlated with the Bankart and bony Bankart lesions. k for physiotherapists, orthopedic surgeons, and trained engineers (in musculoskeletal imaging) were greater

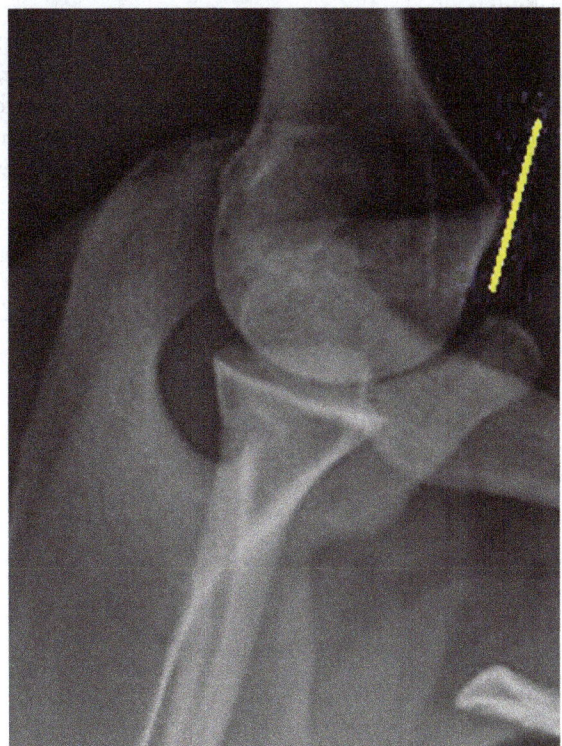

Fig. 2 Traditional radiological image of the shoulder with the Bankart lesions. The yellow line indicates the Bankart lesions. The Grashey view of the patient's shoulder. Images were checked by two radiologists

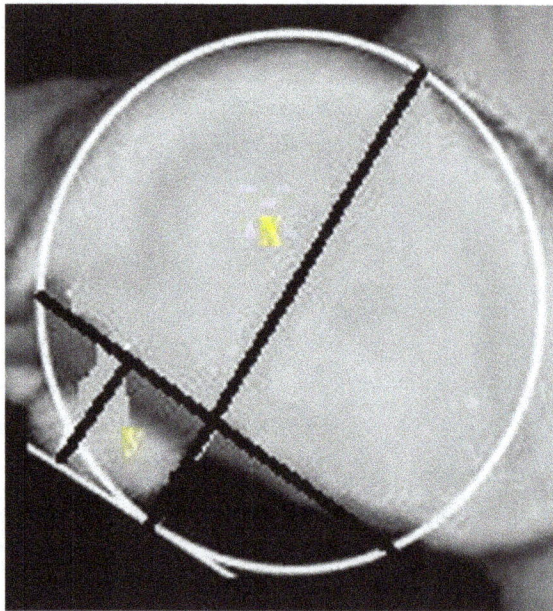

Fig. 3 The Computed Tomography of the patient's shoulder with the Bankart lesions. X: The inferior glenoid circle. Y: The eroded missing area. Images were checked by two engineers (diploma course in musculoskeletal imaging assessments in PR. China after MD radiology) trained in musculoskeletal imaging

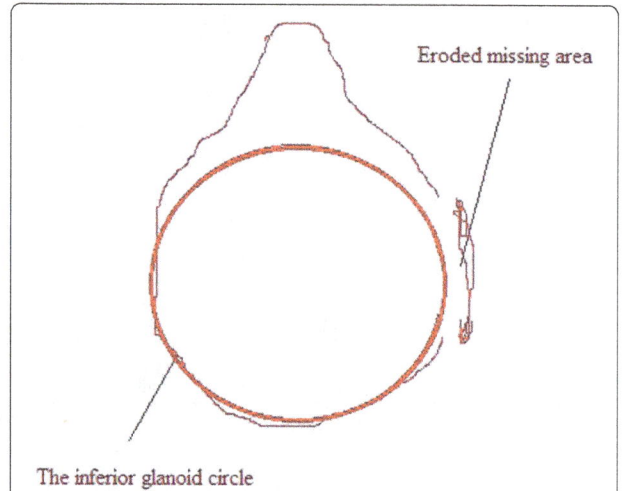

Fig. 5 Surface area method of the simple Computed Tomography in the assessment of patients with shoulder instability and to diagnose the Bankart and bony Bankart lesions. Images were checked by two engineers (diploma course in musculoskeletal imaging assessments in PR. China after MD radiology) trained in musculoskeletal imaging. The Bankart and/or bony Bankart lesions was confirmed if the percentage missing area was minimum 20%

than 0.81 indicated perfect inter-and intra-observer reliabilities (Table 4).

Among clinical examination tests, surprise test has high sensitivity (0.917 ± 0.15) and the anterior drawer test has high accuracy (0.811 ± 0.18). The area under the curve for the clinical examination tests combining the traditional radiological images was fallen down than CT (0.76 ± 0.11 vs.

0.89 ± 0.14, $p < 0.0001$, $q = 9.39$). Overall, the clinical examination tests combining the traditional radiological images had provided limited information for decision making of surgeries (Fig. 6). With respect to CT, sensitivity for the clinical examination tests combining the traditional radiological images had no statistical significance difference (0.972 ± 0.18 vs. 1, $p = 0.11$) even for accuracy there were no statistical significance difference (0.942 ± 0.17 vs. 1, $p < 0.0001$, $q = 3.88$). However, the clinical examination tests combining the traditional radiological images had more inconclusive results (5 vs. 1), false-positive results (6 vs. 5), and false negative results (4 vs. 1) than CT (Table 5). CT was flawless in the decision making of surgeries for the Bankart and bony Bankart lesions than the clinical examination tests combining the traditional radiological images (Table 6).

The area that detects the Bankart and bony Bankart lesions at least one time for CT was higher than that of clinical examination tests combining the traditional radiological images (Table 7). At 0–50% level of diagnostic confidence, orthopedic surgeons had preferred the clinical examination tests combining the traditional radiological images but these tests did not give any sufficient information for decision making of surgery. However, above 50% of the level of diagnostic confidence for the clinical examination tests combining the traditional radiological images, patients had a risk of overdiagnosis and overtreatment. In the range of 0–75% of the level of diagnostic confidence, CT was the most reliable imaging modality and above 75% of the level of diagnostic confidence, CT had a risk of overdiagnosis and overtreatment (Fig. 7).

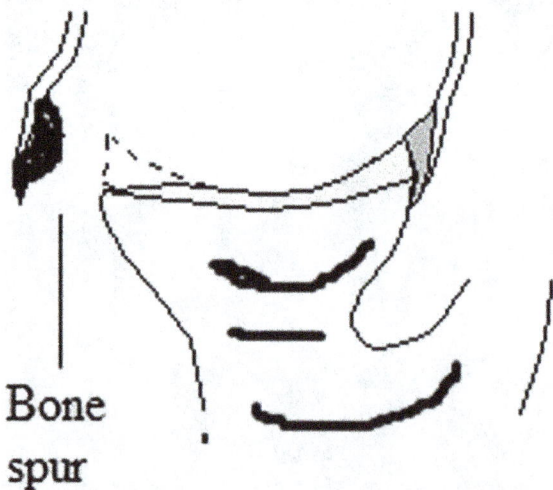

Fig. 4 Traditional radiological images method for detection of the Bankart or bony Bankart lesions. Images were checked by two radiologists. A small bone spur in traditional radiological images of the shoulder was considered as the Bankart or bony Bankart lesions present

Table 4 Reliability of assessments

Parameters	Overall Clinical examination tests	The traditional radiological images	Computed Tomography
Sample size	145	145	145
Evaluators	Physiotherapists	Orthopedic surgeons	[a]Engineers trained in musculoskeletal imaging
Tested Material	Shoulders of subjects	Traditional radiological images	Computed Tomography images
Numbers of evaluators	2	2	2
Numbers of test/images performed	4	1	1
Numbers of test/images analyzed	4	2	2
Tool for decision making	1×1 table	Lightbox	CATIA V5R21 software
[b]The method adopted	Apprehension tests	A small bone spur in images	The glenoid ratio method (% missing area $\geq$ 20%)
kappa value	0.811	0.825	0.891

kappa value ≤ 0.4 low; 0.41–0.6 moderate; 0.61–0.8 substantial; and ≥ 0.81 perfect inter-and intra-observer reliabilities
[a]Diploma course in musculoskeletal imaging assessments in PR. China after MD radiology
[b]for decision making of the Bankart lesion

The costs of clinical examination tests, the traditional radiological images, clinical examination tests combining the traditional radiological images, and CT were 8.59 ± 0.59 \$/patient, 12.64 ± 1.21 \$/patient, 21.11 ± 1.68 \$/patient, and 47.65 ± 4.24 \$/patient respectively. The cost of CT examinations was higher than the clinical examination tests combining the traditional radiological images ($p < 0.0001$, $q = 95.05$, Fig. 8).

After surgeries radiographs showed the union of the grafts and no incidents of re-dislocation during the follow-up period (Fig. 9).

Discussion

In the study, clinical examination tests alone were not provided sufficient information and surgeons were preferred radiological images for decision making of surgeries. There are high varieties of diagnostic modalities available for diagnosis of the instability of shoulders. Among the available methods, apprehension tests are the most frequently used combing traditional radiological images [24]. The Bankart and bony Bankart lesions are difficult to diagnose and there are more chances for failure of surgical procedures [25] because of the low sensitivity of radiological modalities [23]. Moreover, the adoption of the diagnostic method before the surgical procedure for the repair of the bony problem(s) of the shoulder is based on a number of dislocations and prior shoulder trauma [13]. The results of the study were not in line with an available study [13] but in line with the review article [26]. Clinical examination tests combing traditional radiological images

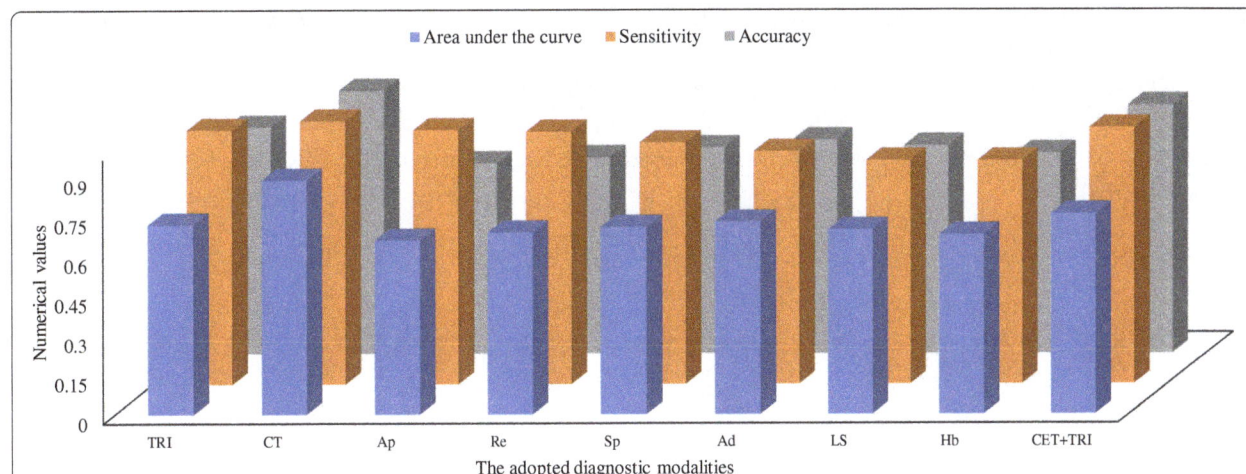

Fig. 6 The analogy of diagnostic modalities for decision making of surgeries of the Bankart and bony Bankart lesions. Accuracy and sensitivity of Computed Tomography were considered as 1. One-way repeated-measures ANOVA following Dunnett Multiple comparisons tests was used for statistical analysis. A p-value < 0.01 and q-value > 4.148 were considered significant. TRI: The traditional radiological images, CT: The Computed Tomography, Ap: Apprehension test, Re: Relocation test, Sp: Surprise test, Ad: Anterior drawer test, LS: Load and shift test, Hb: Hyperabduction test, CET + TRI: Clinical examination tests combining the traditional radiological images

Table 5 Parameters of the adopted diagnostic methods for evaluation of the Bankart and bony Bankart lesions

Parameters	CET						TRI (7)	CET + TRI (9)	CT (10)	SA 9 vs. 10	
	Ap (1)	Re (2)	Sp (3)	Ad (4)	LS (5)	Hb (6)					
Sample size	145	145	145	145	145	145	145	145	145	p	q
BL present	77 (53)	81 (56)	87 (60)	93 (64)	91 (62)	88 (60)	99 (69)	108 (75)	114 (78)	0.136	N/A
BL absent	23 (16)	22 (15)	21 (15)	19 (13)	18 (12)	17 (12)	20 (14)	22 (15)	24 (17)	0.792	N/A
F (+ve)	36 (25)	31 (21)	19 (13)	9 (6)	6 (4)	8 (6)	15 (10)	6 (4)	5 (3)	0.056	N/A
F (−ve)	3 (2)	4 (3)	5 (3)	7 (5)	8 (6)	9 (6)	6 (4)	4 (3)	1 (1)	0.057	N/A
I/C	6 (4)	7 (5)	13 (9)	17 (12)	22 (16)	23 (16)	5 (3)	5 (3)	1 (1)	0.0286	N/A
AUC	0.66 ± 0.08	0.69 ± 0.05	0.71 ± 0.08	0.73 ± 0.04	0.71 ± 0.07	0.68 ± 0.06	0.72 ± 0.1	0.76 ± 0.11	0.89 ± 0.14	< 0.0001	9.39
Sensitivity	0.91 ± 0.16	0.96 ± 0.06	0.917 ± 0.15	0.88 ± 0.08	0.85 ± 0.08	0.68 ± 0.07	0.97 ± 0.15	0.972 ± 0.18	1	0.11	N/A
Accuracy	0.72 ± 0.15	0.75 ± 0.07	0.78 ± 0.05	0.811 ± 0.18	0.79 ± 0.09	0.76 ± 0.07	0.86 ± 0.14	0.942 ± 0.17	1	< 0.0001	3.88

Constant data are represented as number (percentage)

Surgery curative was considered as 'gold standard'

Chi-square independence test for constant data and One-way repeated-measures ANOVA following Dunnett Multiple comparisons tests for continuous data were used for statistical analysis

A p-value < 0.01 was considered significant

A q-value > 4.148 was considered significant

N/A Not applicable, *BL* Accurate the Bankart and bony Bankart lesions, *I/C* Inconclusive results, *AUC* Area under the curve, *Ap* Apprehension test, *Re* Relocation test, *Sp* Surprise test, *Ad* Anterior drawer test, *LS* Load and shift test, *Hb* Hyperabduction test, *TRI* The traditional radiological images, *CET* Clinical Examination Tests, *CET + TRI* Clinical Examination Tests combining the traditional radiological images, *CT* The Computed Tomography, *SA* Statistical analysis

F (+ve): False positive: The Bankart and/or bony Bankart lesions had found in diagnosis, which was led to surgery and actually it was the other bony problem

F (−ve): False negative: A bony problem had found in diagnosis, which was lead arthroscopy or open surgical procedure and actually it was the Bankart and/or bony Bankart lesions

have limited information to guide the surgeons in the decision making of surgeries for repair of the bony problem(s) of the shoulder [15]. In respect to the decisions of surgeons during the study, clinical examination tests combing traditional radiological images are failed in finding limitations of CT for quantification of the Bankart and bony Bankart lesions.

In the study, CT was provided the best visualization and clinical examination tests combing traditional radiological images were provided insufficient details of the Bankart and bony Bankart lesions for decision making of surgeries. This was because clinical examination tests combing traditional radiological images are failed to provide exact loss of the inferior glenoid [27]. These results were in line with available diagnostic studies [3, 28]. A retrospective study [29], literature reviews [4, 5, 25, 27], and a simulated study [30] are also concluded the same. But the published study is on fewer subjects (sample size: 70) [3] and more numbers of observers (four observers) [3, 28], which have less intra-observer and inter-observer reliabilities [22]. However, the results were not in line with the quantitative assessment of radiography and CT [30]. In respect to the results of the twin study, CT assessments have good agreements for decision making of surgeries of the Bankart and bony Bankart lesions.

Table 6 Performance parameters results of the adopted diagnostic methods for evaluation of the Bankart and bony Bankart lesions

Diagnostic modalities	True positive the Bankart and bony Bankart lesions ratio	False positive the Bankart and bony Bankart lesions ratio
Computed Tomography	0.79	0.03
Traditional radiology	0.68	0.10
Without diagnosis images	0.6	0.2
Apprehension test	0.53	0.25
Relocation test	0.56	0.21
Surprise test	0.6	0.13
Anterior drawer test	0.64	0.06
Load and shift test	0.63	0.04
Hyperabduction test	0.61	0.06
Clinical Examination Tests combining the traditional radiological images	0.75	0.15

Table 7 Beneficial score analysis of the adopted diagnostic methods for evaluation of the Bankart and bony Bankart lesions

CP	WF	CT	TRI	WDC	CET						CET + TRI
					Ap	Re	Sp	Ad	LS	Hb	
0	0	0.79	0.68	0.6	0.53	0.56	0.6	0.64	0.63	0.61	0.75
0.1	0.11	0.78	0.67	0.58	0.50	0.53	0.59	0.63	0.62	0.60	0.73
0.2	0.25	0.78	0.66	0.55	0.47	0.51	0.57	0.63	0.62	0.59	0.71
0.3	0.43	0.77	0.64	0.51	0.43	0.47	0.54	0.61	0.61	0.58	0.68
0.4	0.67	0.76	0.61	0.47	0.37	0.42	0.51	0.60	0.60	0.57	0.64
0.5	1	0.75	0.58	0.4	0.28	0.35	0.47	0.60	0.59	0.55	0.59
0.6	1.5	0.74	0.53	0.3	0.16	0.24	0.40	0.55	0.57	0.52	0.51
0.7	2.33	0.71	0.44	0.13	−0.05	0.06	0.29	0.50	0.53	0.48	0.38
0.8	4	0.65	0.27	−0.2	−0.46	−0.3	0.08	0.39	0.46	0.39	0.12
0.9	9	0.48	−0.24	−1.2	−1.70	−1.37	−0.58	0.082	0.26	0.11	−0.67
0.99	99	−2.58	−9.51	−19.2	−24.05	−20.61	−12.37	−5.50	−3.47	−4.86	−14.82

CP A level of diagnostic confidence above its arthroscopy or opens surgical procedure had performed, *WF* Weighting factor (risk of overdiagnosis), *CT* The Computed Tomography, *TRI* The traditional radiological images, *Ap* Apprehension test, *Re* Relocation test, *Sp* Surprise test, *Ad* Anterior drawer test, *LS* Load and shift test, *Hb* Hyperabduction test, *CET* Clinical examination tests, *CET + TRI* Clinical examination tests combining the traditional radiological images, *WDC* Without diagnosis images or Clinical Examination Tests

Weighting factor $= \frac{\text{A level of diagnostic confidence above its arthroscopy or opens surgical procedure had performed}}{1 - \text{A level of diagnostic confidence above its arthroscopy or opens surgical procedure had performed}}$

Decision making of the Bankart and bony Bankart lesions = True positive ratio − (weighting factor × false positive ratio)

CT method was the increased financial burden of the patients. The traditional radiological images and clinical examination tests are cheaper than CT for diagnosis of the Bankart and bony Bankart lesions. However, CT has also prevented the future recurrence and/or failure of surgeries by exact diagnosis [3]. Further research is required to justify the selection of CT for the diagnosis of the Bankart and bony Bankart lesions.

In the limitations of the study, for examples, the study was limited to diagnose the Bankart and bony Bankart lesions only no other type of shoulder

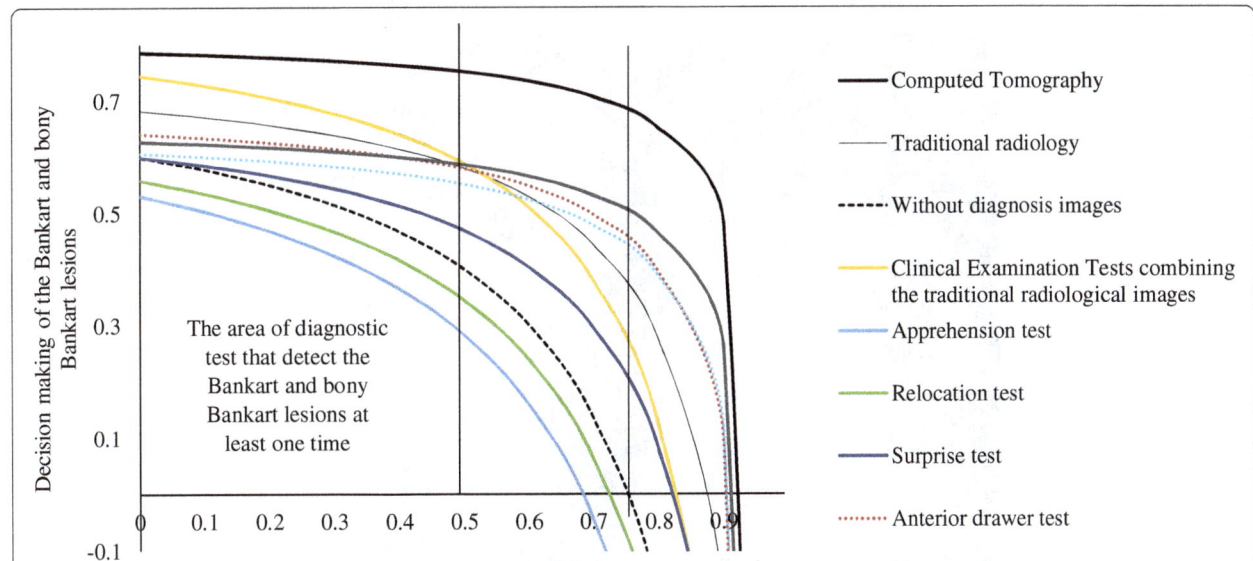

Fig. 7 Decision-making curve analysis for detection of the Bankart and bony Bankart lesions. Radiological images were checked by two radiologists. The Computed Tomographic images were checked by two engineers (diploma course in musculoskeletal imaging assessments in PR. China after MD radiology) trained in musculoskeletal imaging. Two physiotherapists evaluated clinical examination tests twice

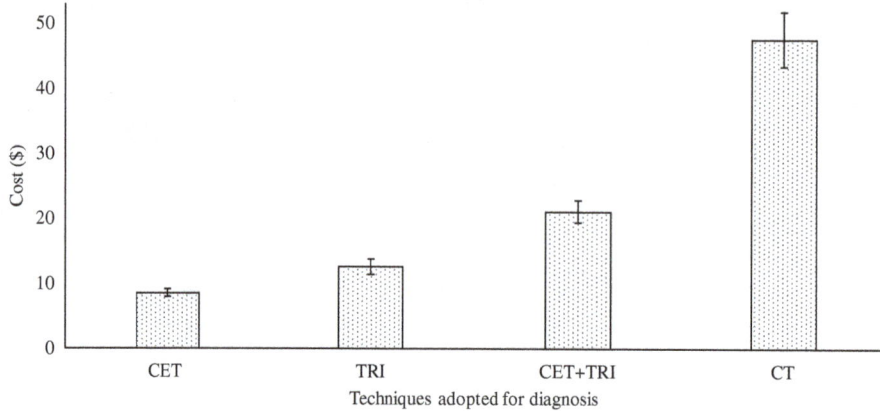

Fig. 8 Costs of techniques for the diagnosis of the Bankart and bony Bankart lesions. CET: Clinical examination tests, TRI: The traditional radiological images, CET + TRI: Clinical examination tests combining the traditional radiological images, CT: The Computed Tomography. Data were represented as mean ± SD. Patients enrolled in the study (sample size: n): 145. One-way ANOVA following the Dunnett Multiple comparisons tests was used for statistical analysis. A p-value < 0.01 and q-value > 4.148 were considered significant

delocalization was addressed in the study. The study was not differentiated the Bankart and bony Bankart lesions. The evaluators of clinical examination tests were not blind to the demographic parameters of the enrolled patients. Imaging modalities like CT arthrography, MRI, MRI arthrography provide better soft tissue details compare to CT alone. The lack of 'gold standard' or further MRI. The possible justification is that further MRI only for head-to-head comparisons of diagnostic methods is vague in clinical practice. Therefore, researchers have not performed Further MRI.

Conclusion
The study concluded that the Computed Tomography has better performance parameters than clinical examination tests combining the traditional radiological images and should be considered for evaluation in patients with shoulder instability and the suspected Bankart and bony Bankart lesions.

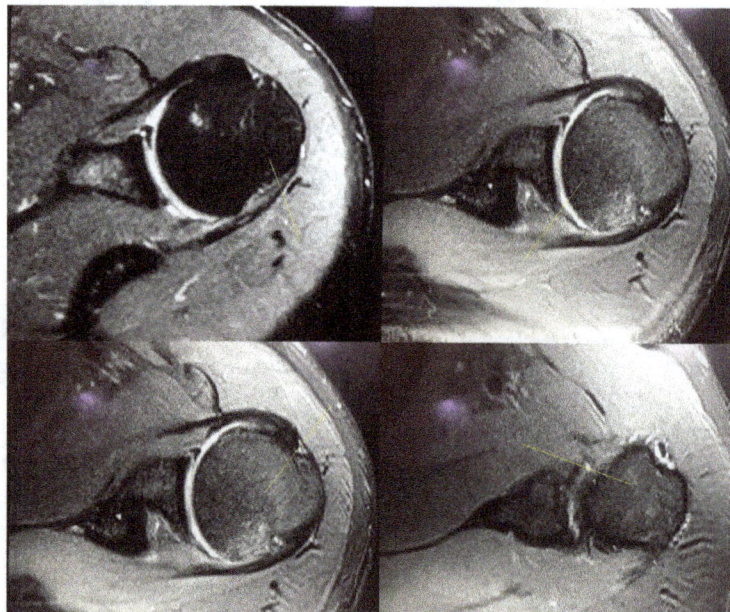

Fig. 9 Postsurgical radiographic images of 29-years female patient with shoulder instability showed the union of the grafts during follow-up. Supine view. The yellow line indicates the union of the Bankart lesions

Abbreviations

ANOVA: Analysis of variance; CT: Computed Tomography; k: kappa value; MRI: Magnetic resonance imaging; STARD: Standards for reporting of diagnostic accuracy studies; STROCSS: The strengthening the reporting of cohort studies in surgery

Acknowledgments

Authors are like to thank for radiological, anesthetic, surgical, medical, and physiotherapist staff of PLA General Hospital, Beijing, China, Affiliated Hospital of Nantong University, Nantong Shi, China, and Dingbian County People's Hospital, Dingbian, China.

Funding

The research did not receive any specific financial motivation from government, non-government, or non-profitable sector to perform research.

Authors' contributions

All authors had read and approved a submission for publication. TL and JM contribute equally to conceptualization and methodology of the study. HC contributed to methodology, data curation, and formal analysis of the study. DH contributed to investigation, resources, and software of the study. LX was project administrator, contributed to data curation, the manuscript preparation, the manuscript editing, and the manuscript review for the intellectual content. The author agrees to be accountable for all aspects of work ensuring integrity and accuracy.

Consent for publication

The enrolled patients signed an informed consent form regarding the publication of the study including patients' personal images (if any) in all formats (hard and/or electronics) irrespective of time and language.

Competing interests

Authors have reported that they have no commercial or associated interest that represents a conflict of interest in connection with results and/or discussion reported the submitted manuscript.

Author details

[1]Department of Medical Imaging, Affiliated Hospital of Nantong University, Shi, Jiangsu Sheng, Nantong 226001, China. [2]Department of Magnetic Resonance Imaging, Dingbian County People's Hospital, Dingbian, Yulin 718600, Shaanxi, China. [3]Department of Radiology, PLA general hospital, No.28 Fuxing Road, Haidian District, Beijing 100000, China.

References

1. Antunes JP, Mendes A, Prado MH, Moro OP, Miro RL. Arthroscopic Bankart repair for recurrent shoulder instability: a retrospective study of 86 cases. J Orthop. 2016;13:95–9.
2. Auffarth A, Mayer M, Kofler B, Hitzl W, Bogner R, Moroder P, Korn G, Koller H, Resch H. The interobserver reliability in diagnosing osseous lesions after first-time anterior shoulder dislocation comparing plain radiographs with computed tomography scans. J Shoulder Elb Surg. 2013;22:1507–13.
3. Delage RA, Balg F, Bouliane MJ, Canet-Silvestri F, Garant-Saine L, Sheps DM, Lapner P, Rouleau DM. Indication for computed tomography scan in shoulder instability: sensitivity and specificity of standard radiographs to predict bone defects after traumatic anterior glenohumeral instability. Orthop J Sports Med. 2017;5. https://doi.org/10.1177/2325967117733660.
4. Auffarth A, Matis N, Koller H, Resch H. An alternative technique for the exact sizing of glenoid bone defects. Clin Imaging. 2012;36:574–6.
5. Skupinski J, Piechota MZ, Wawrzynek W, Maczuch J, Babinska A. The bony Bankart lesion: how to measure the glenoid bone loss. Pol J Radiol. 2017;82: 58–63.
6. Weel H, Tromp W, Krekel PR, Randelli P, van den Bekerom MP, van Deurzen DF. International survey and surgeon's preferences in diagnostic work-up towards treatment of anterior shoulder instability. Arch Orthop Trauma Surg. 2016;136:741–6.
7. Ho AG, Gowda AL, Michael WJ. Evaluation and treatment of failed shoulder instability procedures. J Orthopaed Traumatol. 2016;17:187–97.
8. Wang L, Liu Y, Su X, Liu S. A meta-analysis of arthroscopic versus open repair for treatment of bankart lesions in the shoulder. Med Sci Monit. 2015; 21:3028–35.
9. Bois AJ, Fening SD, Polster J, Jones MH, Miniaci A. Quantifying glenoid bone loss in anterior shoulder instability: reliability and accuracy of 2-dimensional and 3-dimensional computed tomography measurement techniques. Am J Sports Med. 2012;40:2569–77.
10. Provencher MT, Bhatia S, Ghodadra NS, Grumet RC, Bach BR Jr, Dewing CB, LeClere L, Romeo AA. Recurrent shoulder instability: current concepts for evaluation and management of glenoid bone loss. J Bone Joint Surg Am. 2010;92:133–51.
11. Hendry JH, Simon SL, Wojcik A, Sohrabi M, Burkart W, Cardis E, Laurier D, Tirmarche M, Hayata I. Human exposure to high natural background radiation: what can it teach us about radiation risks? J Radiol Prot. 2009;29: A29–42.
12. Agha RA, Borrelli MR, Vella-Baldacchino M, Thavayogan R, Orgill DP, STROCSS Group. The STROCSS statement: strengthening the reporting of cohort studies in surgery. Int J Surg. 2017;46:198–202.
13. van Kampen DA, van den Berg T, van der Woude HJ, Castelein RM, Terwee CB, Willems WJ. Diagnostic value of patient characteristics, history, and six clinical tests for traumatic anterior shoulder instability. J Shoulder Elb Surg. 2013;22:1310–9.
14. van der Linde JA, van Kampen DA, van Beers LW, van Deurzen DF, Terwee CB, Willems WJ. The Oxford shoulder instability score; validation in Dutch and first-time assessment of its smallest detectable change. J Orthop Surg Res. 2015;10. https://doi.org/10.1186/s13018-015-0286-5.
15. Kumar K, Makandura M, Leong NJ, Gartner L, Lee CH, Ng DZ, Tan CH, Kumar VP. Is the apprehension test sufficient for the diagnosis of anterior shoulder instability in young patients without magnetic resonance imaging (MRI)? Ann Acad Med Singap. 2015;44:178–84.
16. Ebrahimzadeh MH, Moradi A, Zarei AR. Minimally invasive modified latarjet procedure in patients with traumatic anterior shoulder instability. Asian J Sports Med. 2015;6. https://doi.org/10.5812/asjsm.26838.
17. Lizzio VA, Meta F, Fidai M, Makhni EC. Clinical evaluation and physical exam findings in patients with anterior shoulder instability. Curr Rev Musculoskelet Med. 2017;10:434–41.
18. Park JY, Kim Y, Oh KS, Lim HK, Kim JY. Stress radiography for clinical evaluation of anterior shoulder instability. J Shoulder Elb Surg. 2016;25: e339–47.
19. Morita W, Tasaki A. Intra- and inter-observer reproducibility of shoulder laxity tests: comparison of the drawer, modified drawer and load, and shift tests. J Orthop Sci. 2018;23:57–63.
20. Barchilon VS, Kotz E, Barchilon Ben-Av M, Glazer E, Nyska M. A simple method for quantitative evaluation of the missing area of the anterior glenoid in anterior instability of the glenohumeral joint. Skelet Radiol. 2008;37:731–6.
21. Fitzgerald M, Saville BR, Lewis RJ. Decision curve analysis. JAMA. 2015;13: 409–10.
22. Dixon SN, Donner A, Shoukri MM. Adjusted inference procedures for the interobserver agreement in twin studies. Stat Methods Med Res. 2016;25: 1260–71.
23. Thomazeau H, Courage O, Barth J, Veillard D, Boileau P, Society FA. Can we improve the indication for Bankart arthroscopic repair? A preliminary clinical study using the ISIS score. Orthop Traumatol Surg Res. 2010;96:S77–88.
24. Bushnell BD, Creighton RA, Herring MM. Bony instability of the shoulder. Arthroscopy. 2008;24:1061–73.

25. Arciero RA, Parrino A, Bernhardson AS, Diaz-Doran V, Obopilwe E, Cote MP, Golijanin P, Mazzocca AD, Provencher MT. The effect of a combined glenoid and hill-Sachs defect on glenohumeral stability: a biomechanical cadaveric study using 3-dimensional modeling of 142 patients. Am J Sports Med. 2015;43:1422–9.

26. Hanchard NC, Lenza M, Handoll HH, Takwoingi Y. Physical tests for shoulder impingements and local lesions of bursa, tendon or labrum that may accompany impingement. Cochrane Database Syst Rev. 2013. https://doi.org/10.1002/14651858.CD00742.

27. Sugaya H. Techniques to evaluate glenoid bone loss. Curr Rev Musculoskelet Med. 2014;7:1–5.

28. Milano G, Saccomanno MF, Magarelli N, Bonomo L. Analysis of agreement between computed tomography measurements of glenoid bone defects in anterior shoulder instability with and without comparison with the contralateral shoulder. Am J Sports Med. 2015;43:2918–26.

29. Loh B, Lim JB, Tan AH. Is clinical evaluation alone sufficient for the diagnosis of a Bankart lesion without the use of magnetic resonance imaging? Ann Transl Med. 2016;4. https://doi.org/10.21037/atm.2016.11.22.

30. Itoi E, Lee SB, Amrami KK, Wenger DE, An KN. Quantitative assessment of classic anteroinferior bony Bankart lesions by radiography and computed tomography. Am J Sports Med. 2013;31:112–1128.

17

Reliability of computed tomography measurements in assessment of thigh muscle cross-sectional area and attenuation

Sören Strandberg[1], Marie-Louise Wretling[1], Torsten Wredmark[2], Adel Shalabi[1*]

Abstract

Background: Advancement in technology of computer tomography (CT) and introduction of new medical imaging softwares enables easy and rapid assessment of muscle cross-sectional area (CSA) and attenuation. Before using these techniques in clinical studies there is a need for evaluation of the reliability of the measurements. The purpose of the study was to evaluate the inter- and intra-observer reliability of ImageJ in measuring thigh muscles CSA and attenuation in patients with anterior cruciate ligament (ACL) injury by computer tomography.

Methods: 31 patients from an ongoing study of rehabilitation and muscle atrophy after ACL reconstruction were included in the study. Axial CT images with slice thickness of 10 mm at the level of 150 mm above the knee joint were analyzed by two investigators independently at two times with a minimum of 3 weeks between the two readings using NIH ImageJ. CSA and the mean attenuation of individual thigh muscles were analyzed for both legs.

Results: Mean CSA and mean attenuation values were in good agreement both when comparing the two observers and the two replicates. The inter- and intraclass correlation (ICC) was generally very high with values from 0.98 to 1.00 for all comparisons except for the area of semimembranosus. All the ICC values were significant (p < 0,001). Pearson correlation coefficients were also generally very high with values from 0.98 to 1.00 for all comparisons except for the area of semimembranosus (0.95 for intraobserver and 0.92 for interobserver).

Conclusion: This study has presented ImageJ as a method to monitor and evaluate CSA and attenuation of different muscles in the thigh using CT-imaging. The method shows an overall excellent reliability with respect to both observer and replicate.

Background

Injury of the anterior cruciate ligament (ACL) is a common injury especially in younger people involved in different kinds of sport activity [1,2]. It is well known that atrophy of the quadriceps femoris muscle is linked to disuse both pre- as well as postsurgical in patients with ACL and/or meniscal damage. Several strategies for treatment, both conservative and surgical, have been used [3]. Different surgical strategies have been applied and there is still an ongoing development of the surgical techniques [2,4]. For evaluation of outcome and follow-up there is a need for a reliable method for measuring muscle size. There is also a need for evaluating of atrophy of the different muscles of the thigh especially as some of the techniques involve the use of grafts either from gracilis and/or semitendinosus tendons or the use of Bone-Patellar Tendon-Bone (BTB) graft. Improvements in digital imaging and imaging software have made it possible to perform such measurements easily. However, it is important to ensure that there is a good reproducibility. In an ongoing study of the outcome of ACL-surgery we had the ethics committee approvement to perform CT examinations and we therefore decided to use these examinations to evaluate the reliability of one method.

Many different methods both radiological and others have been used for evaluation of body composition. A review of the different methods was published by

* Correspondence: adel.shalabi@ki.se
[1]Department of Radiology, Karolinska University Hospital, Karolinska Institutet, Stockholm, Sweden
Full list of author information is available at the end of the article

Mattson and Thomas in 2006 [5]. The methods used to evaluate cross-sectional area (CSA) of skeletal muscle are mainly computer tomography (CT), magnetic resonance imaging (MRI) and ultrasonography (US). There are some studies comparing two or all three of these methods, some of them also correlating the measurements with anatomical studies [6-8]

Several methods have been used to measure CSA. Most of the studies have used some kind of planimetry where the borders of the muscles are manually traced. Some have used the CT-scanners' own computer to measure the area within certain limits of attenuation. Steiger et al [9] have developed an autocontouring technique which semiautomatically delineates the muscles. Lemieux et al [10] have used a technique with imaging densitometer used on X-ray films.

Since the first CT-studies there has been a rapid improvement of the CT-scanners. The image acquisition is much faster and the images have a higher spatial resolution often with a lower radiation dose. The use of new medical imaging softwares, which made it possible to measure areas within specified attenuation limits, has made it possible to exclude interspersed adipose tissue which was generally not possible when CSA was measured with planimetry. Moreover it makes it easy to record the mean attenuation, which reflects functionality of the muscle. The software used in this study, ImageJ, is a free-ware open-source medical imaging software which can run on major computer operating systems. It can be used for images stored in DICOM standard which makes it independent on the CT-scanner used. In this study CSA and attenuation for the individual muscles in the thigh were measured from CT-examinations with ImageJ, which to our knowledge has not been done before.

The aim of the study was to evaluate the inter- and intraobserver reliability of ImageJ in measuring thigh muscles CSA and attenuation in patients with ACL injury by CT.

Methods
To evaluate the measuring method we used subjects selected from an already existent study of rehabilitation and muscle atrophy after ACL-reconstruction with semitendinosus and gracilis tendon graft. The Ethics Committee at the Karolinska Institutet approved the design of the study, and the patients gave their informed consent of the planned procedures. For our reliability study we included the first 31 examined patients (22 men and 9 women). The median age of these patients was 27 years with a range from 16 to 45 years. All the CT-examinations included in this study were performed before surgery.

Axial CT images were acquired at three levels. At the level of, as well as 50 mm and 150 mm above the knee joint with the patients in a supine position. For assessing the reproducibility it was, according to our opinion,

enough to evaluate the level of 150 mm above the knee joint which is best suited for evaluation of muscle CSA of the levels examined. The scans were performed by a Philips Tomoscan SR 7000 (single slice helical CT-scanner, 100 kV and 75 mAs) for 26 patients and with a Siemens Volume Zoom (4 slice MDCT-scanner, 120 kV and 40 mAs) for 5 patients. The use of two different CT-scannerswas due to change of equipment at our department during the study period. Slice thickness in all images was 10 mm. The images were saved as DICOM-images in the departments PACS-system for later analysis.

The images were analyzed by two investigators (MLW and SS) independently using NIH ImageJ version 1.38× software http://rsbweb.nih.gov/ij/ packages. All images were analyzed by both investigators at two times with a minimum of 3 weeks between the two readings.

Both the leg with the ACL-injury and the contralateral leg were analyzed. The muscles identified and measured were: quadriceps, sartorius, gracilis, semimembranosus, semitendinosus and biceps femoris. No attempt was made to separate the different parts of quadriceps (vastus medialis, vastus intermedius, vastus lateralis and rectus femoris) or the two heads of biceps femoris (caput longum and caput breve). Even when analyzing anatomical dissection in cadaver studies it is not always possible to separate the different parts of e.g. quadriceps [11]. On most of the images a small part of the muscles of the adductor group was also present but not measured.

CSA of the individual muscles was measured by outlining the borders of the muscles with the polygon selection tool. This was made after adjusting the image to level 50 and window width to 400 to obtain as good visual discrimination between adipose tissue and muscle as possible. CSA was measured as the area inside the borders with attenuation values from 1 to 101 Hounsfield units (HU) (figure 1). When outlining the borders we tried to avoid nerves and vessels as they have attenuation values within the chosen limits.

Apart from CSA the mean attenuation of the individual muscles was also measured. For some subjects the distribution of attenuation values between -29 HU to 150 HU was also registered to test the validity of the chosen limits of attenuation (figure 2). In this case a line was drawn just inside the border of the muscle to avoid volume averaging at the border affecting attenuation values.

To improve the speed of the process we used the ability of ImageJ to use self-defined macros that reduced the amount of clicking necessary for each measurement.

Statistical methods and data management
The test-retest reliability and the reliability based on the internal consistency was analyzed according to the method described by Bland and Altman, which yields inter- and intraclass correlation, ICC, [12,13]. The Pearson

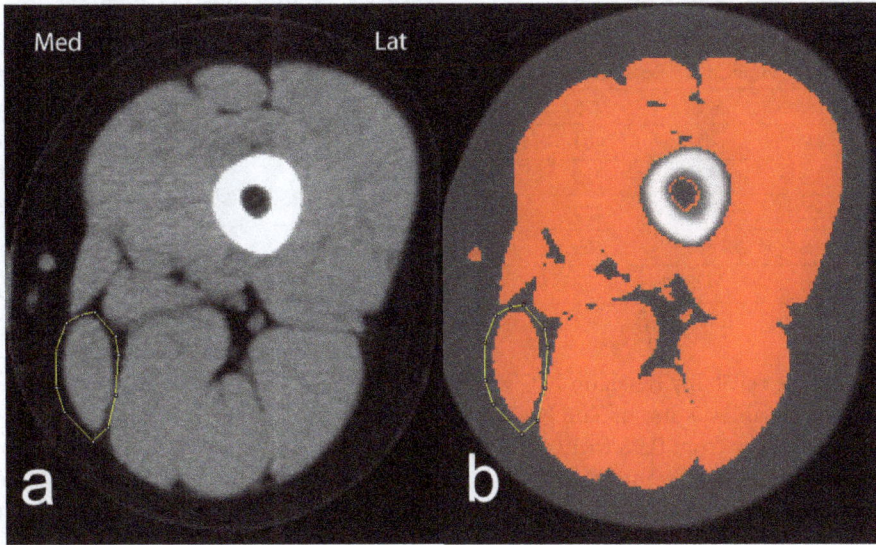

Figure 1 CT image of left thigh viewed with ImageJ. Musculus gracilis encircled. a) with level 50 HU and width 400 HU used when encircling the muscle and b) after highlighting areas with attenuation between 1 and 101 HU.

correlation coefficient was used in order to test independence between variables. In addition to that, descriptive statistics and graphical methods were used to characterize the data. All analyses were carried out by use of the SAS system, and the 5%-level of significance was considered.

Results

Tables 1 and 2 summarize the results for the different muscles with left and right side lumped together. This means that both the healthy side and the side affected by the ACL-injury are lumped together. The differences between the healthy and affected side will be the subject of a future study.

Mean CSA and mean attenuation values were in good agreement both when comparing the two observers and the two replicates but there was a difference between the different muscles with a slightly less good agreement for the area of semimembranosus.

The mean values combine men and women with different age, weight, physical condition and ACL-injury. The

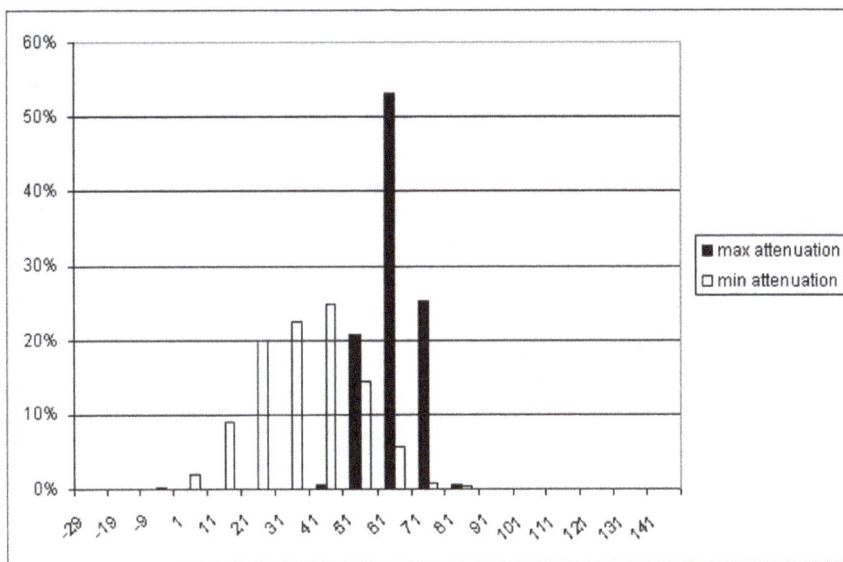

Figure 2 Relative distribution of attenuation values in HU of gracilis. Two examples chosen, with the highest and lowest mean attenuation included in the study respectively. Both are measured by drawing a line just inside the border of the muscle to avoid volume averaging at the border affecting the result.

Table 1 CSA of individual muscles (n = 62)

| | Observer 1 | | Observer 2 | |
	Replicate1	Replicate2	Replicate1	Replicate2
Quadriceps	5787	5784	5726	5705
Sartorius	404	403	404	404
Gracilis	323	322	323	323
Semimembranosus	1420	1422	1400	1420
Semitendinosus	609	609	603	603
Biceps femoris	1739	1739	1732	1741

Mean values in mm^2

test-retest reliability and the reliability based on ICC were analyzed and illustrated in tables 3 and 4. The ICC was generally very high with values from 0.98 to 1.00 for all comparisons except for the area of semimembranosus. All the ICC values were significant (p < 0,001).

The Pearson correlation coefficients were also generally very high with values from 0.98 to 1.00 for all comparisons except for the area of semimembranosus. The reliability can also be measured as coefficient of variation (CV). The mean intra-observer CV, both observers combined, was 0.93% for CSA and 0.23% for attenuation and the mean inter-observer CV, both replicates combined, was 1.61% for CSA and 0.42% for attenuation.

The inter- and intraobserver reliability is also illustrated with scatterplots given in figure 3 and figure 4.

Discussion

The main finding in the present study was the excellent overall reliability with respect to both observer and replicate in evaluation CSA and attenuation of different muscles in the thigh with the methods and equipment described above.

As noted above the method used in this study to evaluate muscle CSA and density gives results with very good reliability with respect both to inter- and intraobserver comparisons. When deciding the usefulness of the results it is also important to discuss the delimitation of muscle tissue and the interpretation of muscle density.

Table 2 Attenuation of individual muscles (n = 62)

| | Observer 1 | | Observer 2 | |
	Replicate1	Replicate2	Replicate1	Replicate2
Quadriceps	58,5	58,5	58,6	58,6
Sartorius	48,9	49,0	48,7	48,7
Gracilis	51,2	51,2	50,9	50,9
Semimembranosus	51,2	51,2	51,3	51,2
Semitendinosus	54,3	54,3	54,2	54,2
Biceps femoris	50,4	50,4	50,5	50,4

Mean values in HU

Table 3 Intraobserver reliability for area and attenuation (n = 62)

| | Observer 1 | | Observer 2 | |
	Area	Attenuation	Area	Attenuation
Quadriceps	1	1	0,997	0,998
Sartorius	0,999	0,999	0,994	0,999
Gracilis	0,999	0,999	0,996	0,997
Semimembranosus	0,999	0,999	0,944	0,998
Semitendinosus	1	0,999	0,996	0,995
Biceps femoris	0,999	1	0,984	0,999

ICC comparing replicate 1 and 2

The definition of "skeletal muscle" in terms of HU differs. Chowdhury et al [14] used -190 to -30 HU for adipose tissue and 152 to 2500 for skeleton and manually circumscribed other organs in the range from -29 to 152. The range of -29 to 150 for skeletal muscle has later been used for example by Mitsiopoulos et al [8] and Irving et al [15].

Kelley et al [16] used -200 to -1 for adipose tissue, 0 to 100 HU for "lean tissue" and >200 for bone. They introduced the concept of "low-density lean tissue" (LDLT) for the range 1-34 HU and measured "normal-density muscle" (NDM) between 35 and 100 HU. They discussed the nature of this LDLT as it in some respects differed from normal muscle. In obese subjects there was a marked increase in LDTD but not in NDM. They discussed the possibility that this LDLT could at least partly be another tissue comprising connective tissue elements but other findings suggested that it was mostly altered skeletal muscle with higher lipid content.

Goodpaster and colleagues have used the term "low-density muscle" (LDM) for tissue with attenuation between 0 and 30 HU in several works [17-19]. Relatively higher proportion of LDM is a typical finding in obese subjects and the lower attenuation is associated with increased lipid content in muscle tissue but CT examinations cannot differ between intracellular lipid deposits and extracellular deposits as far as they has a size smaller than the pixels of the CT image [20].

Table 4 Interobserver reliability for area and attenuation (n = 62)

| | Replicate1 | | Replicate2 | |
	Area	Attenuation	Area	Attenuation
Quadriceps	0,993	0,997	0,994	0,998
Sartorius	0,990	0,996	0,994	0,997
Gracilis	0,992	0,992	0,995	0,992
Semimembranosus	0,970	0,997	0,922	0,997
Semitendinosus	0,985	0,994	0,988	0,995
Biceps femoris	0,985	0,998	0,992	0,998

ICC comparing observer 1 and 2

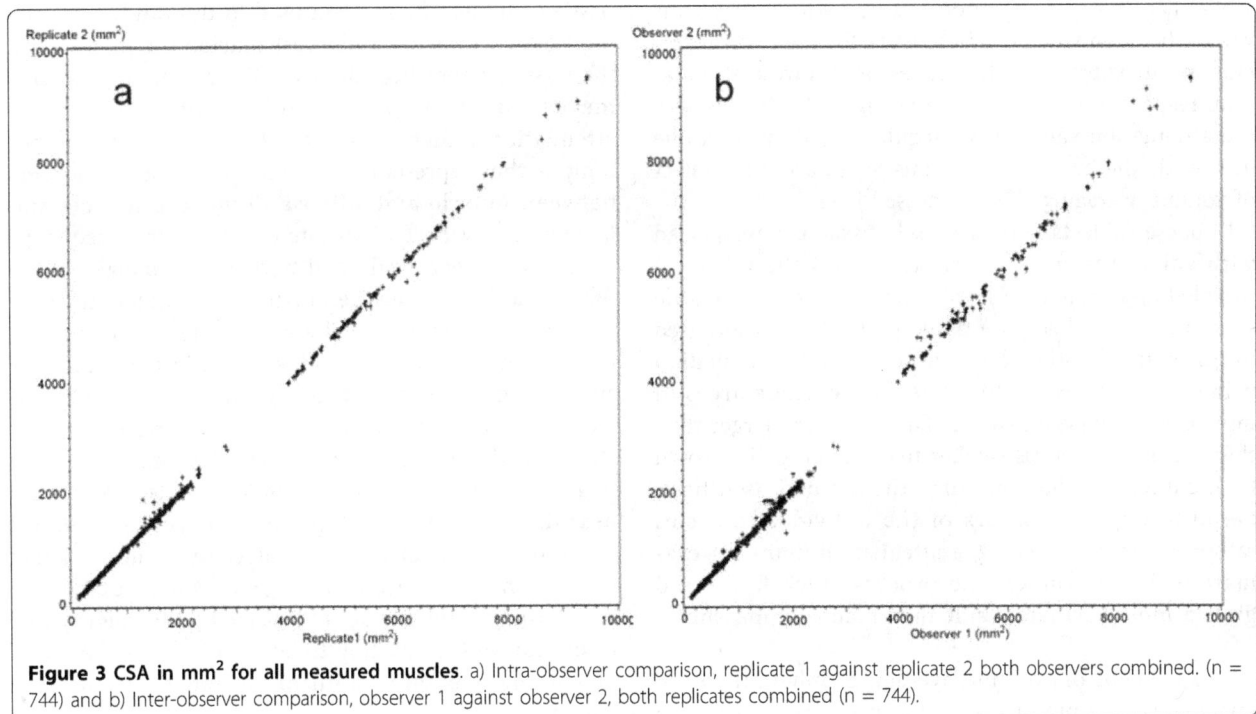

Figure 3 CSA in mm² for all measured muscles. a) Intra-observer comparison, replicate 1 against replicate 2 both observers combined. (n = 744) and b) Inter-observer comparison, observer 1 against observer 2, both replicates combined (n = 744).

Probably other factors have an effect on attenuations as well for example perfusion and difference in intra- and extracellular water content.

Reduced skeletal muscle attenuation is a typical finding in obese subjects but it is also associated with atrophy in for example rotator cuff muscles [21] and hip and knee muscles in osteoarthritis [22] where it is an independent factor apart from reduced muscular CSA, associated with reduced strength.

In this study we used attenuation from 1 to 101 HU for the measurements of the muscles. This included both LDM and NDM as defined by Goodpaster et al

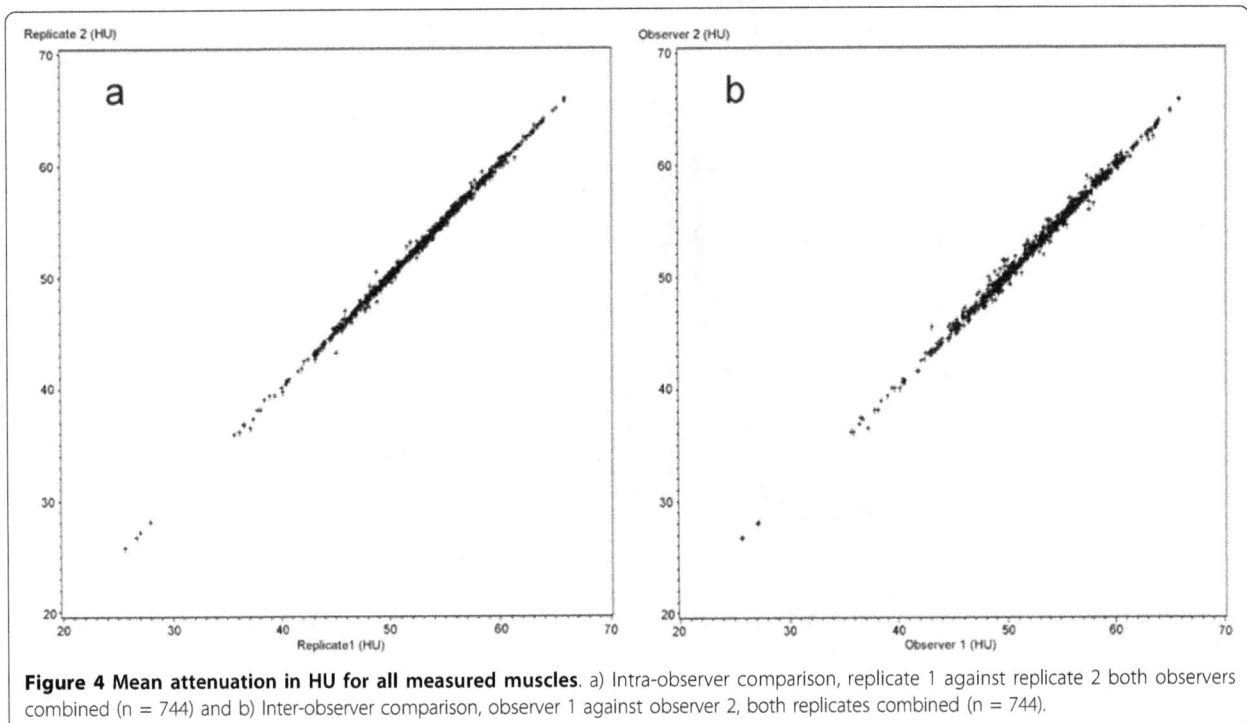

Figure 4 Mean attenuation in HU for all measured muscles. a) Intra-observer comparison, replicate 1 against replicate 2 both observers combined (n = 744) and b) Inter-observer comparison, observer 1 against observer 2, both replicates combined (n = 744).

1999 [17]. It was also supported by own observations where the attenuation characteristics for the two m. gracilis in our study with the highest and lowest attenuation, respectively, were compared (figure 2). In this case the attenuation values were acquired by drawing a line just inside the borders of the muscles to avoid the effect of volume averaging effect discussed later.

In obese subjects normal muscle tissue is interspersed with adipose tissue in a way that gives the muscle a marbled appearance. In lean subjects there is very little such interspersed adipose tissue [18]. The method used in this study, limiting the measured area to attenuation values between HU 1 to 101 would exclude areas of interspersed adipose tissue as far as they are larger than the pixel size but areas smaller than the pixel size would be included. At the same time the method used here, i.e. outlining the borders of the individual muscles rather roughly and then use attenuation limits for evaluation the area makes the process much faster and gives a more accurate result than manually measuring CSA.

The concept of "volume averaging" inherent to CT imaging, i.e. if a pixel (or actually voxel) includes tissues of different attenuations, the resulting attenuation value will be an average of the different tissues, will affect the measurements. If there is a lot of interspersed adipose tissue, it can affect the resulting mean attenuation. Volume averaging also affects the outer borders of the muscles. The muscles are mostly bordered by adipose

tissue or bone. The method used in this study, measuring CSA by drawing a line just outside the muscle and then using a specified range of HU to measure the area means that there will always be some pixels with attenuation values both at the lower and at the upper limit as they represent volume averaging at the borders between muscle and adipose tissue and muscle and bone respectively. To illustrate this, the same quadriceps muscle has been evaluated both in the usual way by drawing a line outside the muscle (i.e. including the borders) and by drawing a line just inside the borders of the muscle (i.e. excluding the borders). In both cases the attenuation has been evaluated from -29 HU to 150 HU and the relative distribution of attenuation values is shown in figure 5. As can be seen, the method used in this study (i.e. including the borders) adds some pixels near the lower and the upper limit but most additions are of pixels with attenuation values that will not affect CSA or the mean attenuation as they are outside the range used for muscle i.e. 1 to 101 HU. The high spatial resolution of CT-imaging today also reduces the effect of volume averaging both on attenuation and area measuring.

With lean subjects there is very little adipose tissue between the muscles which sometimes makes it difficult to delimit the individual muscles. This accounts for some of the variation of area measurements, although as shown by the very high correlation coefficients this is not a major problem. In case of semimembranosus, the

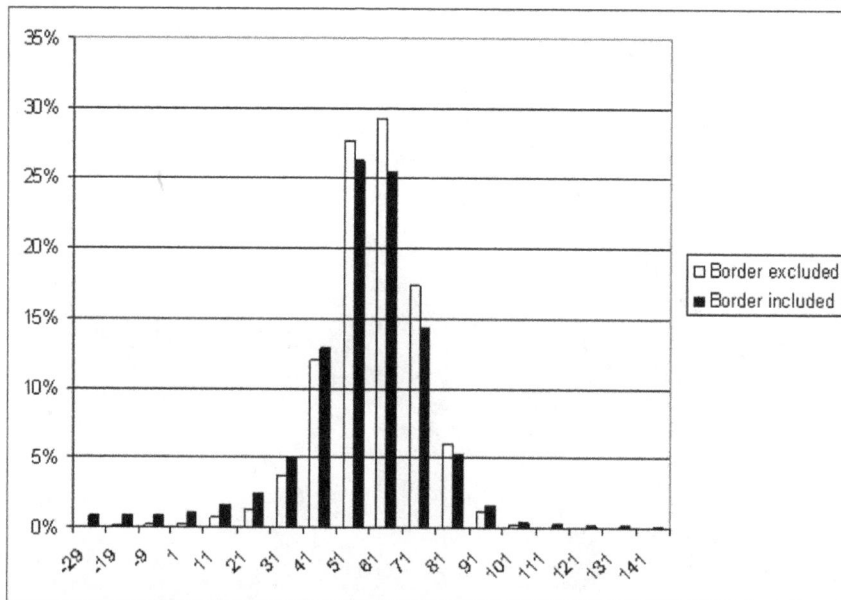

Figure 5 Relative distribution of attenuation values in HU for quadriceps. One example evaluated in two different ways by drawing a line just inside the border of the muscle (border excluded) and by drawing a line just outside the border of the muscle (border included) Relative distribution of attenuation values in HU for quadriceps One example evaluated in two different ways by drawing a line just inside the border of the muscle (border excluded) and by drawing a line just outside the border of the muscle (border included).

main reason for the slightly bigger differences is on the other hand probably that anatomical variation sometimes makes it difficult to delimit semimembranosus from the adductor muscles that are present in some of the patients at this level of the thigh. For longitudinal studies this problem could possibly be overcome by evaluating different examinations of the same patient at the same time.

To obtain reproducible results it is also important to control the time the patient remains in supine position as the change in hydrostatic pressure when the patient moves from upright to supine position has been shown to affect CSA and attenuation [23]. We have not standardized the time in supine position which is a limitation in our study. However, the examination time is generally short. Furthermore, a recent study showed that the effect of changing position can be minimized by examining the patient within 10 min from taking the supine position [24].

Another limitation of the study is that it was designed to test the reliability of measurements from a single set of CT images. Repeated examinations might introduce errors both from technical aspects of the CT-scanner and probably more important from the repositioning of the patient. However a study published by Goodpaster et al [20] has shown these errors to be small with a coefficient of variation for the measurement of attenuation of thigh muscle to be 0.51% We also believe that the use of two different CT-scanners does not effect the results in a significant way.

Not having made repeated examinations of the same patient at the same time is a weakness of this study but it was chosen mainly to keep the radiation dose to the patients low. In a planned longitudinal study of rehabilitation and muscle atrophy after ACL-surgery the contralateral thigh will serve as a control and thus at least reduce this problem.

Conclusion

This study has presented ImageJ as a method to monitor and evaluate CSA and attenuation of different muscles in the thigh using CT-imaging. It has proved to give excellent overall reliability with respect to both observer and replicate.

Author details
[1]Department of Radiology, Karolinska University Hospital, Karolinska Institutet, Stockholm, Sweden. [2]Department of Orthopaedic Surgery, Karolinska University Hospital, Karolinska Institutet, Stockholm, Sweden.

Authors' contributions
SS carried out measurements, participated in statistical analysis, drafted the manuscript. MLW participated in the design of the study, coordination of the examinations, carried out measurements and in drafting of the manuscript. TW participated in the design of the study and coordination of the patients. AS participated in the design of the study, coordination of the examinations and in drafting of the manuscript. All authors read and approved the final manuscript.

Competing interests
The authors declare that they have no competing interests.

References
1. Eriksson KO: **On the semitendinosus tendon in anterior cruciate ligament reconstructive surgery.** *PhD thesis* Karolinska Institutet, Stockholm 2001.
2. Marrale J, Morrissey M, Haddad F: **A literature review of autograft and allograft anterior cruciate ligament reconstruction.** *Knee Surg Sports Traumatol Arthrosc* 2007, 15:690-704.
3. Hurd W, Axe M, Snyder-Mackler L: **Management of the athlete with acute anterior cruciate ligament deficiency.** *Sports Health: A Multidisciplinary Approach* 2009, 1:39-46.
4. Aglietti P, Giron F, Losco M, Cuomo P, Ciardullo A, Mondanelli N: **Comparison between single-and double-bundle anterior cruciate ligament reconstruction: A prospective, randomized, single-blinded clinical trial.** *Am J Sports Med* 2010, 38:25-34.
5. Mattsson S, Thomas BJ: **Development of methods for body composition studies.** *Phys Med Biol* 2006, 51:203-228.
6. Beneke R, Neuerburg J, Bohndorf K: **Muscle cross-section measurement by magnetic resonance imaging.** *Eur J Appl Physiol* 1991, 63:424-429.
7. Engstrom CM, Loeb GE, Reid JG, Forrest WJ, Avruch L: **Morphometry of the human thigh muscles. A comparison between anatomical sections and computer tomographic and magnetic resonance images.** *J Anat* 1991, 176:139-156.
8. Mitsiopoulos N, Baumgartner RN, Heymsfield SB, Lyons W, Gallagher D, Ross R: **Cadaver validation of skeletal muscle measurement by magnetic resonance imaging and computerized tomography.** *J Appl Physiol* 1998, 85(1):115-122.
9. Steiger P, Block JE, Friedlander A, Genant HK: **Precise determination of paraspinous musculature by quantitative CT.** *J Comput Assist Tomogr* 1988, 12:616-620.
10. Lemieux S, Lesage M, Bergeron J, Prud'Homme D, Després JP: **Comparison of two techniques for measurement of visceral adipose tissue cross-sectional areas by computed tomography.** *Am J Hum Biol* 1999, 11:61-68.
11. Engstrom CM, Loeb GE, Reid JG, Forrest WJ, Avruch L: **Morphometry of the human thigh muscles. A comparison between anatomical sections and computer tomographic and magnetic resonance images.** *J Anat* 1991, 176:139-156.
12. Bland J, Altman D: **Statistical methods for assessing agreement between two methods of clinical measurement.** *Lancet* 1986, 1:307-310.
13. Bland J, Altman D: **Agreement between methods of measurement with multiple observations per individual.** *J Biopharm Stat* 2007, 17:571-582.
14. Chowdhury B, Sjöström L, Alpsten M, Kostanty J, Kvist H, Löfgren R: **A multicompartment body composition technique based on computerized tomography.** *Int J Obes Metab Disord* 1994, 18(4):219-234.
15. Irving BA, Weltman JY, Brock DW, Davis CK, Gaesser GA, Weltman A: **NIH ImageJ and Slice-o-matic computed tomography imaging software to quantify soft tissue.** *Obesity* 2007, 15:370-376.
16. Kelley DE, Slasky BS, Janosky J: **Skeletal muscle density: effects of obesity and non-insulin-dependent diabetes mellitus.** *Am J Clin Nut* 1991, 54:509-515.
17. Goodpaster BH, Kelley DE, Wing RR, Meier A, Thaete FL: **Effects of weight loss on regional fat distribution and insulin sensitivity in obesity.** *Diabetes* 1999, 48(4):839-847.
18. Goodpaster BH, Thaete FL, Kelley DE: **Thigh adipose tissue distribution is associated with insulin resistance in obesity and in type 2 diabetes mellitus.** *Am J Clin Nutr* 2000, 71(4):885-892.
19. Goodpaster BH, Thaete FL, Kelley DE: **Composition of skeletal muscle evaluated with computed tomography.** *Ann N Y Acad Sci* 2000, 904:18-24.
20. Goodpaster BH, Kelley DE, Thaete FL, He J, Ross R: **Skeletal muscle attenuation determined by computed tomography is associated with skeletal muscle lipid content.** *J Appl Physiol* 2000, 89(1):104-110.
21. Van de Sande MA, Stoel BC, Obermann WR, Tjong a Lieng JG, Rozing PM: **Quantitative assessment of fatty degeneration in rotator cuff muscles**

determined with computed tomography. *Invest Radiol* 2005,
40(5):313-319.

22. Rasch A, Byström AH, Dalen N, Berg HE: **Reduced muscle radiological
density, cross-sectional area, and strength of major hip and knee
muscles in 22 patients with hip osteoarthritis.** *Acta Orthop* 2007,
78(4):505-510.

23. Berg HE, Tedner B, Tesch PA: **Changes in lower limb muscle cross-
sectional area and tissue fluid volume after transition from standing to
supine.** *Acta Physiol Scand* 1993, **148(4)**:379-385.

24. Cerniglia LM, Delmonico MJ, Lindle R, Hurley BF, Rogers MA: **Effects of
acute supine rest on mid-thigh cross-sectional area as measured by
computed tomography.** *Clin Physiol Funct Imaging* 2007, **27(4)**:249-253.

18

Exposure of the Swiss population to computed tomography

Abbas Aroua[1*], Eleni-Theano Samara[1], François O Bochud[1], Reto Meuli[2] and Francis R Verdun[1]

Abstract

Background: The frequency of CT procedures has registered a significant increase over the last decade, which led at the international level to an increasing concern on the radiological risk associated with the use of CT especially in paediatrics. This work aimed at investigating the use of computed tomography in Switzerland, following the evolution of CT frequency and dose data over a decade and comparing it to data reported in other countries.

Methods: The frequency and dose data related to CT are obtained by means of a nationwide survey. National frequencies were established by projecting the collected data, using the ratio of the number of CT units belonging to the respondents to the total number of CT units in the country. The effective doses per examination were collected during an auditing campaign.

Results: In 2008 about 0.8 Million CT procedures (~ 100 CT examinations / 1000 population) were performed in the country, leading to a collective effective dose of more than 6000 man.Sv (0.8 mSv/caput). In a decade the frequency of CT examinations averaged over the population and the associated average effective dose per caput increased by a factor of 2.2 and 2.9 respectively.

Conclusions: Although the contribution of CT to the total medical X-rays is 6% in terms of the frequency, it represents 68% in terms of the collective effective dose. These results are comparable to those reported in a number of countries in Europe and America with similar health level.

Keywords: Diagnostic radiology, Computed tomography (CT), Medical radiation, X-rays, Population collective dose, Average effective dose

Background

Medical X-rays represent a major source of man-made irradiation of the population. In its 2010 Report, the United Nations Scientific Committee on the Effects of Atomic Radiation (UNSCEAR) indicated that although diagnostic radiology represents at the global level only 20% of the total annual per caput effective dose, it accounts for more than 94% of the man-made component [1]. In Switzerland diagnostic radiology was responsible in 2009 for 30% of the dose received by the population, but more that 92% of man-made irradiation [2]. This is why the exposure of the population by radiodiagnostics is periodically monitored (each 5–10 years) both at global and national level by UNSCEAR and national radiation protection authorities respectively. In Switzerland

this monitoring has been guaranteed for decades by the Federal Office of Public Health (FOPH) and delegated to a research institute [3-6].

The frequency of computed tomography (CT) procedures has registered a significant increase over the last decade. This is due not only to evolution of the demographics and the ageing of the population, but may be attributed also to the technology advance in CT devices, particularly the introduction of multi-slice CT, which opened a new field of vascular investigations and led to the change of medical practice by often replacing fluoroscopy guided procedures with CT scans and to the proliferation of CT units in emergency departments.

CT is now contributing significantly to the total collective dose due to medical X-rays. UNSCEAR [1] estimates the CT dose contribution for developed countries (health level I) to 47% during the period of the study (1997–2007), while recent works reported in six European

* Correspondence: abbas@aroua.com
[1]Institute of Radiation Physics, Lausanne University Hospital, Lausanne, Switzerland
Full list of author information is available at the end of the article

Table 1 2008 Swiss annual frequency and dose data for CT and all X-ray modalities (rounded values)

	CT	All X-ray modalities
Number of examinations (in thousands)	780	13'000
Number of examinations/1000 population	100	1700
Collective dose (man.Sv)	6150	9100
Effective dose/caput (mSv)	0.8	1.2

countries and the USA indicate CT dose contributions ranging from 46% up to 80% of the total collective dose for the years 2006 to 2008 [7-13]. In parallel to the widespread of CT, there has been an increasing concern at the international level on the radiological risk associated the use of this radiological modality especially in paediatrics reflected in scientific literature [14].

The aim of this work was to investigate the use of CT in Switzerland, to assess the evolution of this modality in terms of frequency of examinations and associated collective dose over the past decade and to compare the Swiss situation with other countries of similar health level.

Materials and methods

All healthcare providers running an X-ray unit in Switzerland were addressed. This corresponds to 8,247 practices, radiology institutes and hospital departments, and 17,391 X-ray units authorized by the Regulatory Authority (FOPH). The participants were requested to provide their frequencies of examinations for the year 2008 in paper form by post mail, or in electronic form by email or by registration online. For this purpose, a dedicated website was developed (www.raddose.ch).

The Dose Datamed methodology explained in the European Guidance No 154 [15] was used. The X-ray examinations were grouped into seven radiological modalities: radiography, conventional fluoroscopy, diagnostic interventional radiology, therapeutic interventional radiology, computed tomography, dental radiology, mammography, and bone densitometry. Concerning CT, the participants were asked to give the annual number of procedures related to over 50 types, or in case this was not possible, for about 20 broader categories. The participants were also allowed to provide data in their own format.

Table 3 CT examinations performed in different healthcare providers in 2008

Healthcare providers	N	Ratio
	(in thousands)	(%)
University hospitals	211	27.1
Canton hospitals	137	17.6
Regional hospitals and clinics	301	38.7
Radiology institutes	118	15.2
Dental clinics	11.5	1.5

The data received in local categories were redistributed over the reference categories.

National frequencies were established by projecting the collected data to the whole population. The results corresponding to the participants in the survey were multiplied by the ratio of the number of CT units belonging to the participants to the total number of CT units in the country. The projection was performed separately for each category of healthcare provider (hospitals, practices, radiology institutes).

The effective doses associated to CT procedures were reviewed in an auditing campaign [16]. The tissue weighting factors (w_T) provided by the International Commission on Radiological Protection in its Publication 60 [17] were used for the calculation of the effective dose. The effective dose was also calculated using w_T provided by ICRP Publication 103 [18], for the purpose of comparison. For CT modality, the new w_T resulted in a 2% increase of the collective dose. In the most recent investigation performed in the UK [9] a 2-3% decrease in the collective dose was registered for CT when using the new set of w_T.

It is important to note here that for this survey no CT scans associated to SPECT/CT examinations or PET/CT examinations were taken into account, as they will be considered in a specific survey dedicated to the dose delivered in nuclear medicine [19].

Results

The overall response rate was 45% in terms of number of X-ray units. It was 49% for radiology institutes and 63% for hospital departments.

Table 2 Frequency and dose data for the main CT examinations in terms of frequency and dose

	Number of procedures/1000 population	Effective dose (mSv)/ examination	Effective dose/ caput (mSv)
Full abdomen	19.7	11.7	0.230
Chest	13.1	5.4	0.708
Cerebrum	10.8	2.14	0.231
CT angiography	2.49	39	0.973

Table 4 Comparison of 2008 frequency and dose data with previous surveys

Year	Number of examinations/ 1000 population		N_{CT}/N_{Total}	E (mSv/caput)		E_{CT}/E_{Total}
	Total	CT	(%)	Total	CT	(%)
1998	1340	46.2	3.4	1.0	0.28	28
2003	1470	76.7	5.2	1.2	0.56	47
2008	1680	100	6.0	1.2	0.80	68

Table 5 2008/1998 CT frequency and dose ratios

Ratio	N/1000 population	E (mSv/caput)
2003/1998	1.66	2.00
2008/2003	1.32	1.43
2008/1998	2.19	2.86

Table 1 gives the frequency and dose data obtained in the survey concerning CT and all X-ray modalities. It shows the annual number of examinations performed in Switzerland in 2008 (7.7M population), the number per thousand population, as well as the associated annual collective dose and the average per caput effective dose. Over the 13 Million X-ray examinations performed 0.78 M are CT procedures, which corresponds to 6%. However, the CT contribution to the collective dose is revealed to be as high as 68%.

Table 2 lists the most frequent and/or most irradiating CT procedures and presents the associated frequency and dose data. Full abdomen (upper and lower parts) is the most frequent (19% of total number of CT examinations) and most irradiating (29% of total CT dose) procedure. Chest procedure is the second most frequent (13%) and the third most irradiating (9%) procedure. Cerebrum procedure comes as the third most frequent (11%) and CT angiography as the second most irradiating (12%) procedures. For the latter procedure, although the frequency is low, the relatively high effective dose per procedure (up to 40 mSv in cardiac CT for example) leads to a high contribution to the collective dose.

Table 3 shows the contribution of the different healthcare providers in terms of the frequency of CT procedures. Hospitals undertake 83.3% of the CT examinations, while radiology institutes perform 15.2% of the procedures. The remaining 1.5% is due to dental practices. Table 3 shows also that 11 big-size hospitals (university and canton) perform 44.7% while about 300 small-size hospitals and clinics (regional) perform

38.7 of the CT examinations. In terms of dose, hospitals are responsible of 83.5% and radiology institutes of 16.4% of the CT collective effective dose. The contribution of dental clinics is very low (0.1%).

Discussion

A study was conducted to assess the use of CT in Switzerland in the framework of a nationwide survey aiming at estimating the exposure of the population to medical X-rays. The 5–10 years periodic survey is a robust tool for radiation protection in medicine and the good response rates obtained guaranty statistically significant results.

Table 4 presents the number of all examinations and the number of CT examinations (/1000 population), the average effective dose due to radiodiagnostics and the average effective dose due to CT, for 1998 [4], 2003 [6] and 2008 [this work]. In one decade, the contribution of CT to the total medical X-rays increased from 3.4% to 6% in terms of the frequency and from 28% to 68% in terms of the collective effective dose.

Table 5 compares the CT frequency and dose data obtained in the present study with the data established in Switzerland in 1998 and 2003. Both the frequency of CT examinations and the associated collective effective dose registered a steady increase since 1998: respectively a factor of 2.2 and 2.9 in a decade. It should be noted that the increase was higher between 1998 and 2003 than between 2003 and 2008.

The increase in the number of CT examinations may be attributed partly to the 27% increase in the number of CT units in a decade (187 in 1998 and 238 in 2008), and partly to the technology advance in CT scanners that led to the change of medical practice with new indications for CT and the replacement of some fluoroscopy guided procedures with CT scans. In fact, the increase of the frequency of CT procedures is accompanied by a reduction in the number of diagnostic interventional

Table 6 Number of CT examinations (N_{CT}) and effective dose due to CT (E_{CT}) in various countries

Country	N_{CT} /1000 population	% of total number of X-ray examinations	E_{CT}/caput (mSv)	% of total effective dose	Reference
Switzerland (2008)	100	6	0.8	68	This work
France (2007)*	115	10	0.8	65	[7]
Germany (2008)	132	8	1.0	60	[8]
United Kingdom (2008)	53	7	0.3	67	[9]
The Netherlands (2008)	62	11	0.4	46	[10]
Norway (2008)**	194	29	0.9	80	[11]
Finland (2008)	60	8.3	0.3	58	[12]
USA (2006)	226	18	1.5	66	[13]
UNSCEAR (1997–2007)	129	8	0.9	47	[1]

* Therapeutic interventional procedures excluded.
** Dental radiology is excluded in the total frequency.

procedures and radiography [20]. On the other hand the increase of the average effective dose per caput is due not only to the increase of the frequency of CT examinations, but also to the increase of the average effective dose per CT procedure.

Table 6 compares the number of CT examinations per 1000 population and the per caput average effective dose due to CT in Switzerland and in other countries of similar health level. The Swiss frequency (100/1000 population) and per caput average effective dose (0.8 mSv) are comparable to the French ones (115/1000 population, 0.8 mSv) and to those reported by UNSCEAR for countries of health level I (129/1000 population, 0.9 mSv). They lay in the range of frequencies (53-226/1000 population) and the range effective doses (0.3-1.5 mSv) reported in other countries. Table 6 reveals 3 categories of countries: low, medium and high consumers of CT. The first category is represented by the UK, the Netherland and Finland, the second category by France, Germany, Switzerland and to some extent Norway, and the third one by the USA. Table 6 shows also the contribution of CT examinations to the total number of examinations and to the collective effective dose in Switzerland with that reported in other countries. It shows clearly that the same pattern observed in Switzerland is registered elsewhere: a 10-20% contribution in terms of frequencies is reflected into up to a 2/3 contribution in terms of collective effective dose. In the case of Norway the CT frequency contribution is even higher (29%), since dental radiology is not considered.

Conclusion

This investigation revealed that in 2008 the annual frequency of CT examinations performed in Switzerland was 0.78 Million, corresponding to 100 examinations per 1000 population. This is responsible for a collective effective dose of 6150 man.Sv or an average effective dose of 0.8 mSv/caput. From 1998 to 2008 the CT average frequency of examinations registered an increase of a factor 2.2 and the associated average effective dose increased by a factor 2.9. Computed tomography contributes 6% to the frequency of all medical X-rays and 68% to the total collective effective dose. This makes of CT the most irradiating radiological modality and the main contributor to the population dose due to radiodiagnostics, which is the case in other countries of similar health level. Compared to those countries, Switzerland appeared to be a medium consumer of CT and the efforts already engaged in radiation protection, notably the justification and optimisation of CT procedures should be maintained and consolidated; this is so important since an increase of the number of CT procedures is expected in the future due to the ageing of the population and the increase in healthcare needs.

Keypoints

- In 2008 about 0.8 Million computed tomography procedures (~ 100 CT examinations / 1000 population) were performed in Switzerland.
- CT is the most irradiating radiological modality and the main contributor to the population dose due to radiodiagnostics.
- Justification and optimisation of CT procedures should be maintained and consolidated.

Competing interests
Financial competing interests
- In the past five years have you received reimbursements, fees, funding, or salary from an organization that may in any way gain or lose financially from the publication of this manuscript, either now or in the future? Is such an organization financing this manuscript (including the article-processing charge)? If so, please specify. **NO**
- Do you hold any stocks or shares in an organization that may in any way gain or lose financially from the publication of this manuscript, either now or in the future? If so, please specify. **NO**
- Do you hold or are you currently applying for any patents relating to the content of the manuscript? Have you received reimbursements, fees, funding, or salary from an organization that holds or has applied for patents relating to the content of the manuscript? If so, please specify. **NO**
- Do you have any other financial competing interests? If so, please specify. **NO**

Non-financial competing interests
- Are there any non-financial competing interests (political, personal, religious, ideological, academic, intellectual, commercial or any other) to declare in relation to this manuscript? If so, please specify. **NO**

The authors declare that they have no competing interests in submitting this paper.

Authors' contributions
AA and ETS contributed in the conception and design of the study, in the acquisition of data, in the analysis and interpretation of data as well as in drafting the manuscript. FOB, RM and FRV contributed in the conception and design of the study and in revising the manuscript critically. All authors read and approved the final manuscript.

Acknowledgements
This research project was jointly funded by the Swiss Federal Office of Public Health and the Swiss National Science Foundation.

Author details
[1]Institute of Radiation Physics, Lausanne University Hospital, Lausanne, Switzerland. [2]Department of Diagnostic and Interventional Radiology, Lausanne University Hospital, Lausanne, Switzerland.

References
1. United Nations Scientific Committee on the Effects of Atomic Radiation: *UNSCEAR Report 2008: Sources of Ionizing Radiation*. New York: United Nations; 2010.
2. Federal Office of Public Health: *2009 Annual Report of the Radiological Protection Division*. Bern: FOPH; 2010.
3. Mini RL: *Dosisbestimmungen in der medizinischen Röntgendiagnostik*. Kerzers: Verlag Max Huber; 1992.
4. Aroua A, Burnand B, Decka I, Vader JP, Valley JF: **Nationwide survey on radiation doses in diagnostic and interventional radiology in Switzerland in 1998**. *Health Phys* 2002, 83(1):46–55.
5. Aroua A, Decka I, Burnand B, Vader JP, Valley JF: **Dosimetric aspects of a national survey of diagnostic and interventional radiology in Switzerland**. *Medical Phys* 2002, 29(10):2247–2259.

6. Aroua A, Vader JP, Valley JF, Verdun FR: **Exposure of the Swiss population by radiodiagnostics: 2003 review.** *Health Phys* 2007, **92**(5):442–448.

7. Etard C, Sinno-Tellier S, Aubert B: *Exposure of French Population by Ionizing Radiation due to Medical Diagnostic Examinations in 2007 (in French). Joint Report of the Institut de Radioprotection et de Sûreté Nucléaire and the Institut de Veille.* Paris: Sanitaire; 2010.

8. Bernhard-Ströl C, Hachenberger C, Trugenberger-Schnabel A, Peter J: *Jahresbericht 2009 Umweltradioaktivität und Strahlenbelastung.* Salzgitter: Bundesamt für Strahlenschutz; 2010.

9. Hart D, Wall BF, Hiller MC, Shrimpton PC: *Frequency and Collective Dose for Medical and Dental X-ray Examinations in the UK, 2008.* Chilton: Health Protection Agency. HPA-CECE-012; 2010.

10. De Waard IR, Stoop P: *Information System on Medical Radiation Applications: Data from the Reporting year 2008 (in Dutch).* Bilthoven: Rijksinstituut voor Volksgezondheid en Milieu; 2010. RIVM Report 300081005.

11. Norwegian Radiation Protection Authority: *Radiology in Norway Anno 2008. Trends in examination frequency and collective effective dose to the population. StrålevernRapport 2010:12. Østerås:. Language: Norwegian.* Oslo: NRPA; 2010.

12. Järvinen H: *Finnish Radiation and Nuclear Safety Authority (STUK). Personal Communication.* Helsinki: STUK; 2011.

13. National Council on Radiation Protection and Measurements: *Ionizing Radiation Exposure of the Population of the United States. NCRP Report No. 160.* Bethesda; 2009.

14. Brenner DJ: **Should we be concerned about the rapid increase in CT usage?** *Rev Environ Health* 2010, **25**(1):63–68.

15. European Commission: *European Guidance on Estimating Population Doses from Medical X-ray Procedures. Radiation protection no. 154.* Brussels: Directorate General for Energy and Transport; 2008.

16. Treier R, Aroua A, Verdun FR, Samara E, Stuessi A, Trueb PR: **Patient doses in CT examinations in Switzerland: implementation of national diagnostic reference levels.** *Radiat Prot Dosimetry* 2010, **142**(2–4):244–254.

17. International Commission on Radiological Protection: **The 1991 Recommendations of the ICRP. Publication 60.** *Ann ICRP* 1991, **21**(1):3.

18. International Commission on Radiological Protection: **The 2007 Recommendations of the ICRP. Publication 103.** *Ann ICRP* 2007, **37**(2):4.

19. Roser H: *University Hospital of Basel. Personal communication.* Basel; 2011.

20. Aroua A, Samara ET, Bochud FO, Vader JP, Verdun FR: *Exposure of the Swiss population by Medical X-rays: 2008 Review. Joint Report.* Lausanne: University Institute of Applied Radiation Physics and University Institute of Social and Preventive Medicine; 2011.

Evaluation of living liver donors using contrast enhanced multidetector CT – The radiologists impact on donor selection

Kristina Imeen Ringe[1][*], Bastian Paul Ringe[2], Christian von Falck[1], Hoen-oh Shin[1], Thomas Becker[3], Eva-Doreen Pfister[4], Frank Wacker[1] and Burckhardt Ringe[5]

Abstract

Background: Living donor liver transplantation (LDLT) is a valuable and legitimate treatment for patients with end-stage liver disease. Computed tomography (CT) has proven to be an important tool in the process of donor evaluation. The purpose of this study was to evaluate the significance of CT in the donor selection process.

Methods: Between May 1999 and October 2010 170 candidate donors underwent biphasic CT. We retrospectively reviewed the results of the CT and liver volumetry, and assessed reasons for rejection.

Results: 89 candidates underwent partial liver resection (52.4%). Based on the results of liver CT and volumetry 22 candidates were excluded as donors (31% of the cases). Reasons included fatty liver (n = 9), vascular anatomical variants (n = 4), incidental finding of hemangioma and focal nodular hyperplasia (n = 1) and small (n = 5) or large for size (n = 5) graft volume.

Conclusion: CT based imaging of the liver in combination with dedicated software plays a key role in the process of evaluation of candidates for LDLT. It may account for up to 1/3 of the contraindications for LDLT.

Keywords: LDLT, Transplantation, Living donor, Recipient, CT

Background

Since the first report of successful living donor liver transplantation (LDLT) in 1990 [1], LDLT has become a valuable treatment for patients with end-stage liver disease who cannot receive deceased donor livers. Particularly in children who need a small sized graft, the use of liver transplantation is limited due to shortage of deceased donor organs.

Since the safety of volunteer living donors in LDLT has always been considered paramount, evaluation of potential candidates plays a crucial role to confirm suitability and to identify possible contraindications. Each transplant center has its own protocol for living donor evaluation, which typically includes a comprehensive medical and psychosocial examination as well as non-invasive imaging and other studies to assess size, anatomy and function of the liver.

Both, contrast enhanced computed-tomography (CT), and magnetic resonance imaging (MRI) have been shown to be suitable diagnostic tools, and are being used concurrently in different centers throughout the world. Imaging in a living liver donor has three objectives: (1) to identify any intraparenchymal lesions or abnormalities like fatty changes; (2) to visualize the extra- and intrahepatic vascular and biliary anatomy; and (3) to determine the size of the whole liver and calculate the graft and remnant liver volumes. The main advantage of CT over MRI is based on a higher spatial resolution and manifold post-processing possibilities [2,3].

The preoperative imaging process in LDLT is demanding and conscientious. Radiologists play a key role in filtering and providing the required information to surgeons. In addition, they may help to identify unsuitable donors and avoid unnecessary or invasive studies and procedures. The purpose of our study was thus to

* Correspondence: ringe.kristina@mh-hannover.de
[1]Department of Diagnostic and Interventional Radiology, Hannover Medical School, Carl-Neuberg Str. 1, 30625, Hannover, Germany
Full list of author information is available at the end of the article

evaluate the significance of multidetector CT in this process, and therefore to reflect the radiologists impact on donor selection.

Materials and methods

This retrospective study was approved by the ethics committee of Hannover Medical School with a waiver of consent granted.

Candidate donors and recipients

Between May 1999 and October 2010 170 candidate donors (92 female, 78 male, mean age 39 years, range 18-61 years) underwent biphasic CT of the liver (Table 1). In addition, all donors had routine ultrasound examination. Further, biliary anatomy was assessed intraoperatively. The recipients were 143 patients (53 female, 90 male; 99 children, 44 adults) with a mean age of 15.3 years (4 months-71 years) (Table 2). In 121 recipients one donor was evaluated by means of CT, in 19 recipients two donors, in 1 recipient three donors, and in 2 recipients four donors, respectively. Most common underlying diseases were biliary atresia in children (n = 69), liver cirrhosis (n = 19), and hepatocellular carcinoma respectively hepatoblastoma (n = 22). We retrospectively reviewed the results of the CT and liver volumetry, and reasons for rejection were assessed.

Image acquisition

Until October 2005 CT was performed using a 4-channel multi-detector row CT (Somatom Plus 4A, Siemens, Erlangen, Germany). To keep radiation dose levels as low as possible, a native CT scan was not acquired. 150 ml of a nonionic iodinated contrast agent (Ultravist 300®, Bayer Schering Pharma, Berlin) followed by a 40 ml saline flush (NaCl 0.9%) were injected at a flow of 3-5 ml /sec. Biphasic image acquisition of the liver started 5 seconds after bolus detection in the abdominal aorta for the arterial phase. Portal-venous phase scanning followed after an interscan delay of 15 seconds. The parameters were identical for both scans: 3 mm slice collimation, a table feed of 5 mm per gantry rotation, and 2 mm reconstruction interval. Starting in October 2005 CT was performed using a 64-channel scanner (Lightspeed VCT, GE

Table 1 Candidate donor demographic data

Number of potential donors	170	
Donor age (years)	18-61 (mean 39)	
Donor sex (male / female)	78 / 92	
Performed LDLT	89	*Mean graft volume [ml]*
Left lateral	57	277 (SD 63)
Full left lobe	1	414
Right lobe	31	1134 (SD 317)

LDLT = living donor liver transplantation; SD = standard deviation.

Table 2 Recipient demographic data

Number of potential recipients	143
Patient age	4 months - 71 years (mean 15.3 years)
Patient sex (male / female)	90 / 53
Underlying disease	
Biliary atresia	69
Liver cirrhosis	19
Tumour (HCC, Hepatoblastoma)	22
PSC, PBC	7
α1-Antitrypsin deficiency	6
Alagille syndrome	4
Acute liver failure	2
Other	14

Medical Systems, USA). Multiphase scanning was performed after intravenous injection of 120 ml of a nonionic iodinated contrast medium (Imeron 400®, Nycomed GmbH, Germany) followed by a 50 ml saline flush (NaCl 0,9%) at a rate of 5 ml/sec. Arterial dominant phase images were obtained 15 seconds after bolus detection in the abdominal aorta, portal-venous scanning followed after an interscan delay of 25 seconds. Again, the parameters were identical for both scans: 1.25 mm slice collimation, a table feed of 39.37 mm per gantry rotation, and 1 mm reconstruction interval.

Image analysis and postprocessing

Postprocessing was performed on a commercially available workstation (ADW 2.2-4.4, GE Healthcare, USA). In addition to multiplanar reformations, maximum intensity projections (MIP) and 3D volume rendered (VR) images were used for evaluation of the vascular anatomy and identifying relevant anatomic variants. Relevant steatosis was suspected when pronounced liver-spleen attenuation was observed or the attenuation of the liver parenchyma was less than the attenuation of the muscle, as suggested by previous studies [4,5]. In the relevant donors, liver biopsy was performed in order to confirm the degree of steatosis. Volume calculations of liver segments were performed using dedicated software (Hepa-Vision®: MeVis, Germany) (Figures 1 and 2) [6,7]. Liver volumetry and segmentation was performed by an experienced radiologist, and subsequent drawing of the resection plane in agreement with the respective transplant surgeon.

Results

After completion of the evaluation process living donor liver transplantation was realized in 89 cases, respectively 52.4% (Figure 3). These included transplantation of the left lateral liver (segments 2 and 3) in 57 patients, transplantation of a full left lobe (segments 1-4) in one

remaining candidates surgery was not carried out either because a graft from a deceased donor became available (n = 28), death of the recipient before transplantation (n = 9) or because the donor was rejected for LDLT (n = 35). In 9 patients the evaluation process is still in progress and LDLT is planned.

Based on the results of contrast enhanced CT scan and liver volumetry, 22 candidates were excluded as donors. Reasons included signs of a fatty liver (n = 9) which was later on confirmed by biopsy, vascular anatomical variants (n = 4), coincidental finding of hemangioma and focal nodular hyperplasia (n = 1) or small for size (n = 5) or large for size (n = 5) graft volume, respectively. In this context small for size was defined as GRBR (graft weight to recipient to recipient body weight ratio; synonym GRWR) <0.8%. In the five potential donors calculated as large for size the relevant grafts were left lateral segments designated for children aged 5 months to 5 years with a calculated graft volume of 345 to 511 ml. The vascular variants encountered were as follows: right hepatic artery arising from the superior mesenteric artery, left hepatic artery arising from the celiac trunk in combination with a right hepatic artery arising from the superior mesenteric artery (Figure 5), and atypical venous drainage of segment 5. Candidates were further excluded in the course of the evaluation process as donors due to medical reasons, such as profound arterial hypertension and unexplained elevation of transaminases, as well as social or respectively ethical reasons (e.g. poor prognosis of the recipient).

Discussion

To meet the need of increasing potential liver transplant recipients, alternative procedures have been developed, such as reduced-size, split and living donor liver transplantation [8]. LDLT has two major advantages over transplantation from a brain-dead donor: excellent graft quality and reduced ischemia-reperfusion injury [9].

On the other hand, donor safety is the first priority. It is important to keep in mind that LDLT should only be performed if the risk to the donor is justified by expectation of an acceptable outcome in the recipient. Overall donor morbidity is estimated to be approximately 35%, including bile leakage, wound infection and ileus [10]. A recent survey identified 33 living liver donor deaths, including 3 donors who succumbed after an attempted rescue with a liver transplant [11].

Preoperative imaging of the liver is essential in order to identify and minimize the individual risk of the potential donor. It is further determining for graft survival and in preventing vascular complications. The implementation of imaging studies of the liver, the choice of the imaging modality (CT, MRI, ultrasound, angiography, e.g.) as well as the timing of imaging (early in the

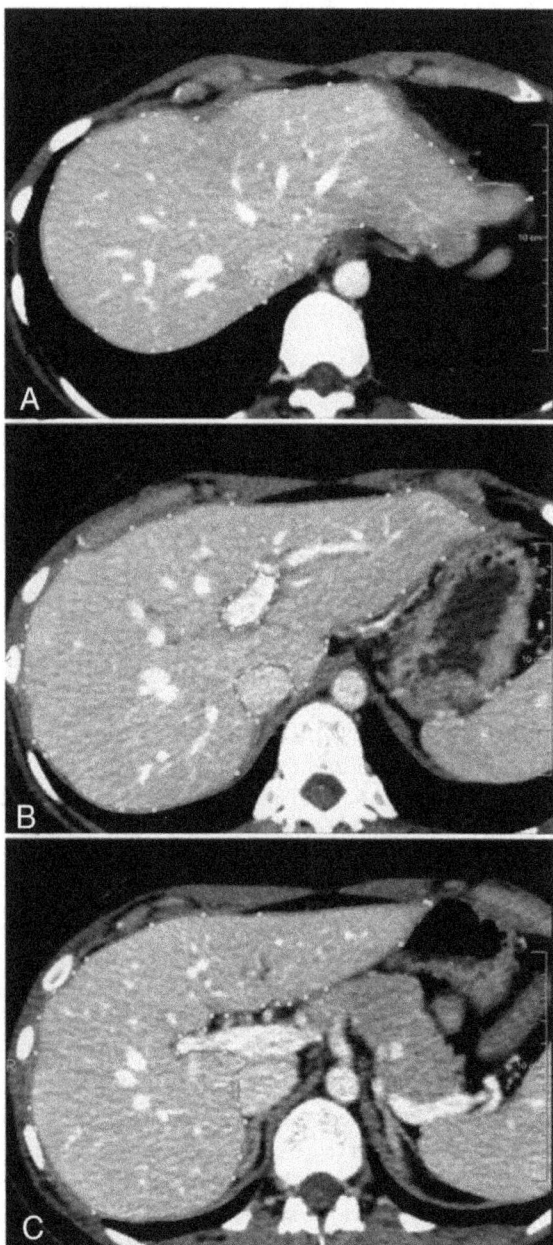

Figure 1 Total liver volume was calculated using dedicated software (HepaVision®, MeVis, Germany) by tracing around the margins of the hepatic parenchyma on selected transversal slices. Slices in between were interpolated. Large vessels as the inferior vena cava and extrahepatic portal vein were excluded. The cross sectional area (cm²) within the region of interest was determined, and all individual areas were summed yielding the total liver volume (cm³).

patient, and transplantation of the right lobe (segments 5-8) in 31 patients (Table 1). For the right liver graft the resection line ran approximately 1 cm to the right of the middle hepatic vein. In one donor, a focal nodular hyperplasia was resected simultaneously, which was incidentally detected on the CT scan (Figure 4). In the

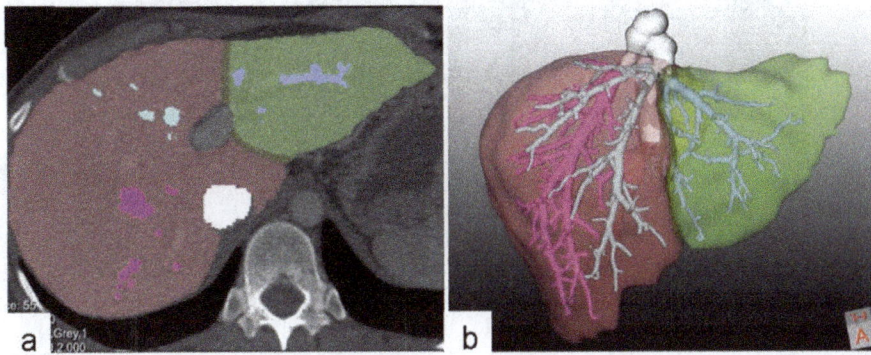

Figure 2 Calculation of graft and remnant liver volume after virtual resection using HepaVision® software (MeVis, Germany). Visualization of the resection line on transversal slices (**a**) and in 3D including hepatic veins (**b**).

evaluation process vs. in the end) varies in different transplant centers.

MRI is undoubtedly becoming more significant in the course of living donor liver evaluation, due to the development of hepatobiliary-specific contrast agents and new imaging techniques (such as chemical shift imaging, MR spectroscopy), opening up new possibilities for comprehensive imaging of the liver [12,13]. However, availability of MR is still an issue.

The purpose of this retrospective study was therefore to review the radiologist's contribution to the process of evaluation of donors for LDLT by means of contrast enhanced CT, especially since we can look back on a large group of donors being evaluated with this technique over a significant period of time. Based on the results of the CT scan and liver volumetry in our study 22 candidates were excluded as donors, which accounts for nearly one third (31%) of the cases in which LDLT was not carried out. This relatively high number could be an argument to perform CT imaging early rather than late in the process of donor evaluation. The overall costs for complete donor evaluation have been estimated

in previous studies to be in the range from 1383-2569€ [14], in some centers even as high as 4589€ [15]. Early implementation of CT imaging (estimated costs of approximately 400-600€) in the evaluation process might therefore prevent further studies in unsuitable donors and reduce costs.

Nine candidate donors were excluded because CT indicated steatosis of the liver, which was confirmed with ultrasound and liver biopsy. Fatty infiltration in hepatic grafts is known to be an important risk factor for primary graft nonfunction in deceased donor liver transplantation as well as in LDLT [16,17]. Liver grafts with a mild degree of fatty changes can be used for liver transplantation without ill effect, but liver grafts with moderate or severe degree of fatty changes have been found to have a negative effect on post transplant graft function and patient survival [17,18]. Marcos et al estimated that 1% of hepatic steatosis can decrease the functional graft mass by 1% [19]. More recently the same group published a series in which no impairment in function was found in either the living donor or the recipient using grafts containing less than 30% steatosis [20]. In our

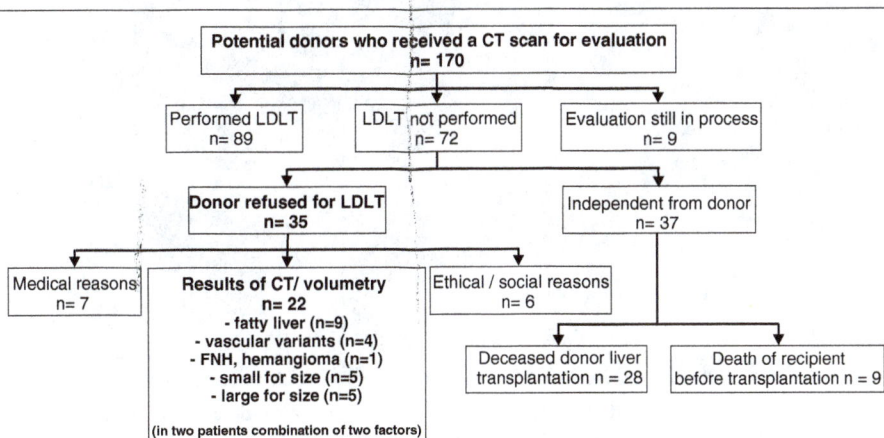

Figure 3 Follow-up of candidate donors being evaluated for LDLT by means of contrast enhanced CT.

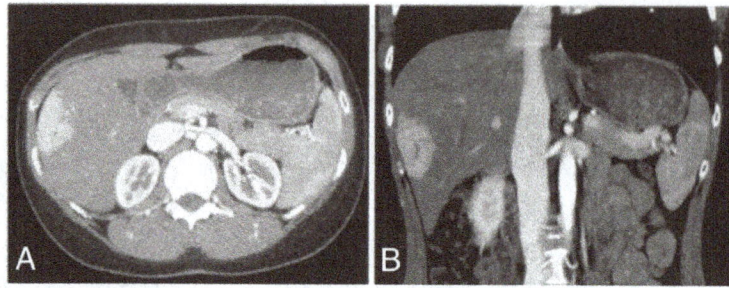

Figure 4 Donor candidate in whom the left lateral segments where resected for LDLT. Simultaneously, a FNH in the right lobe, incidentally detected in the CT scan, was resected.

own institution the acceptable upper limit of fatty changes in the liver graft is 30%.

10 candidate donors were excluded because of the results of liver volumetry, depicting either small (n = 5) or large for size (n = 5) graft volume. Preoperative assessment of total, graft and remnant liver volume is of utmost importance, since inadequate liver mass can influence patient and graft survival. There are several formulas for calculating total liver volume depending on the body weight, body surface and gender [21,22]. Results do not always correlate and liver volume is often overestimated [23]. Depending on the individual method used, it is considered acceptable when the ratio between graft weight and recipient body weight or between graft volume and the estimated standard liver volume of the recipient are at least 0,8% and 40%, respectively [24].

In case of left lateral donation remnant liver volume is usually safe for the donor, whereas graft size might be too large in small children. In our study this led to the

exclusion of five donors. Especially in case of right liver donation remnant liver volume might be too small (risking acute liver failure of the donor), whereas graft size might as well be too small resulting in a "small-for-size -syndrome" in the recipient, characterized by hepatocyte ballooning, steatosis, centrilobular necrosis and parenchymal cholestasis [25]. This led to the exclusion of three donors who were evaluated for donation of the right lobe.

CT is further important in assessment of vascular hepatic anatomy. Certain anomalies may require modification of the surgical procedure, while others might be a contraindication for surgery [26]. Other vascular variants may even be advantageous, e.g. a displaced right artery arising from the superior mesenteric artery in case of right donation. Due to the greater variability of the right hepatic vascular anatomy right hepatectomy can be one of the most challenging surgical procedures. In addition to the arterial supply of the graft and the

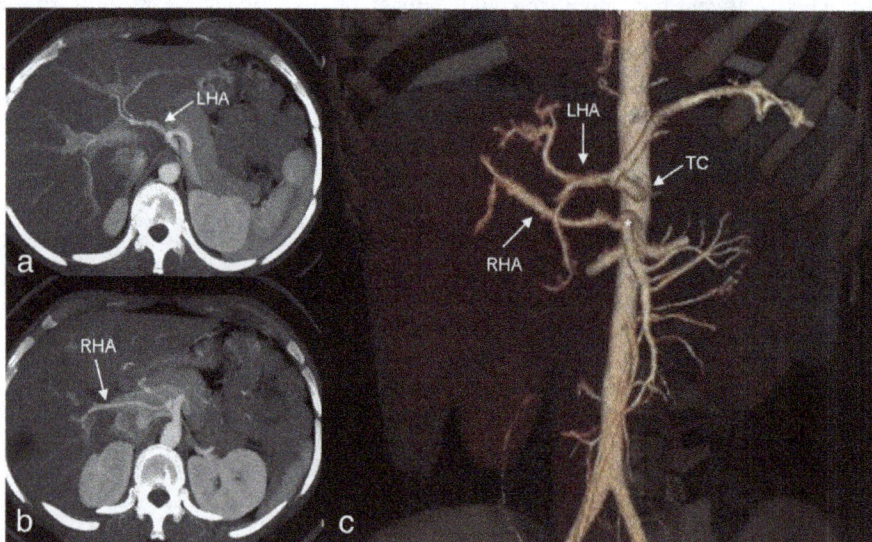

Figure 5 Maximum Intensity Projections (a,b) and 3D volume rendered image (c) in a candidate with a left hepatic artery (LHA) arising from the celiac trunk (TC) and a right hepatic artery (RHA) arising from the superior mesenteric artery (*). LDLT was not carried out, as graft volume was large for size.

remnant liver attention has to be paid to the venous drainage in order to prevent venous congestion. In our study 4 candidate donors were excluded from LDLT because of various vascular anatomic variants. Even though our reported vascular variants do not present absolute contraindications, in these specific cases LDLT would have been involved with an increased surgical complexity and an increased risk of graft failure respectively complications in the donor as well as in the recipient. It is important that anatomic vascular variants are assessed in context with the planned resection, and the decision whether a specific donor is suited for a specific recipient is in the end up to the responsible transplant surgeon.

Conclusions

The use of imaging studies in the process of liver donor evaluation, specifically the choice of the imaging modality (CT, MRI, ultrasound, or angiography) as well as the timing of imaging (early in the evaluation process vs. in the end) has significant implications for the subsequent evaluation process. In our long-term experience, CT based imaging of the liver in combination with dedicated software plays a key role in the process of evaluation of candidates for LDLT. In this series almost 1/3 of donor candidates were rejected because of CT findings. CT can help to reduce the risk for donor and recipient by exclusion of unsuitable donor livers. If performed early during the evaluation process it can also prevent unnecessary studies, further reducing the risks and costs.

Competing interests
The authors declare that they have no competing interests.

Authors' contributions
KIR and BR conceived and designed the experiments. KIR, CF, BPR, TB, HS and EDP performed the experiments and acquisition of data. KIR, BPR and BR analyzed and interpreted the data. TB and FW contributed materials and analysis tools. All authors participated in drafting and revising the manuscript. All authors read and approved the final manuscript.

Acknowledgements
None.

Author details
[1]Department of Diagnostic and Interventional Radiology, Hannover Medical School, Carl-Neuberg Str. 1, 30625, Hannover, Germany. [2]Department of General, Visceral and Transplantation Surgery, Hannover Medical School, Carl-Neuberg Str.1, 30625, Hannover, Germany. [3]Department of General and Thoracic Surgery, University Hospital Schleswig-Holstein, Arnold-Heller Str.1, 24105, Kiel, Germany. [4]Department of Pediatric Gastroenterology and Hepatology, Hannover Medical School, Carl-Neuberg Str. 1, 30625, Hannover, Germany. [5]Drexel University, College of Medicine, 216 N Broad Street, Philadelphia, PA 19102, USA.

References
1. Strong RW, Lynch SV, Ong TH, Matsunami H, Koido Y, Balderson GA: Successful liver transplantation from a living donor to her son. N Engl J Med 1990, 322:1505–1507.
2. Prokop M, Shin H, Schanz A, Schaefer-Prokop CM: Use of maximum intensity projections in CT angiography: a basic review. Radiographics 1997, 17:433–451.
3. Sahani D, Saini S, Pena C, Nichols S, Prasad SR, Hahn PF, Halpern EF, Tanabe KK, Mueller PR: Using multidetector CT for preoperative vascular evaluation of liver neoplasms: technique and results. AJR Am J Roentgenol 2002, 179:53–59.
4. Johnston RJ, Stamm ER, Lewin J, Hendrick RE, Archer PG: Diagnosis of fatty infiltration of the liver on contrast enhanced CT: limitations of liver-minus-spleen attenuation difference measurements. Abdom Imaging 1998, 23:409–415.
5. Panicek DM, Giess CS, Schwartz LH: Qualitative assessment of liver for fatty infiltration on contrast-enhanced CT: is muscle a better standard of reference than spleen? J Comput Assist Tomogr 1997, 21:699–705.
6. Frericks BB, Caldarone FC, Nashan B, Savellano D, Stamm G, Kirchhoff TD, Shin HO, Schenk A, Selle D, Spindler W, Klempnauer J, Peitgen HO, Galanski M: 3D CT modeling of hepatic vessel architecture and volume calculation in living donated liver transplantation. Eur Radiol 2004, 14:326–333.
7. Frericks BB, Kirchhoff TD, Shin HO, Stamm G, Merkesdal S, Abe T, Schenk A, Peitgen HD, Klempnauer J, Galanski M, Nashan B: Preoperative volume calculation of the hepatic venous draining areas with multi-detector row CT in adult living donor liver transplantation: Impact on surgical procedure. Eur Radiol 2006, 16:2803–2810.
8. Alonso-Torres A, Fernandez-Cuadrado J, Pinilla I, Parron M, de Vicente E, Lopez-Santamaria M: Multidetector CT in the evaluation of potential living donors for liver transplantation. Radiographics 2005, 25:1017–1030.
9. Kawasaki S, Makuuchi M, Matsunami H, Hashikura Y, Ikegami T, Nakazawa Y, Chisura H, Terada M, Miyagawa S: Living related liver transplantation in adults. Ann Surg 1998, 27:269–274.
10. Barr LM, Belghiti J, Villamil FG, Pomfret EA, Sutherland DS, Gruessner RW, Langnas AN, Delmonico FL: A report of the Vancouver forum on the care of the live organ donor: lung, liver, pancreas, and intestine data and medical guidelines. Transplantation 2006, 81:1373–1385.
11. Ringe B, Strong RW: The dilemna of living liver donor deaths: to report or not to report? Transplantation 2008, 85:790.
12. Ma X, Holalkere NS, Kambadakone RA, Mino-Kenudson M, Hahn PF, Sahani DV: Imaging-based quantification of hepatic fat: methods and clinical applications. Radiographics 2009, 29:1253–1277.
13. Seale MK, Catalano OA, Saomo S, Hahn PF, Sahani DV: Hepatobiliary-specific MR contrast agents: role in imaging of the liver and biliary tree. Radiographics 2009, 29:1725–1748.
14. Sagmeister M, Mullhaupt B, Kadry Z, Kullak-Unlick GA, Clavien PA, Renner EL: Cost-effectiveness of cadaveric and living-donor liver transplantation. Transplantation 2002, 73:616–622.
15. Valentin-Gamazo C, Malago M, Karliova M, Lutz JT, Frilling A, Nadalin S, Testa G, Ruehm SG, Erim Y, Paul A, Lang H, Gerken G, Broelsch CE: Experience after the evaluation of 700 potential donors for living donor liver transplantation in a single center. Liver Transpl 2004, 10:1087–1096.
16. Todo S, Demetris AJ, Makowka L, Teperman L, Podesta L, Shaver T, Tzakis A, Starzl TE: Primary nonfunction of hepatic allografts with preexisting fatty infiltration. Transplantation 1989, 47:903–905.
17. D'Alessandro AM, Kalayoglu M, Sollinger HW, Hoffmann RM, Reed A, Knechtle SJ, Pirsch JD, Hafez GR, Lorentzen D, Belzer FO: The predictive value of donor liver biopsies for the development of primary nonfunction after orthotopic liver transplantation. Transplantation 1991, 51:157–163.
18. Moon D, Lee S, Hwang S, Kim K, Ahn C, Park K, Ha T, Song G: Resolution of severe graft steatosis following dual-graft living donor liver transplantation. Liver Transpl 2006, 12:1156–1160.
19. Marcos A, Ham JM, Fisher RA, Fisher RA, Olzinski AT, Posner MP: Single-center analysis of the first 40 adult-to-adult living donor liver transplants using the right lobe. Liver Transpl 2000, 6:296–301.
20. Marcos A, Fisher RA, Ham JM, Shiffman ML, Sanyal AJ, Luketic VA, Sterling RK, Fulcher AS, Posner MP: Liver regeneration and function in donor and recipient after right lobe adult to adult living donor liver transplantation. Transplantation 2000, 69:1375.
21. Urata K, Kawasaki S, Matsunami H, Hasikura Y, Ikegami T, Ishizone S, Momose Y, Komiyama A, Makuchi M: Calculation of child and adult standard liver volume for liver transplantation. Hepatology 1995, 21:1317–1321.

22. DeLand FH, North WA: **Relationship between liver size and body size.** *Radiology* 1968, **91**:11951–1198.

23. Kamel IR, Kruskal JB, Warmbrand G, Goldberg SN, Pomfret EA, Raptopoulos V: **Accuracy of volumetric measurements after virtual right hepatectomy in potential donors undergoing living adult liver transplantation.** *Am J Roentegnol AJR* 2001, **176**:483–487.

24. Chen YS, Cheng YF, De Villa VH, De Villa VH, Wang CC, Lin CC, Huang TL, Jawan B, Chen CL: **Evaluation of living liver donors.** *Transplantation* 2003, **75**(3 Suppl):S16–19.

25. Emond JC, Renz JF, Ferrell LD, Rosenthal P, Lim RC, Roberts JP, Lake JR, Ascher NL: **Functional analysis of grafts from living donors. Implications for the treatment of older recipients.** *Ann Surg* 1996, **224**:544–552.

26. Catalano OA, Singh AH, Uppot RN, Hahn PF, Ferrone, Sahani DV: **Vascular and biliary variants in the liver: implications for liver surgery.** *Radiographics* 2008, **28**:359–378.

20

Acute pulmonary embolism in the era of multi-detector CT: a reality in sub-Saharan Africa

Joshua Tambe[1], Boniface Moifo[1*], Emmanuel Fongang[2], Emilienne Guegang[1,2] and Alain Georges Juimo[1,2]

Abstract

Background: The advantages of multi-detector computed tomography (MDCT) have made it the imaging modality of choice for some patients with suspected cardiothoracic disease, of which pulmonary embolism (PE) is an exponent. The aim of this study was to assess the incidence of PE in patients with clinical suspicion of acute PE using MDCT in a sub-Saharan setting, and to describe the demographic characteristics of these patients.

Methods: Consecutive records of patients who underwent MDCT pulmonary angiography for suspected acute PE over a two-year period at the Radiology Department of a university-affiliated hospital were systematically reviewed. All MDCT pulmonary angiograms were performed with a 16-detector computed tomography (CT) scanner using real-time bolus tracking technique. Authorization for the study was obtained from the institutional authorities.

Results: Forty-one MDCT pulmonary angiograms were reviewed of which 37 were retained. Of the 4 excluded studies, 3 were repeat angiograms and 1 study was not technically adequate. Twelve of 37 patients (32.4%) had CT angiograms that were positive for PE, of which 7 were males. The mean age of these patients was 47.6±10.5 years (age range from 33 to 65 years). Twenty five patients out of 37 (67.6%) had CT angiograms that were negative for PE. Eleven PE-positive patients (91.7%) had at least 1 identifiable thromboembolic risk factor whilst 5 PE-negative patients (20%) also had at least a thromboembolic risk factor. The relative risk of the occurrence of PE in patients with at least a thromboembolic risk factor was estimated at 14.4.

Conclusion: Acute PE is a reality in sub-Saharan Africa, with an increased likelihood of MDCT evidence in patients with clinical suspicion of PE who have at least a thromboembolic risk factor. The increasing availability of MDCT will help provide more information on the occurrence of PE in these settings.

Keywords: Acute pulmonary embolism, multi-detector CT angiography, sub-Saharan Africa, thromboembolic risk factors

Background

Multi-detector computed tomography (MDCT) pulmonary angiography is increasingly being used to evaluate patients with suspected pulmonary embolism (PE) [1]. This is largely due to its many advantages over conventional angiography whose place as a diagnostic standard of reference has been increasingly challenged [2]. MDCT angiography is non-invasive, results in shorter acquisition times with improved contrast enhancement, thinner collimation hence superior image resolution and improved visualization of the pulmonary arterial tree [3-5]. Some studies have shown MDCT pulmonary angiography to have a high diagnostic yield and to be more cost-effective than conventional angiography in investigating patients with suspected PE [6,7]. The diagnostic usefulness of MDCT pulmonary angiography is further enhanced by its ability to detect concurrent or other cardiothoracic diseases mimicking PE. These combined advantages of MDCT angiography make it very appropriate for some patients with suspected cardiothoracic disease [1,8].

Little is known about the occurrence of acute pulmonary embolism (PE) in sub-Saharan settings. Considered rare, it has often been diagnosed based on clinical symptoms in patients with or without evidence of deep vein thrombosis on Doppler ultrasound [9]. This has largely been due to the lack of diagnostic facilities over the

* Correspondence: bmoifo@yahoo.fr
[1]Department of Radiology and Radiation Oncology, University of Yaounde 1, Yaounde, Cameroon
Full list of author information is available at the end of the article

years. With the introduction of MDCT, it has proved to be a useful diagnostic tool in investigating suspected cases of acute PE. The purpose of this study therefore was to assess the incidence of PE in patients with clinical suspicion of acute PE using MDCT in a sub-Saharan setting, and to describe the demographic characteristics of these patients.

Results

A total of 41 CT pulmonary angiograms were reviewed, of which 37 were retained. Of the 4 excluded studies, 3 were repeat CT angiograms, and in 1 study the pulmonary arteries were not sufficiently opacified.

Patient demographics

The mean age of the study population was 48.5±12.7 years (mean±SD) with range from 23 to 74 years, and sex-ratio 1:1. Twelve of 37 patients (32.4%) had CT angiograms that were positive for PE, with a mean age of 47.6±10.5 years (range 33 to 65 years). Table 1 summarizes the demographic characteristics of the study population.

Risk factors

The specific thromboembolic risk factors identified in the study population with their associated frequencies are shown in Table 2.

Of the 12 patients with CT angiograms positive for PE, 11 (91.7%) had at least one identifiable thromboembolic risk factor. One patient had no identifiable thromboembolic risk factor. Five patients with PE-negative scans (20%) had at least 1 identifiable thromboembolic risk factor. The relative risk of the occurrence of PE with respect to the thromboembolic risk factors was 14.4 $(RR =11/16 \times 21 = 14.4)$ (Figure 1).

Ancillary and other significant CT angiographic findings of PE-positive and PE-negative patients

Ancillary findings were observed in some PE-positive patients: they included 4 cases of wedge-shaped opacities

Table 1 Demographic characteristics of the study population

	All Patients	PE positive	PE negative
Age (years)*			
All	48.5±12.7	47.6±10.6	48.9±13.8
Male	52.5±11.2	46.1±10.1	57.0±13.5
Female	45.1±13.1	49.6±12.0	43.6±10.1
Age range	23 – 74	33 – 65	23 – 74
Sex, no./total no.(%)			
Male	17/37 (45.9)	7/12 (58.3)	10/25 (40.0)
Female	20/37 (54.1)	5/12 (41.7)	15/25 (60.0)

* Plus-minus values are mean±standard deviation (SD).

Table 2 Identified thromboembolic risk factors and frequencies

Risk factor	PE-positive	PE-negative
Age ≥ 65 years	1	3
Postoperative state	5	2
Known DVT†	3	0
Malignancy	1	0
Immobilisation for medical reasons	4	2

DVT† stands for deep vein thrombosis.

with pleural effusions and 2 cases of pleural effusions only. Significant findings in PE-negative patients included 5 cases of lung consolidation, 2 cases of ground glass opacities, 4 cases of pleural effusions, a case of pericardial effusion, 3 cases of aneurysms of the thoracic aorta and a case of aneurysm of the main pulmonary artery (Figures 2 and 3).

Discussion

From these results acute PE is not as rare a finding in sub-Saharan African populations as previously reported [9], after obtaining as high as 32% MDCT angiograms that were positive for PE. This positivity rate exceeds that of the multicentre PIOPED II (prospective investigation of pulmonary embolism diagnosis) study which recorded 23.3% positive scans for PE [10,11]. Mamlouk et al. and Prologo et al. working in the United States recorded even lower rates of 9.8% and 10.4% respectively [12,13] whilst Karabulut and Kiroglu in Turkey obtained 38% [14]. This study was carried out in just one hospital setting which alone had the available diagnostic imaging facility (16-detector CT) in the locality. This relative unavailability of diagnostic imaging facilities imposes a geographic selection as eligible patients with clinical suspicion of PE in settings without this facility would not have had access to MDCT. Also, some eligible patients in the setting where this facility is available might not have had access due to the cost (the direct cost of a CT angiogram at the study setting is about 250 US dollars). With MDCT being more and more available and accessible in sub-Saharan settings, many cases of PE that could have remained undiagnosed would be depicted, and hence provide more information on the subject.

MDCT evidence for acute PE was more likely to occur in patients with at least one of the following identifiable thromboembolic risk factors: age 65 years and above, known deep vein thrombosis, immobilization due to surgery (mostly caesarean section) or medical reasons and malignancy, with a calculated relative risk of 14.4. Mamlouk et al. had earlier arrived at a similar conclusion [11,12]. On the other hand patients who do not have these risk factors and yet have symptoms indicative of

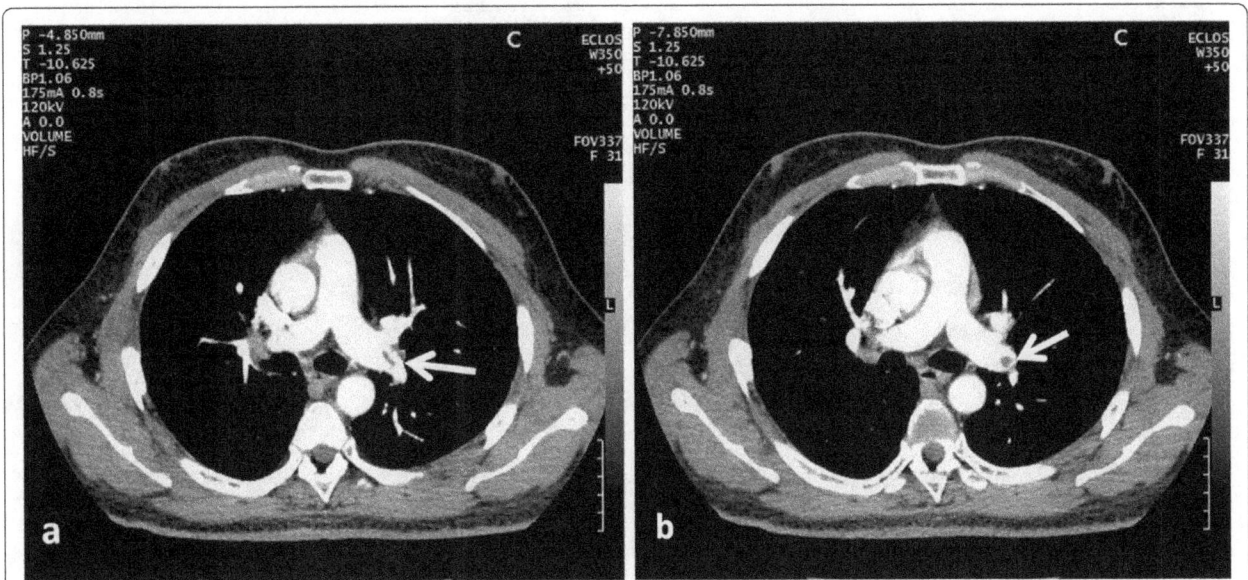

Figure 1 A 41-year-old man, with dyspnea of sudden onset. CT angiogram shows a typical embolus in the left pulmonary artery (arrow). No thromboembolic risk factor was found.

acute PE would be unlikely to have CT pulmonary angiographic findings consistent with acute PE. This might help reduce unnecessary MDCT angiography requests, which would be vital especially in resource-limited settings where patients are often required to pay directly for diagnostic procedures. However, the possibility of depicting any cardiothoracic condition in patients without acute PE or occurring concomitantly with PE may continue to justify routine MDCT angiography in suspected cases of acute PE [14,15]. Symptoms of acute

PE may be mild or absent, particularly in patients with PE only in the segmental pulmonary branches, and even in patients with severe PE [11]. Furthermore, symptoms of acute PE are not specific, as other conditions such as lung parenchyma, pleural, cardiac and thoracic vascular abnormalities can equally manifest in the same way. Nevertheless some conditions that mimic acute PE such as occlusion of the coronary arteries remain undiagnosed in the absence of an optimal scanning technique involving ECG-gating. Although the predictive value of

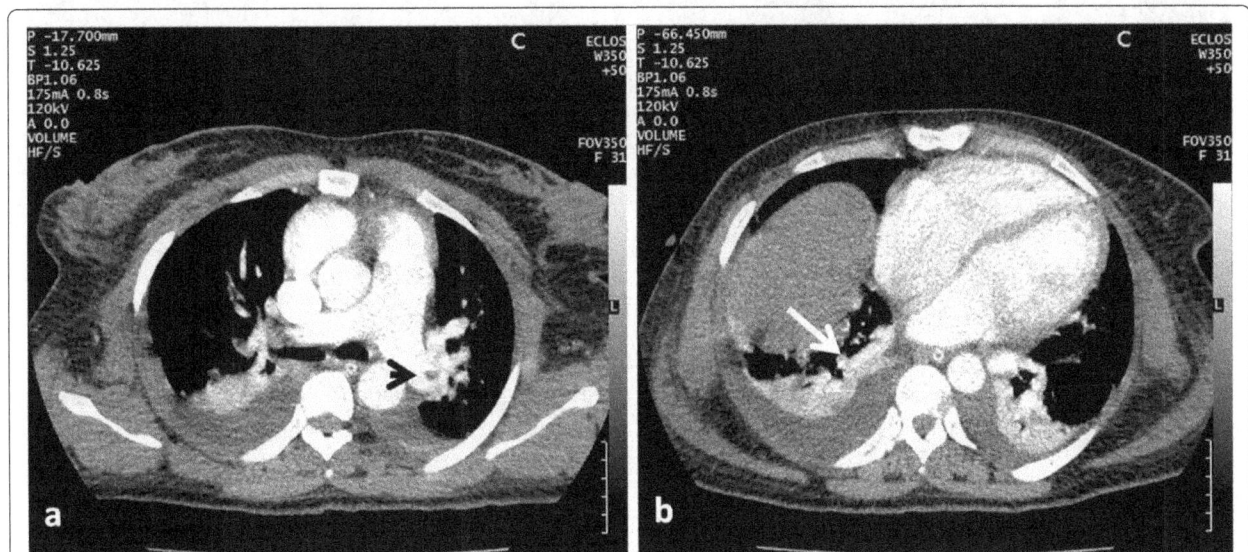

Figure 2 CT angiogram of a 33-year-old woman with clinical suspicion of PE three days after surgery (Caesarean section) shows an embolus in the left pulmonary artery (2a, arrowhead) and in the right postero-basal pulmonary artery (2b, white arrow). Note bilateral pleural effusion and peripheral wedge-shaped opacity.

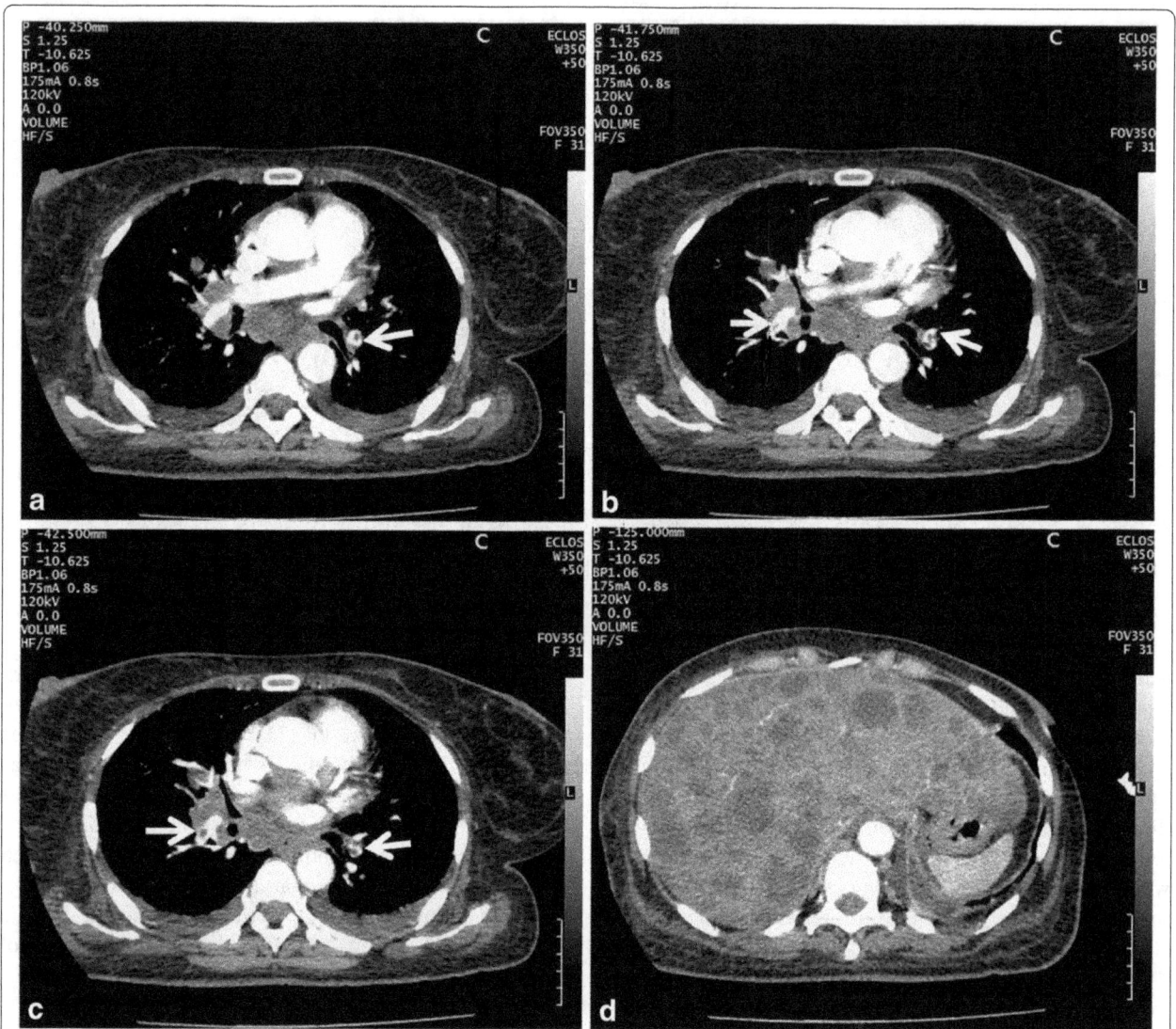

Figure 3 CT angiogram in a 50-year-old woman with sudden and unexplained shortness of breath, who was also restless, shows multiple and bilateral emboli (3a, 3b, 3c, white arrow) associated with multiple enlarged mediastinal and hilar lymph nodes. The liver is enlarged with multiple hypodense and non-enhancing nodules suggestive of metastases (3d).

normal MDCT is high, normal MDCT angiography does not absolutely rule out pulmonary embolism, thus additional testing is necessary especially when the clinical probability is inconsistent with the imaging results [10].

High radiation exposure with MDCT has been documented [12], and in the absence of other diagnostic techniques in this study setting such as the D-dimer test with a high positive predictive value [12] and perfusion scans, we are left with the patient's symptoms, thromboembolic risk factors and CT. This emphasizes the need to carefully select patients for MDCT and thus minimize unnecessary patient irradiation [16].

Some aspects that have served as limitations to this study include retrospective data collection and a small sample size. Also no other diagnostic test was performed

besides MDCT angiography to further confirm or ascertain the nature of the emboli.

Conclusion

This study shows that acute PE is a reality in sub-Saharan Africa. The rare occurrence earlier reported can only be associated to the long-term absence of appropriate diagnostic imaging modalities which are sophisticated and costly, requiring trained professionals for optimum results. Patients with clinical suspicion of acute PE with at least a thromboembolic risk factor are more likely to have CT evidence of PE on MDCT pulmonary angiograms. MDCT also retains its unique role in diagnosing concomitant conditions besides PE and will often provide an alternative diagnosis to PE.

Methods

Patients

Consecutive records of patients who had MDCT pulmonary angiography performed at the Radiology Department of a university-affiliated hospital (Yaounde General Hospital) from September 2009 to August 2011 were systematically reviewed. Authorization for the study was obtained from the institutional authorities (Yaounde General Hospital Ethics Committee). The MDCT angiograms were requested based on clinical suspicion of acute PE. Wells criteria included leg or calf pain (11%), "an alternative diagnosis is less likely than PE" (24%), tachycardia (19%), recent surgery or immobilization (35%), previous deep vein thrombosis (8%), and malignancy (3%). The most common clinical symptoms were sudden and/or unexplained chest pain, malaise, syncope or shortness of breath.

MDCT angiography technique

All CT angiograms were performed with a 16-row detector computed tomography (CT) scanner (ECLOS, Hitachi Medical Corporation, Tokyo, Japan). No special patient preparation was required prior to the exam. The patients were positioned head first with both arms raised above the head. Scanning was done in the cephalo-caudal direction in one breath-hold from the thoracic inlet to the upper abdomen with a display field of view (FOV) from rib-to-rib. About 95–97 ml of iodinated contrast material (370 mg I/ml) was administered preferably through an antecubital vein at a rate of 2.5 to 3.5 ml/s using an 18- or 20- gauge cannula and an automated power injector (VISTRON CT™ Injection System). Real-time bolus tracking technique was used with no saline flushes. Scanning parameters were as follows: collimation 0.625 mm ×16; pitch of 1.06; reconstruction index 0.75 mm; peak voltage 120 kV; tube current 175 mA. The images were transferred to a workstation and viewed using the software Hitachi Image Explorer 4.5.1 (Hitachi Medical Corporation). Standard mediastinal and lung windows with real-time ability to modify the window width and level settings were used to optimize vessel visualization. Multiplanar reformation was used when necessary to help differentiate PE from possible artifacts.

The MDCT pulmonary angiographic diagnostic criteria of acute pulmonary embolism consisted of direct visualisation of an endoluminal, low-attenuating non enhancing filling defect in the main pulmonary artery or a primary-, secondary-, or tertiary-order pulmonary artery branch [4]. This filling defect should be complete or partial forming an acute angle with the arterial wall or centrally located [17]. All the CT angiograms were reviewed by two radiologists with over five to thirty-five years of experience. Repeat and technically inadequate MDCT pulmonary angiograms were excluded from the study.

Data collection and statistical analysis

A questionnaire was used to collect data. Thromboembolic risk factors were assessed from the clinicians' documentation where available and recorded: age 65 years or older, postoperative state, known deep vein thrombosis DVT), immobilization due to medical reasons and malignancy [10-12]. The presence of PE and other MDCT findings were also noted. Statistical analysis was performed using the software PASW® Statistics 17.0 (SPSS Inc., Chicago, Illinois, USA).

Abbreviations

FOV: field of view; I: iodine; kV: kilo volts; mA: milli Ampere; MDCT: multi-detector computed tomography; mg: milli gramme; ml: milli litre; mm: milli metre; PE: pulmonary embolism; s: second; SD: standard deviation; SPSS: statistical package for social sciences.

Competing interests

The authors declare that they have no competing interests.

Authors' contributions

JT conceived the study and participated in its design, data collection, statistical analysis and drafting of the manuscript. BM participated in the study design, review of the images, statistical analysis and the drafting of the manuscript. EF participated in the review of the images and proof-reading of the manuscript. EG participated in the review of the images and proof-reading of the manuscript. AGJ participated in the study design and proof-reading of the manuscript. All authors read and approved the final manuscript.

Acknowledgements

The authors wish to thank Mrs Olomo Virginie for helping with the patients' records, Dr Fointama and Pr Gonsu for proof-reading the final version of the manuscript.

Author details

¹Department of Radiology and Radiation Oncology, University of Yaounde 1, Yaounde, Cameroon. ²Yaounde General Hospital, Yaounde, Cameroon.

References

1. Wittram C, Meehan MJ, Halpern EF, Shepard JA, McLoud TC, Thrall JH: Trends in thoracic radiology over a decade at a large academic medical center. *J Thorac Imaging* 2004, 19:164–170.
2. Stein PD, Henry JW, Gottschalk A: Reassessment of pulmonary angiography for the diagnosis of pulmonary embolism: relation of interpreter agreement to the order of the involved pulmonary arterial branch. *Radiology* 1999, 210:689–691.
3. Remy-Jardin M, Remy J, Baghaie F, Fribourg M, Artaud D, Duhamel A: Clinical value of thin collimation in the diagnostic workup of pulmonary embolism. *Am J Roentgenol* 2000, 175:407–411.
4. Schoepf UJ, Holzknecht N, Helmberger TK, Crispin A, Hong C, Becker CR, et al: Subsegmental pulmonary emboli: improved detection with thin-collimation multi-detector row spiral CT. *Radiology* 2002, 222:483–490.
5. Patel S, Kazerooni EA, Cascade PN: Pulmonary embolism: optimization of small artery visualization at multi-detector row CT. *Radiology* 2003, 227:455–460.
6. van Erkel AR, van Rossum AB, Bloem JL, Kievit J, Pattynama PM: Spiral CT angiography for suspected pulmonary embolism: a cost-effectiveness analysis. *Radiology* 1996, 201:29–36.

7. Rosen MP: **Spiral CT, angiography for suspected pulmonary embolism: a cost-effectiveness analysis.** *Acad Radiol* 1999, **6**:72–75.

8. Prologo JD, Gilkeson RC, Diaz M, Asaad J: **CT pulmonary angiography: a comparative analysis of the utilization patterns in emergency department and hospitalized patients between 1998 and 2003.** *Am J Roentgenol* 2004, **183**:1093–1096.

9. Kingue S, Tagny-Zukam D, Binam F, Nouedoui C, Teyang A, Muna WFT: **Venous thromboembolism in Cameroon (description of 18 cases).** *Med Trop* 2002, **62**:47–50. French.

10. Stein PD, Fowler SE, Goodman LR, Gottschalk A, Hales CA, Hull RD, *et al*: **Multidetector computed tomography for acute pulmonary embolism.** *N Engl J Med* 2006, **354**:2317–2327.

11. Stein PD, Beemath A, Matta F, Weg JG, Yusen RD, Hales CA, *et al*: **Clinical Characteristics of Patients with Acute Pulmonary Embolism: Data from PIOPED II.** *Am J Med* 2007, **120**:871–879.

12. Mamlouk MD, vanSonnenberg E, Gosalia R, Drachman D, Gridley D, Zamora JG, *et al*: **Pulmonary Embolism at CT Angiography: Implications for Appropriateness, Cost, and Radiation Exposure in 2003 Patients.** *Radiology* 2010, **256**:525–632.

13. Prologo JD, Gilkeson RC, Diaz M, Cummings M: **The Effect of Single-Detector CT Versus MDCT on Clinical Outcomes in Patients with Suspected Acute Pulmonary Embolism and Negative Results on CT Pulmonary Angiography.** *Am J Roentgenol* 2005, **184**:1231–1235.

14. Karabulut N, Kıroğlu Y: **Relationship of parenchymal and pleural abnormalities with acute pulmonary embolism: CT findings in patients with and without embolism.** *Diagn Interv Radiol* 2008, **14**:189–196.

15. Richman PB, Courtney DM, Friese J, Matthews J, Field A, Petri R, Kline JA: **Prevalence and Significance of Nonthromboembolic Findings on Chest Computed Tomography Angiography Performed to Rule Out Pulmonary Embolism: A Multicenter Study of 1,025 Emergency Department Patients.** *Acad Emerg Med* 2004, **11**:642–647.

16. Costantino MM, Randall G, Gosselin M, Brandt M, Spinning K, Vegas CD: **CT angiography in the evaluation of acute pulmonary embolus.** *Am J Roentgenol* 2008, **191**:471–474.

17. Wittram C, Maher MM, Halpern EF, Shepard JA: **CT Angiography of Pulmonary Embolism: Diagnostic Criteria and Causes of Misdiagnosis.** *Radiographics* 2004, **24**:1219–1238.

21

Estimating radiation effective doses from whole body computed tomography scans based on U.S. soldier patient height and weight

Robert D Prins[1,2*], Raymond H Thornton[1†], C Ross Schmidtlein[1†], Brian Quinn[1†], Hung Ching[1†] and Lawrence T Dauer[1†]

Abstract

Background: The purpose of this study is to explore how a patient's height and weight can be used to predict the effective dose to a reference phantom with similar height and weight from a chest abdomen pelvis computed tomography scan when machine-based parameters are unknown. Since machine-based scanning parameters can be misplaced or lost, a predictive model will enable the medical professional to quantify a patient's cumulative radiation dose.

Methods: One hundred mathematical phantoms of varying heights and weights were defined within an x-ray Monte Carlo based software code in order to calculate organ absorbed doses and effective doses from a chest abdomen pelvis scan. Regression analysis was used to develop an effective dose predictive model. The regression model was experimentally verified using anthropomorphic phantoms and validated against a real patient population.

Results: Estimates of the effective doses as calculated by the predictive model were within 10% of the estimates of the effective doses using experimentally measured absorbed doses within the anthropomorphic phantoms. Comparisons of the patient population effective doses show that the predictive model is within 33% of current methods of estimating effective dose using machine-based parameters.

Conclusions: A patient's height and weight can be used to estimate the effective dose from a chest abdomen pelvis computed tomography scan. The presented predictive model can be used interchangeably with current effective dose estimating techniques that rely on computed tomography machine-based techniques.

Background

This research was driven by the need to estimate the radiation dose from computed tomography scans given to soldiers and civilians injured in austere environments. Nearly 50% of all injuries to United States Army soldiers in Operation Iraqi Freedom and Operation Enduring Freedom occurred in the head/neck, abdomen, and thorax region of the body [1,2]. Injuries in these regions are most commonly assessed using diagnostic x-ray scanning modalities such as computed tomography (CT). Current CT machines are able to scan an entire body in as little as 30 seconds making them particularly advantageous for diagnosing the extent of injuries sustained in traumatic events [3]. As a result, CT scanning is an integral part of the medical treatment schema from patient initial diagnosis through rehabilitation. In fact, because of this, CT scanning usage has steadily increased since its inception in 1972 [4]. While CT scanners have traditionally been used in fixed large hospital facilities technological advancements have made deployable CT machines a reality on battlefield environments [5].

While CT imaging as many advantages over other diagnostic modalities for diagnosing trauma injuries, it does have some drawbacks. CT procedures give patients more radiation dose than traditional x-ray imaging modalities.

* Correspondence: robert.prins@us.army.mil
† Contributed equally
[1]Department of Medical Physics, Memorial Sloan-Kettering Cancer Center, 1275 York Ave. New York, NY 10021, USA
Full list of author information is available at the end of the article

Because of this and CT's increased use, patients are exposed to more dose which may result in unintended health effects. As such, trade-offs exist between risk and benefit in the use of CT. In order to manage the risks associated with CT effectively, healthcare providers need to be able to estimate and track the dose these patients receive from their CT scan(s). Additionally, CT generates an order of magnitude more information than traditional medical imaging modalities.

The Joint Patient Tracking Application was developed to allow users to get real-time information on the status of their injured troops [6]. However, the trauma record does not show how many radiographic procedures were performed in the trauma diagnosis. Furthermore, advances in diagnostic imaging have not made the management of patient imaging records easier. This is illustrated by the fact that for a brief time period, one combat hospital switched from film radiography to digital radiography and then back to film radiography because of increased throughput during trauma situations and the inability of outside facilities to read the compact disks with the films saved on them [7].

The probability of repeat diagnostic scanning procedures increases when failure to transfer relevant understandable radiographic information along with the patient occurs. Additionally, as the level of integrated hospital care increases, the radiographic technology also increases resulting in multiple diagnostic procedures on the same area with different diagnostic modalities. Increasing numbers of radiographic procedures are not unique to military medicine. Victims of trauma receive multiple diagnostic scans and thus are at an increased risk of detrimental health risks from cumulative radiation dose [3,8,9].

Quantification of the risk derived from the repeated use of CT scans is needed in order to assess the consequences of the increased dose to these soldiers. A common metric for estimating the dose from CT scans, effective dose, describes the relationship between the probability of stochastic effects from radiation and equivalent dose for a mathematical reference phantom [10]. Estimating the effective dose is usually performed using machine-based parameters and derived conversion coefficients [4,11].

However, if the CT machine-based parameters for the scan are unknown because the requisite information is lost as a patient is transferred from one hospital to another, the only other means of estimating the effective dose from a CT scan is through the use of broad estimates based on published nominal values [12]. We propose an alternate method that estimates the chest abdomen pelvis scan effective dose to a mathematical phantom based upon the patient's height and weight at the time of the scan.

Methods

The approach we took to develop the alternate method for estimating effective dose involved three steps. The first step required the development of a mathematical model based upon a fictitious population of phantoms representing a range of body parameters common for U.S. Army soldiers. The second step verified the model by comparison of absorbed doses to organs using anthropomorphic phantoms. Finally, the third step validated the model with a real patient dataset. The development of estimating the effective dose model differs from the current method of estimation which uses machine-based parameters.

The most common method of estimating the effective dose when machine-based parameters from a CT scan are available involves multiplying the dose-length-product (DLP), a product of the volume computed tomography dose index ($CTDI_{vol}$) and the scanning length, by a conversion coefficient. The DLP is available by referencing the dose report generated by most commercial scanners at the end of the CT scanning procedure. Conversion coefficients have been derived using Monte Carlo simulations and experimental measurements.

Commercial CT scanners provide an estimate of the DLP in the dose report generated at the end of a scanning procedure. The DLP is derived from the $CTDI_{vol}$ which is measured using a 32-cm diameter acrylic cylinder and a 100-mm long pencil shaped ionization chamber [13]. The chamber provides the dosimetry measurements at the center of the cylinder (c) and on the periphery (p) of the cylinder from which the weighted CTDI ($CTDI_w$) is calculated using

$$CTDI_w = \frac{2}{3}CTDI_p + \frac{1}{3}CTDI_c. \qquad (1)$$

$CTDI_{vol}$ is calculated by considering both the $CTDI_w$ and the pitch of the machine given by

$$CTDI_{vol} = \frac{CTDI_w}{pitch}, \qquad (2)$$

where pitch is the table increment travelled per complete rotation of the x-ray tube. DLP is the product of the $CTDI_{vol}$ and the scan length.

$$DLP = CTDI_{vol} \times scan\ length \qquad (3)$$

Effective dose, the primary outcome measure of our study, can be calculated from the CT machine-based parameters and is the product of the DLP (mGy cm) and specific conversion coefficients (CC) (mSv mGy^{-1} cm^{-1}), using

$$E = DLP \times CC \qquad (4)$$

Conversion coefficients are available in several publications including the American Association of Physicists in Medicine (AAPM) Report 96 [11] and the National Council on Radiation Protection and Measurements (NCRP) Report 160 [4]. The conversion coefficient used in our study for a chest abdomen pelvis (CAP) scan is 0.015 mSv mGy^{-1} cm^{-1}[14].

The radiation dose from axial scanning is converted to radiation dose from helical scanning by dividing the axial scanning dose by the CT pitch.

We used a commercially available software program, (PCXMC 2.0.1 (Personal Computing X-ray Monte Carlo), STUK, Finland) [15], for calculating patient average absorbed organ doses in medical x-ray examinations. The software uses mathematical hermaphrodite phantoms.

As the software is primarily designed for projection radiography, four projections (anterior posterior (AP), posterior anterior (PA), right lateral (RLAT), and left lateral (LLAT)) were used to simulate a 360 degree exposure from a CT machine [16]. Each projection had the same slice thickness as a CT axial slice. Calibration factors were developed for effective dose comparison with a commonly used CT software program (ImPACT CT Patient Dosimetry Calculator, version 0.99x; ImPACT, London, England).

Mathematical phantoms of varying sizes were developed to represent the range of sizes of U.S. Army soldiers. Typical-sized U.S. Army soldiers have a body mass index (BMI, kg/m^2) of 20 to 30 [17,18]. Development of the phantom population used BMI, ranging from 18 (underweight) to 36 (obese), as a means of determining the height and weight of a theoretical U.S. Army population. Corresponding heights and weights were calculated from the BMI values. One hundred hermaphrodite mathematical phantoms with height and weight ranging from 5 feet 1 inch up to 6 feet 7 inches and 95 pounds up to 317 pounds were configured for use within the software. The methodology for determining the number of phantoms of varying height and weight was based on common guidelines that suggest the use of ten observations for each predictor [19,20].

In our study, all dose calculations per slice were simulated with 1×10^6 photons. Anode angle was set at 7 degrees with a beam quality half-value layer of 7.4 mm aluminum [21]. X-ray tube voltage was set at 120 kV for all calculations and software-required entrance air kerma values were obtained from measurements of the four projections at the center point of a typical chest abdomen pelvis scan using an anthropomorphic phantom. Averaged absorbed doses to organs were generated and recorded.

Multivariate regression analysis was performed using the R Project for Statistical Computing statistical program [22] in order to determine a best-fit model using height and weight as predictors of the effective dose. Full regression models were generated that identified effective dose as the dependent variable and the independent variables as height (cm), height^2 (cm^2), weight (kg), and weight^2 (kg^2). Bayesian information criterion techniques were used for

variable selection. Statistical significance was defined as $p < 0.05$.

Experimental verification measurements were performed using two adult anthropomorphic phantoms (CIRS, Inc., Norfolk, Virginia). The female adult anthropomorphic phantom (height 160 cm and weight 55 kg) and male adult anthropomorphic phantom (height 173 cm and weight 73 kg) were manufactured with dosimetry verification plugs enlarged to accommodate optically stimulated luminescent dosimeters utilizing an Al_2O_3 detector (Landauer Nanodot, Landauer, Inc., Glenwood, IL). All computed tomography scans were performed using a GE LightSpeed 16 (General Electric Healthcare, Waukesha, WI) (Figure 1). Manufacturer recommended calibration procedures were followed prior to irradiation [23]. For the purposes of this study, an 80 kVp calibration set was used and final dosimeter readings were adjusted to account for CT scanning (at 120 kVp) by multiplying each final reading by 1.15 based upon an experimentally determined energy response curve corresponding to the manufacturer calibration and usage instructions.

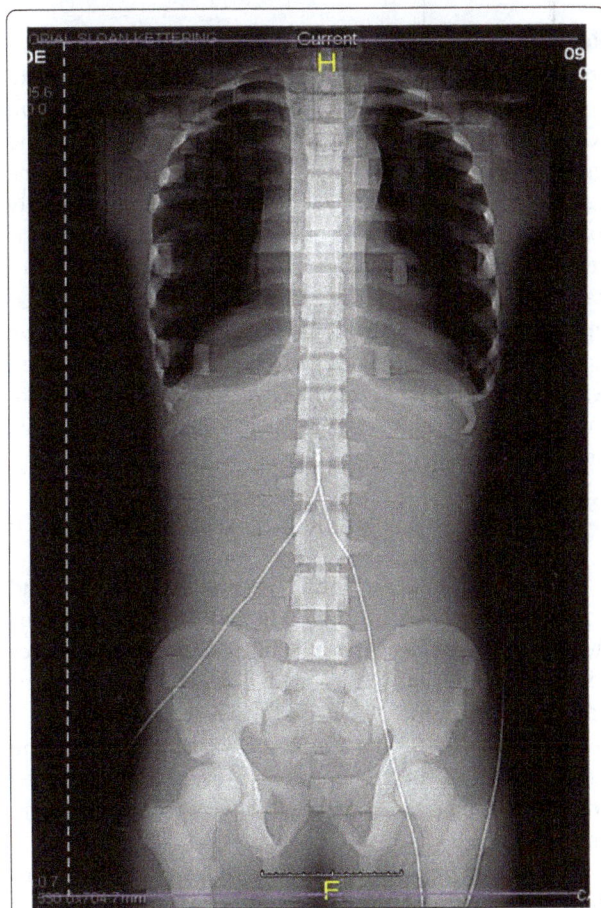

Figure 1 Representative Chest Abdomen Pelvis Scanning Range. Representative scanning range (vertical dashed line) of a chest abdomen pelvis (CAP) scan.

Both phantoms were scanned with the same experimental technique factors: 120 kVp, automatic mA (220 - 380 mA), slice thickness of 10-mm, and a helical scanning pitch 1.375.

The model for estimating effective dose presented in this paper was compared to the method of estimating effective dose using DLP and conversion coefficients because this latter method is the current accepted method [11,24]. An institutional review board approved retrospective study (Memorial Sloan-Kettering Cancer Center WA 0313-10 dated 23 June 2010) (n = 28) was conducted to compare the developed height weight predictive effective dose model with the current effective dose estimation method of multiplying the DLP by a published conversion coefficient. A Bland-Altman plot was used to visually inspect the variation between the two methods of estimating the effective dose. Bland-Altman plots (also known as an average versus difference plot) show the average of the methods on the x-axis and the difference between the methods on the y-axis [25]. This type of plot is effective in visually displaying the potential for systematic differences and method agreements.

Results

In the univariate analysis, patient height (H) (cm) and weight (W) (kg) demonstrated a significant association with effective dose (E) (mSv) and were entered into the multivariable linear regression analysis (equation 5). The variation (R^2 = 0.96) in the effective dose is primarily explained by a patient's height and weight. In the multivariable linear regression analysis, increasing patient height had a positive effect on the effective dose whereas increasing patient weight had a negative effect on the effective dose. A 1-cm increase in a patient's height is associated with a 0.3% increase in the effective dose. Similarly, a 1-kg increase in a patient's weight is associated with a 0.5% decrease in the effective dose given by

$$E \text{ (mSv)} = 18 + 0.067 \text{ H(cm)} - 0.11 \text{ W (kg)}. \quad (5)$$

Since effective dose is not a measurable quantity in and of itself, verification of the model (equation 5) was conducted by comparing experimentally obtained organ doses for eleven different organs which represent important components of effective dose to the organs doses estimated using the Monte Carlo software code. All of the organs listed in the tables (tables 1 and 2) are included within the primary scanning field of view except the brain and eyes.

The percent difference between the effective doses determined using either the mathematical phantom or experimental measurement is 9% for the female anthropomorphic phantom and 5% for male anthropomorphic phantom.

The absolute percent difference of the average effective dose for the IRB-approved population (n = 28) for the two means of calculating the effective doses was 33%. The population average effective dose calculated using the predictive model was 21 ± 2 mSv, while the population average effective dose calculated using the DLP CC method was 15 ± 5 mSv (Figure 2). Three of the four effective dose outliers shown on the predictive model plot are due to the patient BMI being greater than the range of BMIs (18 - 36 kg m^{-2}) used to develop the predictive model. The fourth effective dose outlier shown on the predictive model plot is due to the patient BMI (35 kg m^{-2}) being at the upper range of the BMIs used to develop the predictive model. The two means of calculating the effective doses are significantly different (paired t-test, p < 0.001) so analyzing the average of the effective doses versus the difference of the effective doses was performed.

Figure 3 shows the Bland-Altman plot for the two methods of calculating the effective dose from a chest abdomen pelvis scan. The height weight predictive model has a positive bias compared to the DLP CC method (mean of the differences = 6.38 mSv). The positive bias indicates that the height weight predictive model consistently estimated slightly higher effective doses than the DLP CC method. There is no significant systematic difference because the line of equality is within the ±1.96 standard deviation lines. All plotted values are within two standard deviations (solid heavy horizontal lines) of the mean (dashed horizontal line). Those plotted values that are near the -1.96 standard deviation line are a result of very large DLP values due to the patient BMI being greater than the BMIs used to develop the predictive model (Figure 4).

Discussion

In cardiology scans, it is well known that a patient's BMI is correlated with the effective dose from computed tomography scans [26,27]. Since BMI is a quantity comprising height and weight, the development of a model based upon height and weight will allow for estimating effective dose with minimal information and will result in similar accuracy of effective dose estimates when compared to current methods using CT machine-based parameters and these parameters are unknown. There is currently no known research specifically addressing such a model for chest abdomen pelvis CT scans. This research was designed to address that information gap.

The goal of using height and weight as predictors was to obtain a minimally confounded estimate of the effect of patient dimensions on effective dose from CT trauma protocols. A physician can utilize the predictive model (equation 5) to estimate the effective dose for the CT whole body (chest abdomen pelvis) scan. Specific machine characteristics were not assessed as predictors because this information is often not known for retrospective

Table 1 Organ absorbed doses

Organ	Female				Male		
	Measured Absorbed Dose (mGy)	Calculated Absorbed Dose (mGy)	ABS % Difference		Measured Absorbed Dose (mGy)	Calculated Absorbed Dose (mGy)	ABS % Difference
Adrenals/Gall Bladder	26.90 ± 0.03	25 ± 1	2		27.9 ± 0.4	23 ± 1	5
Brain	0.29 ± 0.02	0.4 ± 0.1	8		0.7 ± 0.3	0.4 ± 0.1	14
Colon	22.3 ± 0.7	21.1 ± 0.8	1		28 ± 5	20 ± 0.8	8
Esophagus	25 ± 1	23 ± 1	2		22.1 ± 0.4	21 ± 1	1
Eye	0.495 ± 0.008	NA			0.74 ± 0.08	NA	
Kidney	24.2 ± 0.5	31.5 ± 0.9	7		24.2 ± 0.8	30.3 ± 0.9	5
Liver	26.0 ± 0.2	29.5 ± 0.3	3		26.3 ± 0.9	28.1 ± 0.3	2
Lung	27 ± 1	33.9 ± 0.7	6		24 ± 1	32.4 ± 0.6	7
Pancreas	25.9 ± 0.4	25.1 ± 0.7	1		28.5 ± 0.2	23.2 ± 0.7	5
Thymus	23.5 ± 0.3	25 ± 5	2		27.0 ± 0.5	24 ± 5	3
Thyroid	12.3 ± 0.4	24 ± 9	16		30.2 ± 0.8	24 ± 9	6
Uterus/Testes	25.6 ± 0.1	21 ± 4	5		8 ± 4	0.8 ± 0.4	41

Organ absorbed doses for a chest abdomen pelvis scan. The measured absorbed dose values are from the anthropomorphic phantoms and the calculated absorbed dose values are from the mathematical phantom.

Table 2 Estimates of the effective dose

Organ	ICRP103 Tissue Weighting Factor	Measured Equivalent Dose (Female) (mSv)	Calculated Equivalent Dose (mSv)	ABS Diff (%)	Measured Equivalent Dose (Male) (mSv)	Calculated Equivalent Dose (mSv)	ABS Diff (%)
Brain	0.01	0.0029 ± 0.0002	0.004 ± 0.001		0.007 ± 0.003	0.004 ± 0.001	
Colon	0.12	2.68 ± 0.08	2.5 ± 0.1		3.4 ± 0.6	2.4 ± 0.1	
Esophagus	0.04	1.00 ± 0.04	0.92 ± 0.04		0.88 ± 0.02	0.84 ± 0.04	
Liver	0.04	1.040 ± 0.008	1.18 ± 0.01		1.05 ± 0.04	1.12 ± 0.01	
Lung	0.12	3.24 ± 0.12	4.07 ± 0.08		2.9 ± 0.1	3.89 ± 0.07	
Thymus	0.04	0.94 ± 0.01	1.0 ± 0.2		1.08 ± 0.02	1.0 ± 0.2	
Thyroid	0.04	0.49 ± 0.02	1.0 ± 0.4		1.21 ± 0.03	1.0 ± 0.4	
Remainder	0.12	3.08 ± 0.08	3.1 ± 0.5		2.7 ± 0.5	2.3 ± 0.2	
Organs:							
Pancreas							
Uterus							
Kidney							
Adrenals/ Gall							
Bladder							
Effective Dose (mSv)		12.5 ± 0.2	13.7 ± 0.7	9%	13.1 ± 0.8	12.5 ± 0.6	5%

Effective dose for a chest abdomen pelvis scan.

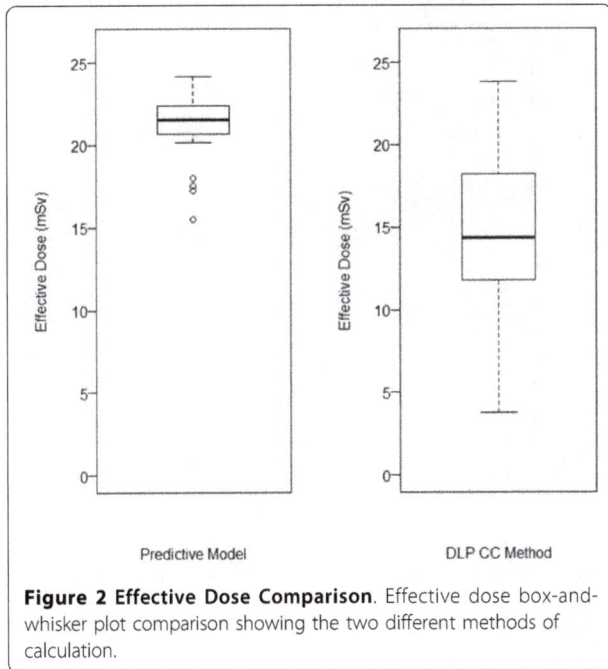

Figure 2 Effective Dose Comparison. Effective dose box-and-whisker plot comparison showing the two different methods of calculation.

assessment of effective dose from CT scans. The coefficient of determination, R^2, was used to describe the variability in the calculated effective dose explained by the linear regression model.

Utilizing Bland-Altman [25,28] plots to compare two methods allow us to determine whether or not the two methods can be used interchangeably. Since both calculations are an estimate of the effective dose the limits of agreement were set to be +/- 2 standard deviations of mean difference of the two methods. Convention allows that when the difference between the two methods lies

within two standard deviations of the difference mean, either method can be used with respect to accuracy [29]. The height weight predictive model is consistent with current literature which suggests that the DLP CC is known to underestimate the effective dose per scan [11,30-32]. Furthermore, literature suggests that experimental measurements of effective dose will often be higher than DLP CC methods for calculating effective dose because DLP CC methods can underestimate the effective dose by up to 37% [31-33]. Part of the reason for this difference is that conversion factors are highly dependent upon the specific size of the phantom used and the assumed scanning length [30].

DLPs can also underestimate the total energy imparted over the scanning length [11]. When scanning lengths are increased or decreased, organs are either brought into the scanning field-of-view or removed from the scanning field-of-view. For scanning regions which include fewer major organs (brain scan and cervical spine scan), differences between various methods of calculating effective doses result from dimensional differences between phantoms and patients. Dose variations between phantoms, physical and mathematical, will be less when organs are small in volume and can be easily represented by an averaged point dose estimate. Dose variations between phantoms will also be less for large organs which receive a fairly uniform absorbed dose throughout its volume [34].

This research was limited in the verification and validation of the model by using only two reference anthropomorphic phantoms and one type of CT scanner. Additional research should be performed verifying the model with other CT scanner types since dose variations

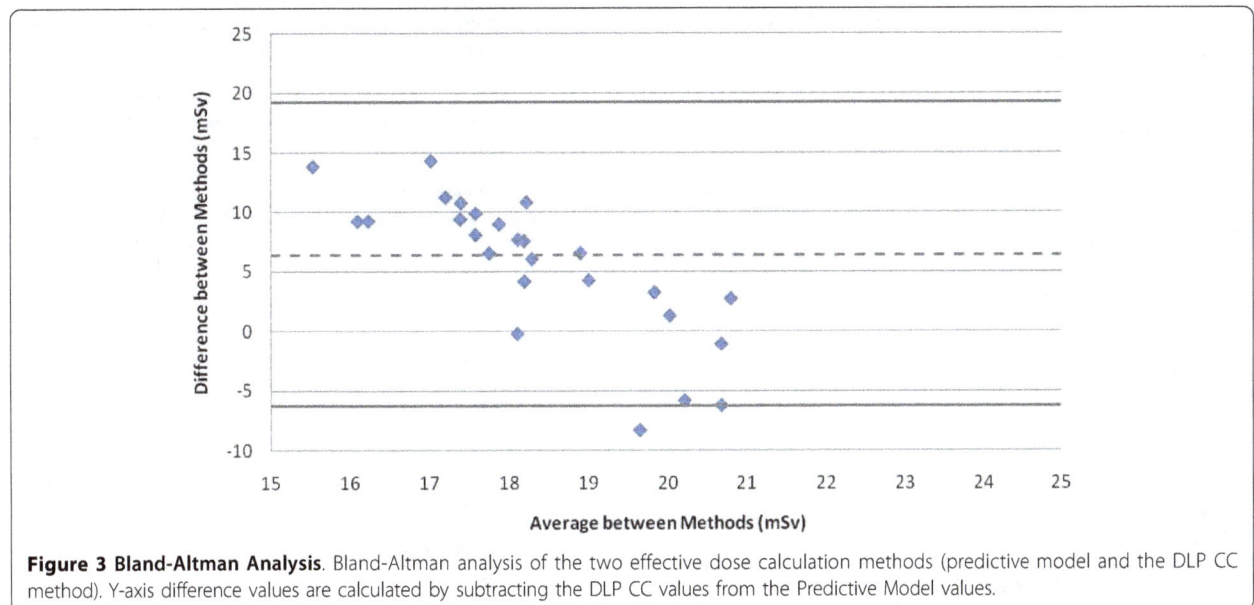

Figure 3 Bland-Altman Analysis. Bland-Altman analysis of the two effective dose calculation methods (predictive model and the DLP CC method). Y-axis difference values are calculated by subtracting the DLP CC values from the Predictive Model values.

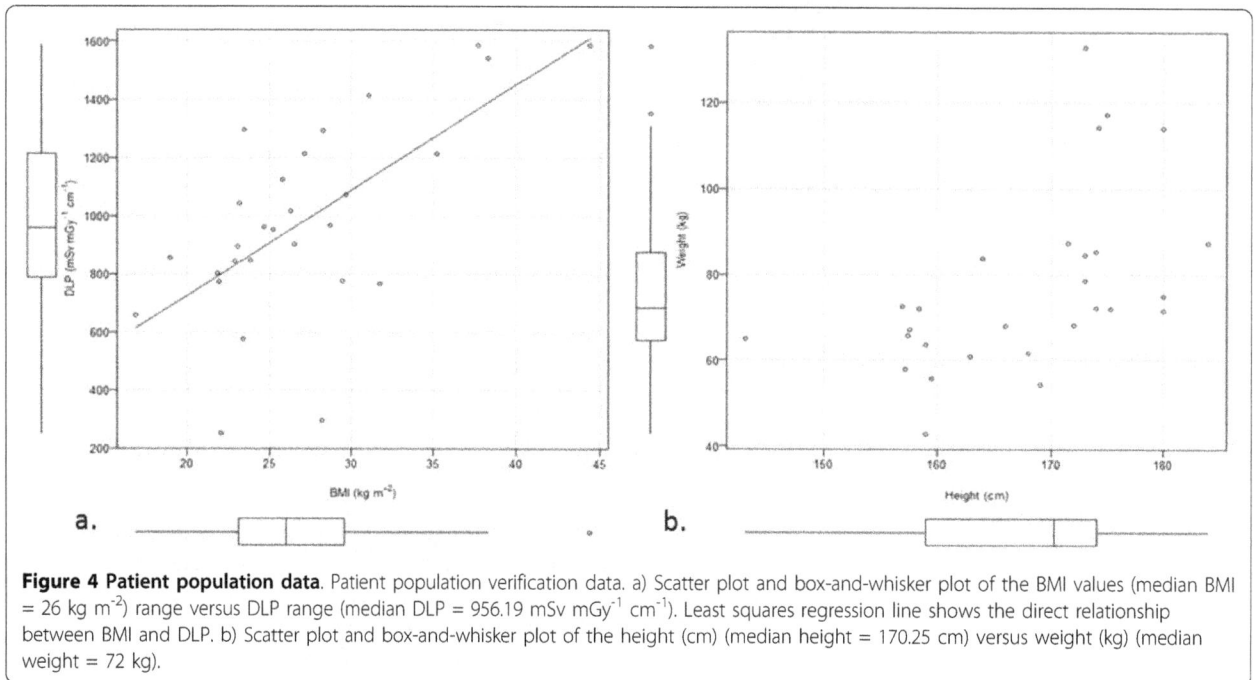

Figure 4 Patient population data. Patient population verification data. a) Scatter plot and box-and-whisker plot of the BMI values (median BMI = 26 kg m^{-2}) range versus DLP range (median DLP = 956.19 mSv mGy^{-1} cm^{-1}). Least squares regression line shows the direct relationship between BMI and DLP. b) Scatter plot and box-and-whisker plot of the height (cm) (median height = 170.25 cm) versus weight (kg) (median weight = 72 kg).

among CT scanners made by different manufacturers is known to occur [35,36].

Conclusions

The model described in this article can be used to estimate the effective dose from a chest abdomen pelvis CT scan to a mathematical phantom based on a patient's height and weight. Effective dose estimation gives the medical professional a means of comparing patient doses from CT with those of other radiation diagnostic modalities. This model allows for retrospective effective dose estimation when the machine parameters are not known for patient populations of similar characteristics with the mathematical and anthropomorphic phantoms.

Acknowledgements
The authors wish to thank the MSKCC Radiology Department for giving us research time on the CT scanner.

Author details
[1]Department of Medical Physics, Memorial Sloan-Kettering Cancer Center, 1275 York Ave. New York, NY 10021, USA. [2]Department of Environmental Health Sciences, Mailman School of Public Health, Columbia University, 722 West 168th Street, New York, NY 10032, USA.

Authors' contributions
RDP and LTD conceived of the study, collected the bulk of the data, and drafted the manuscript. CRS, RHT, BQ, and HC participated in the design and coordination of the study and assisted in the collection of the data. All authors read and approved the final manuscript.

Authors' information
RDP: Lieutenant Colonel Robert D. Prins, United States Army, completed his doctoral program at Columbia University and performed his doctoral research at Memorial Sloan-Kettering Cancer Center.

Competing interests
The authors declare that they have no competing interests.

References
1. Belmont PJ Jr, Goodman GP, Zacchilli M, Posner M, Evans C, Owens BD: Incidence and epidemiology of combat injuries sustained during "the surge" portion of operation iraqi freedom by a U.S. army brigade combat team. *Journal of Trauma - Injury, Infection and Critical Care* 2010, **68**(1):204-210.
2. Owens BD, Kragh JF Jr, Wenke JC, Macaitis J, Wade CE, Holcomb JB: Combat wounds in operation Iraqi Freedom and operation Enduring Freedom. *J Trauma* 2008, **64**(2):295-299.
3. Sodickson A, Baeyens PF, Andriole KP, Prevedello LM, Nawfel RD, Hanson R, Khorasani R: Recurrent CT, cumulative radiation exposure, and associated radiation-induced cancer risks from CT of adults. *Radiology* 2009, **251**(1):175-184.
4. National Council on Radiation Protection and Measurements: Ionizing radiation exposure of the population of the United States. *NCRP Report 160* 2009.
5. Morrison JJ, Clasper JC, Gibb I, Midwinter M: Management of penetrating abdominal trauma in the conflict environment: The role of computed tomography scanning. *World Journal of Surgery* 2011, **35**(1):27-33.
6. Holcomb JB, Stansbury LG, Champion HR, Wade C, Bellamy RF: Understanding combat casualty care statistics. *J Trauma* 2006, **60**(2):397-401.
7. Murray CK, Reynolds JC, Schroeder JM, Harrison MB, Evans OM, Hospenthal DR: Spectrum of care provided at an echelon II Medical Unit during Operation Iraqi Freedom. *Mil Med* 2005, **170**(6):516-520.
8. Tien H, Tremblay L, Rizoli S, Gelberg J, Spencer F, Caldwell C, Brenneman F: Radiation exposure from diagnostic imaging in severely injured trauma patients. *J Trauma* 2007, **62**(1):151-156.
9. Kim PK, Gracias VH, Maidment ADA, O'Shea M, Reilly PM, Schwab CW: Cumulative radiation dose caused by radiologic studies in critically ill trauma patients. *Journal of Trauma - Injury, Infection and Critical Care* 2004, **57**(3):510-514.
10. Quantities used in radiological protection. *Annals of the ICRP* 1991, **21**(1-3):4-11.

11. The Measurement, Reporting, and Management of Radiation Dose in CT, Report 96. In *Report of AAPM Task Group 23 of the Diagnostic Imaging Council CT Committee*. Edited by: American Association of Physicists in Medicine. College Park: AAPM; 2008:.

12. Radiation Exposure in X-ray and CT Examinations. [http://www.radiologyinfo.org].

13. International Electrotechnical Commission: Medical Electrical Equipment. Part 2-44. Particular Requirements for the safety of X-ray equipment for computed tomography. Geneva, Switzerland: IFC: IFC publication number 60601-2-44 amendment 1;, 2 2003.

14. Shrimpton PC, Hillier MC, Lewis MA, Dunn M: National survey of doses from CT in the UK: 2003. *Br J Radiol* 2006, 79(948):968-980.

15. PCXMC version 2.0. [http://www.stuk.fi/sateilyn_kaytto/ohjelmat/PCXMC/en_GB/pcxmc/].

16. Fulea D, Cosma C, Pop IG: Monte Carlo method for radiological X-ray examinations. *Romanian Journal in Physics* 2009, 54(7-8):629-639.

17. Reynolds K, Cosio-Lima L, Bovill M, Tharion W, Williams J, Hodges T: A comparison of injuries, limited-duty days, and injury risk factors in infantry, artillery, construction engineers, and Special Forces soliders. *Military Medicine* 2009, 174(7):702-708.

18. Reynolds KL, White JS, Knapik JJ, Witt CE, Amoroso PJ: Injuries and risk factors in a 100-mile (161-km) infantry road march. *Preventive Medicine* 1999, 28(2):167-173.

19. Peduzzi P, Concato J, Feinstein AR, Holford TR: Importance of events per independent variable in proportional hazards regression analysis II. Accuracy and precision of regression estimates. *Journal of Clinical Epidemiology* 1995, 48(12):1503-1510.

20. Concato J, Peduzzi P, Holford TR, Feinstein AR: Importance of events per independent variable in proportional hazards analysis I. Background, goals, and general strategy. *Journal of Clinical Epidemiology* 1995, 48(12):1495-1501.

21. LightSpeed Series Technical Reference Manual. Edited by: GE Systems 2005, 2nd Revision.

22. The R Development Core Team: R: A Language and Environment for Statistical Computing. Vienna, Austria: R Foundation for Statistical Computing; 2007.

23. MicroStar Specifications. [http://www.osldosimetry.com/documents/MicroStar_Specifications.pdf].

24. McCollough CH, Leng S, Lifang Y, Cody DD, Boone JM, McNitt-Gray MF: CT Dose Index and Patient Dose: They Are Not the Same Thing. *Radiology* 2011, 259(2):6.

25. Bland JM, Altman DG: Comparing methods of measurement: why plotting difference against standard method is misleading. *Lancet* 1995, , 346: 3.

26. Wielandts JY, De Buck S, Ector J, LaGerche A, Willems R, Bosmans H, Heidbuchel H: Three-dimensional cardiac rotational angiography: Effective radiation dose and image quality implications. *Europace* 2010, 12(2):194-201.

27. Mühlenbruch G, Hohl C, Das M, Wildberger JE, Suess C, Klotz E, Flohr T, Koos R, Thomas C, Günther RW, *et al*: Evaluation of automated attenuation-based tube current adaptation for coronary calcium scoring in MDCT in a cohort of 262 patients. *European Radiology* 2007, 17(7):1850-1857.

28. Altman DG, Bland JM: Measurement in Medicine: the Analysis of Method Comparison Studies. *The Statistician* 1983, , 32: 11.

29. LaMantia KR, O'Connor T, Barash PG: Comparing methods of measurement: an alternative approach. *Anesthesiology* 1990, 72(5):781-783.

30. Huda W, Ogden K, Khorasani M: Converting dose-length product to effective dose at CT. *Radiology* 2008, 248(3):995-1003.

31. Fujii K, Aoyama T, Yamauchi-Kawaura C, Koyama S, Yamauchi M, Ko S, Akahane K, Nishizawa K: Radiation dose evaluation in 64-slice CT examinations with adult and paediatric anthropomorphic phantoms. *The British Journal of Radiology* 2009, , 82: 9.

32. Groves AM, Owen KE, Courtney HM, Yates SJ, Goldstone KE, Blake GM: 16-detector multislice CT: dosimetry estimation by TLD measurement compared with Monte Carlo simulation. *The British Journal of Radiology* 2004, , 77: 4.

33. Hurwitz LM, Yoshizumi TT, Goodman PC, Frush DP, Nguyen G, Toncheva G, Lowry C: Effective dose determination using an anthropomorphic phantom and metal oxide semiconductor field effect transistor technology for clinical adult body multidetector array computed tomography protocols. *Journal of Computer Assisted Tomography* 2007, 31(4):544-549.

34. Sessions JB, Roshau JN, Tressler MA, Hintenlang DE, Arreola MM, Williams JL, Bouchet LG, Bolch WE: Comparisons of point and average organ dose within an anthropomorphic physical phantom and a computational model of the newborn patient. *Med Phys* 2002, 29(6):1080-1089.

35. Aldrich J, Bilawich A, Mayo J: Radiation doses to patients receiving computed tomography examinations in British Columbia. *Can Assoc Radiol J* 2006, 57(2):79-85.

36. Smith-Bindman R, Lipson J, Marcus R, Kim KP, Mahesh M, Gould R, Berrington de Gonzalez A, Miglioretti DL: Radiation dose associated with common computed tomography examinations and the associated lifetime attributable risk of cancer. *Arch Intern Med* 2009, 169(22):2078-2086.

Cone-beam computed tomography study of root and canal morphology of mandibular premolars in a western Chinese population

Xuan Yu[1,4†], Bin Guo[2†], Ke-Zeng Li[1], Ru Zhang[1], Yuan-Yuan Tian[1], Hu Wang[3*] and Tao Hu DDS[1*]

Abstract

Background: Traditional radiography is limited in its ability to give reliable information on the number and morphology of root canals. The application of cone-beam computed tomography (CBCT) provides a non-invasive three-dimensional confirmatory diagnosis as a complement to conventional radiography. The aim of this study was to evaluate the root and canal morphology of mandibular premolars in a western Chinese population using CBCT scanning.

Methods: The sample included 149 CBCT images comprising 178 mandibular first premolars and 178 second premolars. The tooth position, number of roots and canals, and canal configuration according to Vertucci's classification were recorded.

Results: The results showed that 98% of mandibular first premolars had one root and 2% had two roots; 87.1% had one canal, 11.2% had two canals and 0.6% had three canals. The prevalence of C-shaped canals was 1.1%. All mandibular second premolars had one root; 97.2% had one canal and 2.2% had two canals. The prevalence of C-shaped canals was 0.6%.

Conclusions: The prevalence of multiple canals in mandibular first premolars was mainly of Type V, and mandibular second premolars had a low rate of canal variation in this western Chinese population. Root canal bifurcation occurred at the middle or apical third in most bicanal mandibular premolars. CBCT scanning can be used in the management of mandibular premolars with complex canal morphology.

Keywords: Cone-beam computed tomography, Mandibular premolar, Morphology, Root canal configuration

Background

A thorough knowledge of root canal morphology is essential for successful endodontic treatment. Neglecting to probe, prepare, and fill all of the canals can lead to failure of endodontic treatment [1]. As a group, the mandibular premolars are among the most difficult teeth to treat endodontically [2], because they have a high incidence of multiple roots or canals. A possible explanation for this difficulty may be the extreme variations in root canal morphology that occur in these teeth. Furthermore, the incidence, location, and morphology of root canal systems may vary in different ethnic or regional populations.

The dimensions of the mandibular premolar root canal system are wider buccolingually than mesiodistally. Two pulp horns are easily detected: a large, pointed buccal horn and a small, rounded lingual horn. At the cervix of the tooth, both the root and canal are oval; this shape tends to become flat or round where the canal approaches the middle of the root. If two canals exist, they are usually circular from the pulp cavity to their apical foramen. In another anatomic variation, a single, broad root canal may bifurcate into two separate root canals at the apex of the root [3]. Direct access to the buccal canal is usually possible, whereas the lingual canal is often very difficult to locate and tends to deviate from the main canal at a sharp angle. In addition, the lingual inclination of the crown tends to direct files

* Correspondence: wanghu200108@163.com; acomnet@263.net
†Equal contributors
[3]Department of Radiology, West China School of Stomatology, Sichuan University, Chengdu, China
Full list of author information is available at the end of the article

Table 1 Number and percentage of roots and canals in 356 mandibular premolars according to location

| | No. of roots | | | | No. of canals | | | | | | | |
| | One-rooted | | Two-rooted | | 1 | | 2 | | 3 | | c-shaped | |
	left	right	left	right	left	right	left	right	left	right	left	right
First premolar	78	96	1	3	68	87	9	11	0	1	1	1
Total	174 (98%)		4 (2%)		155 (87.1%)		20 (11.2%)		1 (0.6%)		2 (1.1%)	
Second premolar	79	99	0	0	76	94	3	4	0	0	0	1
Total	178 (100%)		0 (0%)		173 (97.2%)		4 (2.2%)		0 (0%)		1 (0.6%)	

buccally, making the location of a lingual canal orifice highly challenging [4]. A mandibular first premolar may sometimes have three roots and three canals [5-7] or one root and four canals [8]. One study reported a C-shaped canal anatomy in the mandibular first premolar [9].

Traditional radiography, hard tissue section, and root canal staining or micro-CT scanning *in vitro* are commonly used tools in identifying the configuration of canals. Conventional images compress three-dimensional (3D) anatomy into a two-dimensional image, resulting in some important features of the tooth and its surrounding tissues being visualized only in the mesiodistal plane. Thus, features presenting in the buccolingual dimension may not be fully appreciated. Cone-beam computed tomography (CBCT) scanning was introduced in the field of endodontics in 1990 [10]. This non-invasive, 3D imaging technique has many endodontic applications, including morphologic analysis [11]. Several studies of root canal morphology in permanent maxillary and mandibular first molars have been performed using CBCT, and the reports revealed that the application of CBCT is advantageous in identifying variations in canal configuration [12-15]. Compared with the helical CT scanner, its major advantages are a substantial reduction in radiation exposure [16] and higher-quality image rendering for assessment of dental hard tissues [17]. Many studies of root and canal morphology in mandibular premolars have been conducted because these teeth present complex morphology that often complicates treatment [18,19]. However, most of these studies have been performed *ex vivo* [20,21] and involved complete destruction of the tooth during examination (hard tissue sections) or have acquired only two-dimensional anatomic information (traditional radiography). Thus, the current study was designed to test 3D CBCT imaging as a means of determining root and canal morphology in mandibular first and second premolars as an adjunct to clinical diagnosis and treatment planning.

Methods

All experimental procedures in this study were approved by the West China Stomatology School ethics committee.

The West China Hospital of Stomatology, located in Chengdu, functions as the clinical treatment center for oral diseases and maxillofacial surgery in the Western-China area This area include Sichuan, Yunnan, Guizhou, Tibet etc. provinces, and is the most concentrated area of ethnic minorities in china, there are 44 ethnic minority groups except the Han ethnic, which is the main group. All of the Western population belong to the Asian.We selected 149 CBCT images from the medical imaging center at the West China Hospital of Stomatology, between July 2009 and December 2010. All images were taken using a 3D Accuitomo CBCT machine (MCT-1 [EX-2 F], Morita Manufacturing Corp, Kyoto, Japan) with image capture parameters set at 80 kV and 5.0 mA, and an exposure time of 17 s. The voxel size was 0.125 mm and the slice thickness was 1.0 mm. Samples of fully erupted permanent mandibular first and second premolars were included. Qualifying mandibular premolars each demonstrated fully developed apices and lacked root canal fillings, posts and crown restorations. The CBCT images of 356 mandibular premolars from 149

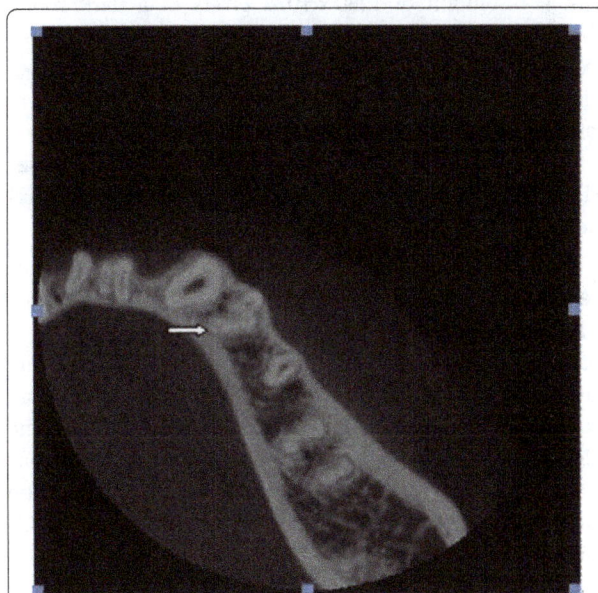

Figure 1 Type VIII canal configuration in mandibular first premolar with three canals. White arrow illustrates three independent canals in the cross-sectional image.

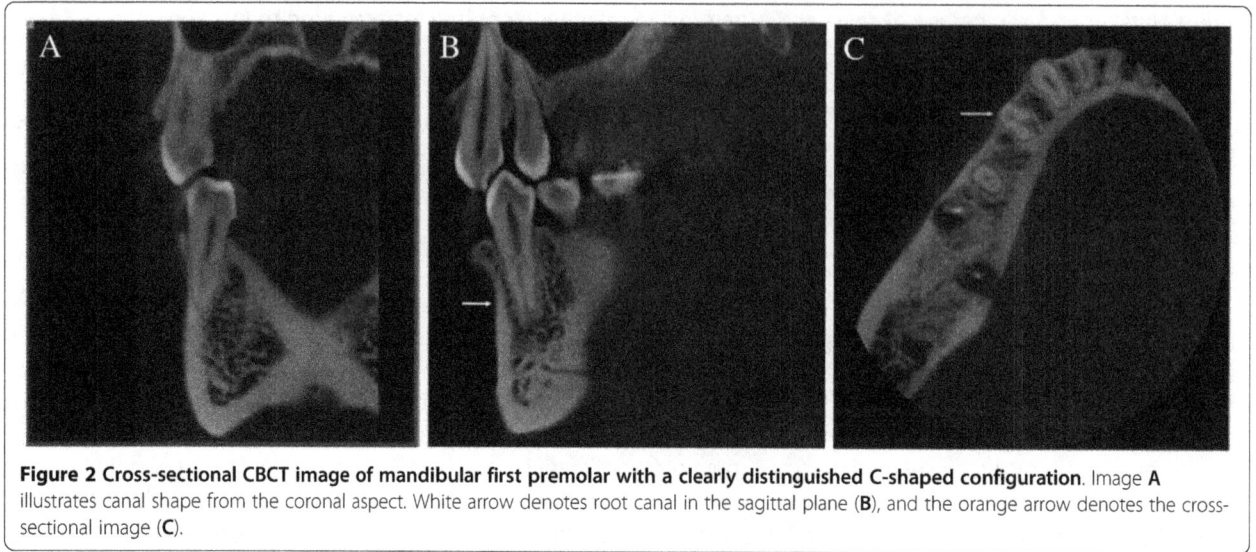

Figure 2 Cross-sectional CBCT image of mandibular first premolar with a clearly distinguished C-shaped configuration. Image **A** illustrates canal shape from the coronal aspect. White arrow denotes root canal in the sagittal plane (**B**), and the orange arrow denotes the cross-sectional image (**C**).

Table 2 Number and percentage of canal system types in 174 single-rooted mandibular first premolars

Root canal configurations

	Type I 1	Type II 2-1	Type III 1-2-1;	Type IV 2	Type V 1-2	Type VI 2-1-2	Type VII 1-2-1-2	Type VIII 1-3	C-shaped
Number	151	0	3	0	17	0	0	1	2
Percentage	86.8	0	1.7	0	9.8	0	0	0.6	1.1

patients of Chinese descent were analyzed with inbuilt software (i-Dixel one volume viewer 1.5.0) using a Dell Precision T5400 workstation (Dell, Round Rock, TX, USA). Axial, coronal, and sagittal two-dimensional sectional images were displayed on a 32-inch Dell LCD screen with a resolution of 1280 × 1024 pixels in a dark room. Two independent endodontists assessed the number of roots and canals, the position where canal bifurcation occurred and the canal configuration using One Data Viewer software (Morita Manufacturing Corp) to reach consensus in the interpretation of radiographic findings. In cases where consensus was not reached, a third professional oral radiologist was asked to perform a decisive evaluation.

Results

Number of roots and canals

Of 178 mandibular first premolars, 174 (98%) had one root and four (2%) had two roots; 87.1% had one canal, 11.2% had two canals, 0.6% had three canals and the prevalence of C-shaped canals was 1.1%. All mandibular second premolars had one root. Of these, 97.2% had one canal and 2.2% had two canals. The prevalence of C-shaped canals was 0.6% (Table 1).

Variations in root canal system morphology

The canal morphology of mandibular first premolars according to Vertucci's classification [22] was as follows:

Type I = 151 (86.8%), Type III = 3 (1.7%), Type V = 17 (9.8%), Type VIII = 1 (0.6%) (Figure 1), while two teeth had a C-shaped configuration (1.1%) (Figure 2). Four of the mandibular first premolars had two roots and two canals (one canal in each root) (Table 2). All 178 mandibular second premolars were single-rooted and the canal configurations of these teeth according to Vertucci's classification were Type I (173 teeth, 97.2%), Type II (one tooth, 0.55%) and Type V (3 teeth, 1.7%); one tooth had a C-shaped configuration (0.55%) (Figure 3, Table 3). In both first and second mandibular premolar teeth exhibiting Type V or Type VIII morphology, the canal bifurcation occurred at the middle-apical part of the

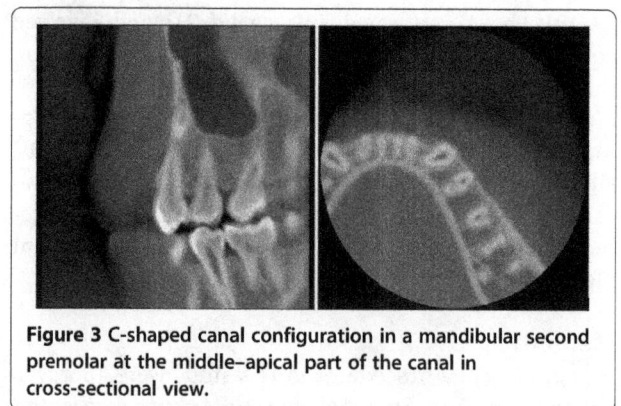

Figure 3 C-shaped canal configuration in a mandibular second premolar at the middle–apical part of the canal in cross-sectional view.

Table 3 Number and percentage of canal system types in 178 mandibular second premolars

Root canal configurations

	Type I 1	Type II 2-1	Type III 1-2-1	Type IV 2	Type V 1-2	Type VI 2-1-2	Type VII 1-2-1-2	Type VIII 1-3	C-shaped
Number	173	1	0	0	3	0	0	0	1
Percentage	97.2	0.55	0	0	1.7	0	0	0	0.55

root, which is where 87% and 75% of the canal system variations occur in mandibular first and second premolars, respectively.

Discussion

Our findings on the number of roots and canals in mandibular first premolars, showing that most had only one root and one canal, are in keeping with the results of previous studies [18,22-25]. In mandibular second premolars, we also found that all had one root and most had only one canal, in agreement with the findings of Miyoshi et al. [26]. However, these results are somewhat different to those reported in other studies. One study of a Chinese population in the Taiwan area found that only 54% of mandibular first premolars exhibited a single canal, whereas 22% contained two canals (vs. 11% in this study) and 18% percent had a C-shaped configuration (vs. 1.1% in this study) [20]. Furthermore, a literature review showed that, on average, 91.0% of mandibular second premolars have a single canal and 9.0% have two or more canals (vs. 97.2% and 2.2%, respectively, in this study) [19]. These divergent results may be explained by methodological differences or by variations in sample size, ethnic and/or regional background of the samples used [9,18,20,27,28].

The cross-sectional morphology of the majority of canals in this study was oval in the coronal third, circular or oval in the middle third and circular in the apical third. Interestingly, the root canal bifurcation tended to occur in the middle or apical third in the vast majority of bicanal mandibular premolars (87% and 75% in first and second premolars, respectively), consistent with previous investigations [3,20,29]. This indicates a high probability of variation in the root canal when the clinician detects a change of shape or direction in the middle-apical sections of the canal.

The complex root canal anatomy of mandibular premolars may be disguised in routine straight-on or even oblique radiography in clinical situations. A previous study [21] has demonstrated the low sensitivity of mesio-distal or buccolingual angulated radiographs in detection of root canal morphology. Conventional intraoral periapical radiographs are an important clinical diagnostic tool for assessing canal morphology, but these radiographs are not completely reliable because of inherent limitations such as distortion and superimposition of dental structures [8]. The application of CBCT has been suggested in these cases to provide a 3D confirmatory diagnosis without causing any tooth damage. It offers high resolution and is well suited for endodontic applications as a complement to conventional radiography [14]. When uncertainty exists in the diagnosis of canal variations, or a change of shape/direction in the middle-apical third of the canal is detected, periapical radiography associated with CBCT can be used to determine or confirm the presence and location of canal bifurcation.

Conclusion

Mandibular first premolars in a western Chinese population exhibited high variability and complexity in their canal systems. The root and canal configuration of mandibular second premolars was less variable than that of mandibular first premolars. Significantly, a CBCT scanner was able to detect these complex variations. This suggests that CBCT has potential as an auxiliary tool in the evaluation of mandibular premolars with complex canal morphology to improve the quality of root canal therapy. The importance of accurately determining the existence of complex canal systems is reflected in the elevated failure rate that occurs when additional canals are missed during root canal therapy. CBCT scanning is of great value in detecting anomalous canal morphology when diagnosis by conventional radiography is inconclusive.

Competing interests
All authors declare that they have no competing interests.

Acknowledgments
This work was supported by the Key Clinical Program of the Ministry of Health of China. The funding body had no role in study design, data collection/analysis, decision to publish, or preparation of the manuscript. We thank Hu Wang for his help with the acquisition of the raw data.

Author details
[1]State Key Laboratory of Oral Diseases, Departments of Operative Dentistry and Endodontics, West China School of Stomatology, Sichuan University, Chengdu, P.R. China. [2]Institute of Stomatology of Chinese PLA General Hospital, Beijing, P.R. China. [3]Department of Radiology, West China School of Stomatology, Sichuan University, Chengdu, China. [4]Department of Stomatology, Yinzhou People's Hospital, Ningbo, Zhejiang, P.R.China.

Authors' contributions
XY, BG, RZ, KZL, YYT, TH and HW participated in the design of the experiment and wrote the manuscript. XY and BG participated in the acquisition, analysis and interpretation of data. All authors read and approved the final manuscript.

References

1. Torabinejad M, Walton RE: *Principles and Practice of Endodontics*. 4th edition. St. Louis: Saunders; 2009:216–218.
2. Slowey RR: Root canal anatomy: road map to successful endodontics. *Dent Clin North Am* 1979, **23**:555–573.
3. Baisden MK, Kulild JC, Weller RN: Root canal configuration of the mandibular first premolar. *J Endod* 1992, **18**:505–508.
4. Vertucci FJ: Root canal morphology and its relationship to endodontic procedure. *Endodontic Topics* 2005, **10**:3–29.
5. Rodig T, Hulsmann M: Diagnosis and root canal treatment of a mandibular second premolar with three root canals. *Int Endod J* 2003, **36**:912–919.
6. De Moor RJ, Calberson FL: Root canal treatment in a mandibular second premolar with three root canals. *J Endod* 2005, **31**:310–313.
7. Cohen S, Burns RC: *Pathways of the Pulp*. 8th edition. St Louis: CV Mosby; 2006:216–219.
8. Tzanetakis GN, Lagoudakos TA, Kontakiotis EG: Endodontic treatment of a mandibular second premolar with four canals using operating microscope. *J Endod* 2007, **33**:318–321.
9. Fan B, Yang J, Gutmann JL, *et al*: Root canal systems in mandibular first premolars with C-shaped root configurations. Part I: micro computed tomography mapping of the radicular groove and associated root canal cross sections. *J Endod* 2008, **34**:1337–1341.
10. Tachibana H, Matsumoto K: Applicability of x-ray computerized tomography in endodontics. *Endod Dent Traumatol* 1990, **6**:16–20.
11. Patel S, Dawood A, Pitt Ford T, *et al*: The potential applications of cone beam computed tomography in the management of endodontic problems. *Int Endod J* 2007, **40**:818–830.
12. Neelakantan P, Subbarao C, Ahuja R, *et al*: Cone-beam computed tomography study of root and canal morphology of maxillary first and second molars in an Indian population. *J Endod* 2010, **36**(10):1622–1727.
13. Huang CC, Chang YC, Chuang MC, *et al*: Evaluation of root and canal systems of mandibular first molars in Taiwanese individuals using cone-beam computed tomography. *J Formos Med Assoc* 2010, **109**:303–308.
14. Matherne RP, Angelopoulos C, Kulild JC, *et al*: Use of cone-beam computed tomography to identify root canal systems in vitro. *J Endod* 2008, **34**:87–89.
15. Zhang R, Yang H, Yu X, *et al*: Use of CBCT to identify the morphology of maxillary permanent molar teeth in a Chinese subpopulation. *Int Endod J* 2011, **44**(2):1620–169.
16. Mozzo P, Procacci C, Tacconi A, *et al*: A new volumetric CT machine for dental imaging based on the cone-beam technique: preliminary results. *Eur Radiol* 1999, **8**:1558–1564.
17. Hashimoto K, Kawashima S, Kameoka S, *et al*: Comparison of image validity between cone beam computed tomography for dental use and multidetector row helical computed tomography. *Dentomaxillofac Rad* 2007, **36**:465–471.
18. Cleghorn BM, Christie WH, Dong CC: The root and root canal morphology of the human mandibular first premolar: a literature review. *J Endod* 2007, **33**:509–516.
19. Cleghorn BM, Christie WH, Dong CC: The root and root canal morphology of the human mandibular second premolar: a literature review. *J Endod* 2007, **33**:1031–1037.
20. Lu TY, Yang SF, Pai SF: Complicated root canal morphology of mandibular first premolar in a Chinese population using the cross section method. *J Endod* 2006, **32**:932–936.
21. Khedmat S, Assadian H, Saravani AA: Root canal morphology of the mandibular first premolars in an Iranian population using cross-sections and radiography. *J Endod* 2010, **36**(2):214–217.
22. Vertucci FJ: Root canal morphology of mandibular premolars. *J Am Dent Assoc.* 1978, **97**:47–50.
23. Pineda F, Kuttler Y: Mesiodistal and buccolingual roengenographic investigation of 7275 root canals. *Oral Surg Med Oral Pathol* 1972, **33**:101–110.
24. Green D: Double canals in single roots. *Oral Surg Oral Med Oral Pathol.* 1973, **35**:689–696.
25. Zillich R, Dawson J: Root canal morphology of mandibular first and second premolars. *Oral Surg Oral Med Oral Pathol.* 1973, **36**:738–744.
26. Miyoshi S, Fujiwara J, Tsuji YT, Yamamoto K: Bifurcated root canals and crown diameter. *J Dent Res* 1977, **56**:1425.
27. Trope M, Elfenbein L, Tronstad L: Mandibular premolars with more than one root canal in different race groups. *J Endod* 1986, **12**:343–345.
28. Sert S, Aslanalp V, Tanalp J: Investigation of the root canal configurations of mandibular permanent teeth in the Turkish population. *Int Endod J* 2004, **37**:494–499.
29. Vertucci FJ: Root canal anatomy of the human permanent teeth. *Oral Surg Oral Med Oral Pathol* 1984, **58**:589–599.

New quantitative classification of the anatomical relationship between impacted third molars and the inferior alveolar nerve

Wei-Quan Wang[1], Michael Y. C. Chen[1,2], Heng-Li Huang[1,3], Lih-Jyh Fuh[1,2], Ming-Tzu Tsai[4] and Jui-Ting Hsu[1,3*]

Abstract

Background: Before extracting impacted lower third molars, dentists must first identify the spatial relationship between the inferior alveolar nerve (IAN) and an impacted lower third molar to prevent nerve injury from the extraction. Nevertheless, the current method for describing the spatial relationship between the IAN and an impacted lower third molar is deficient. Therefore, the objectives of this study were to: (1) evaluate the relative position between impacted lower third molars and the IAN; and (2) investigate the relative position between impacted lower third molars and the IAN by using a cylindrical coordinate system.

Methods: From the radiology department's database, we selected computed tomography images of 137 lower third molars (from 75 patients) requiring removal and applied a Cartesian coordinate system by using Mimics, a medical imaging software application, to measure the distribution between impacted mandibular third molars and the IAN. In addition, the orientation of the lower third molar to the IAN was also measured, but by using a cylindrical coordinate system with the IAN as the origin.

Results: According to the Cartesian coordinate system, most of the IAN runs through the inferior side of the third molar (78.6 %), followed by the lingual side (11.8 %), and the buccal side (8.9 %); only 0.7 % is positioned between the roots. Unlike the Cartesian coordinate system, the cylindrical coordinate system clearly identified the relative position, r and θ, between the IAN and lower third molar.

Conclusions: Using the cylindrical coordinate system to present the relationship between the IAN and lower third molar as (r, θ) might provide clinical practitioners with a more explicit and objective description of the relative position of both sites. However, comprehensive research and cautious application of this system remain necessary.

Keywords: Impacted third molar, Inferior alveolar nerve, Computed tomography, Cartesian coordinate system, Cylindrical coordinate system

Background

In the clinical environment of oral medicine, extraction of the lower third molar is a common surgical procedure. However, various postsurgery complications can occur [1–5]. Among such complications, injury to the inferior alveolar nerve (IAN) is the most severe. Because the IAN occasionally contacts or is near the third molar/root, or molars with a "crooked root," the IAN can be easily damaged during this procedure. Temporary and permanent IAN injury comprises approximately 5.0–7.0 % and 0.5–1.0 % of such incidents, respectively [2, 6–12]. Therefore, information regarding the spatial relationship between the third molars and IAN is critical for preoperative procedures.

Clinically, taking panoramic film is essential for evaluation before extraction. However, because panoramic film is a two-dimensional imaging tool, the image can be distorted or overlapped [13]. Nakagawa et al. [14] stated that this may lead clinicians to misinterpret the results or make incorrect judgments. Therefore, to minimize

* Correspondence: jthsu@mail.cmu.edu.tw
[1]School of Dentistry, College of Medicine, China Medical University, 91 Hsueh-Shih Road, Taichung 40402, Taiwan
[3]Department of Bioinformatics and Medical Engineering, Asia University, Taichung 413, Taiwan
Full list of author information is available at the end of the article

postoperative complications and improve judgments, computed tomography (CT) is introduced to evaluate the spatial relationship between the third molar and IAN canal.

Based on the Cartesian coordinate system concept, Maegawa et al. [15] reported that the probability of the IAN canals being positioned at the buccal, lingual, and inferior sides of the lower third molar and between the roots was 51, 26, 19, and 4 %, respectively. Ghaeminia et al. [16] employed a similar method on Westerners and reported observations on the buccal side (17 %), lingual side (49 %), inferior side (19 %), and between the roots (15 %). In addition, various researchers have reported inconsistent data including the trends of position probability. This is primarily because of measurement position discrepancies among various races; it may also have resulted from differences in the tooth morphology of the mandible structure and lower third molar root, which can cause approximate and imprecise classification of the teeth (such as between the inferior and buccal and between the inferior and lingual), leading to judgment errors and varying results.

Accordingly, this study was conducted to analyze the spatial relationship between impacted third molars and the IAN, the results of which were compared with those of previous studies. Specifically, this study was aimed at (1) establishing the distribution between impacted third molars and the IAN, and (2) investigating the relative position between the lower third molars and IAN by using a cylindrical coordinate system.

Methods
Patient selection
This retrospective study was based on a database of head CT scans for patients presenting to the Radiology Department of the China Medical University Hospital for an evaluation of impacted mandibular third molars and the IAN between July 2009 and January 2011. In this retrospective study, only the mandibles of patients with impacted third molars were selected for measurement. CT scans were performed (LightSpeed, General Electric, Milwaukee, WI) with the following technical parameters: 1.25-mm increments, 240 mm field of view, and 512×512 pixels. Before the position of the IAN was measured, the patient's head was first rotated with the Down's mandibular plane parallel to the horizontal plane in Mimics, then further rotated with the mandible centered on the midsagittal plane of the image perpendicular to the Down's mandibular plane. Subsequently, buccolingual images were created using the "online reslice" function of Mimics to obtain continual slices of the mandibular bone. There was no need to obtain consent because this is a retrospective study. In addition, all the patients were adults. The research protocol was approved by

the institutional research board of China Medical University and Medical Center.

Measurements of the relationship between the IAN and third molar
Cartesian coordinate system
From continuous buccolingual slices, the layer where the IAN and lower third molar were the closest was selected as the reference image to determine their relative position. First the position of the IAN and lower third molar were categorized as either contacting or noncontacting, and then the structural center of the lower third molar was located to serve as the origin in the Cartesian coordinate system. Subsequently, we determined whether the IAN was distributed on the lingual side, buccal side, or inferior side of the lower third molar or between the roots (Fig. 1).

Cylindrical coordinate system
From continuous buccolingual slices, the layer where the IAN and lower third molar were the closest was selected as the reference image to evaluate their relative position. First, the position of the IAN and lower third molar were categorized as contacting or noncontacting, and then the IAN (the structural center of the IAN canal) was located to serve as the origin in the cylindrical coordinate system. A line was drawn from this point to the nearest point on the lower third molar root, and the angle between this line and the inferior–superior axis was measured from 0° to 360° and then divided by 30°. The shortest distance between the lower third molar and the mandible canal was also measured (Fig. 2). The relationship between the IAN and lower third molar can be expressed as (r, θ) in the cylindrical coordinate system, where r is the shortest distance between the mandible and lower third molar, and θ is the orientation of the lower third molar relative to the IAN.

Statistical analysis
Descriptive statistics were computed to classify the probability distribution by using either the Cartesian coordinate system or cylindrical coordinate system.

Results
Based on the selection criteria, mandibular bone CT images of 75 patients (age_{mean} 37.0 + 18.9 years; age_{range} 18–77 years) were used in this study. From the 75 mandibular bones, 137 lower third molars (100 noncontact cases; 37 contact cases) were used for the measurement. For the Cartesian coordinate system (Table 1), the IAN distribution relative to the third molar was 78.8 % (108/137) in the inferior position, 11.7 % (16/137) in the lingual site, 8.8 % (12/137) in the buccal site, and 0.7 % (1/137) between the roots (Table 1).

	Periradicular			Interradicular
	Lingual	Buccal	Inferior	Between roots
Contact				
Non-contact				

Fig. 1 Classification of the position and relationship of the IAC with the right mandibular third molars using the Cartesian coordinate system

Regarding the relationship between the IAN and third molar in an angular distribution, no case between 60° and 270° was observed using the cylindrical coordinate system (Table 2). The highest probability region with 43.8 % was between 330° and 360°, followed by 32.1 % between 0° and 30°, and 21.2 % between 300° and 330°. The lowest probability with 0.8 % was between 270° and 300°. In addition, for the noncontact cases, Table 3 lists the shortest distances between the mandible canal and third molar. Most of them occurred above the 3-mm group, 11 % were in the 1–2-mm group, 11 % were at 1–2 mm, and only 3 % were in the 0–1-mm group.

Discussion

To reduce the risk of IAN injury when extracting the mandibular third molars, the appropriate tools must be used. Therefore, using CT images to accurately identify the relationship between the molars and IAN at the buccolingual section is crucial. In previous studies, the reported probability of various IAN positions relative to the lower third molars has been inconsistent. This is possibly due to the human discrimination affects derived from the subjective judgments of different dentists. The morphologies of the alveolar bone and lower third molar are highly divergent, which easily leads to approximate and imprecise distinguishing and classification (such as

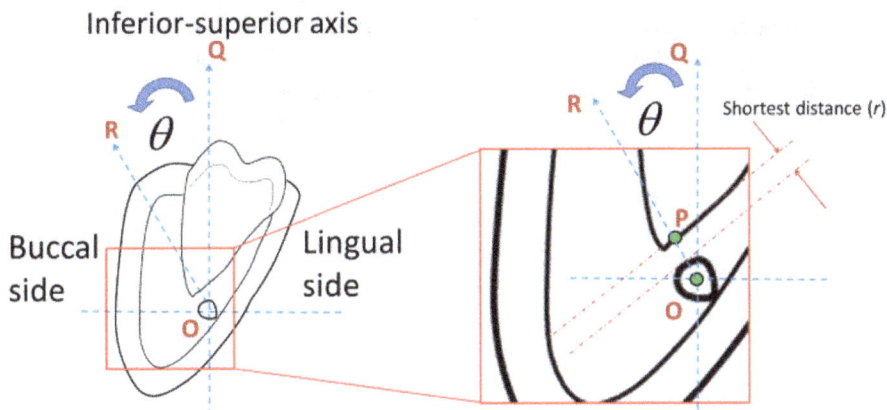

Fig. 2 Classification of the position and relationship of the IAN canal with the right mandibular third molars using the cylindrical coordinate system. This approach can be defined as follows: (1) Use the IAN bundle as the original reference point (point O); (2) find the point on the third molar (point P) closest to the IAN bundle, and draw a line (line OR) from the original reference point (point O) to point P; and (3) determine the angle between the inferior-superior axis (line OQ) and line OR

Table 1 Relationship between the IAN and third molar using the Cartesian coordinate system

Anatomical relationship	Contact	Non-contact	Total	Percentage (%)
Buccal	3	9	12	8.8
Lingual	8	8	16	11.7
Between roots	1	0	1	0.7
Inferior	25	83	108	78.8
Total	37	100	137	100

Table 3 The shortest distance between the mandible canal and the lower third molar for non-contact cases

The nearest distance	Sample number	Percentage (%)
0 ~ 1 mm	3	3
1 ~ 2 mm	11	11
2 ~ 3 mm	11	11
>3 mm	75	75
Total	100	100

between the inferior and buccal sides and between the inferior and lingual sides). This eventually results in judgment errors and inconsistent results. Compared with the traditional Cartesian coordinate system, the anatomical structure can be categorized more objectively and accurately by using the cylindrical coordinate system. This study developed a method that involves using a cylindrical coordinate system to assess the relationship between the IAN and lower third molar for Asian populations.

Previous studies have compared the ability of CT and panoramic filming for evaluating the relative position of the IAN and third molar [15, 17]. These studies have indicated that CT is an efficient tool for determining the relative position between the IAN and lower third molar. Although CT scans were employed in determining the relative position, we varied from other studies [15, 17, 18] in that the Down's mandibular plane was employed because resectioning methods cause the buccolingual section slices to become perpendicular to the mandibular canal.

In recent years, dental cone-beam CT (CBCT) has been prevalently employed in dental surgery [19–21] and basic research [22–25]. In addition to the presurgical orthodontic, orthognathic, and endodontic treatment evaluations, CBCT images also frequently serve as a reference when extracting impacted lower third molars [16, 26]. Therefore, although a CT image database was employed in the present study, the proposed cylindrical coordinate system proposed can also be applied to CBCT images.

The spatial relationships between the IAN and lower third molar identified in this study were compared with

those reported in literature (Table 4). When the Cartesian coordinate system was used, the IAN distribution relative to the third molars was found to be consistent with that reported by Tantanapornkul et al. [26] (Table 4). The highest distribution was on the inferior side, and the probability distribution on the lingual side was slightly higher than that on the buccal side; the lowest distribution was between the roots. Similarly, Monoco et al. [9] also indicated that the probability that the IAN would be located on the inferior side was the highest (Table 4). However, Ueda et al. [27] and Maegawa et al. [15] reported that the probability of the IAN distribution on the buccal side was higher than that on the lingual side (Table 4). Ghaeminia et al. [16], de Melo Albert et al. [28], and Ohman et al. [17] have reported that the probability of the distribution on the lingual side was the highest (Table 4). Variations in the results of previous studies and those of the present study may be due to the differing patient ethnicities of the patients and the various orientations of the mandibular bone in the buccolingual slices.

Regarding the experimental results of previous studies, Maegawa et al. [15], Tantanapornkul et al. [26], and Ueda et al. [27] have investigated conditions in Japan, which is near Taiwan. However, based on the Cartesian coordinate system, the spatial distributions in the experimental results of these studies are inconsistent. Maegawa et al. [15] and Ueda et al. [27] have reported that the highest distribution was on the buccal side, followed by the lingual side, inferior side, and then between the roots. The experimental results of the current study were similar to those reported by Tantanapornkul et al. [26], which indicated that the highest distribution was on the inferior side, followed the lingual side, buccal side, and then between the roots. This difference may have resulted from the ambiguous classification derived from the Cartesian coordinate system, particularly in the buccoinferior and linguoinferior regions.

Although the cylindrical coordinate system is used in orthodontics [29], it is not widely employed for oral surgery. During extraction of the lower third molar, protecting the IAN is critical. This raises questions as to why observations are made from the perspective of the molar to be extracted and why the position of the nerve is categorized relative to the molar. Instead, we propose

Table 2 Orientation of the lower third molar in relation to the IAN using the cylindrical coordinate system

Anatomical relationship	Contact	Non-contact	Total	Percentage (%)
0 ~ 30°	23	21	44	32.1
30° ~ 60°	1	2	3	2.1
60° ~ 270°	0	0	0	0
270° ~ 300°	1	0	1	0.8
300° ~ 330°	6	23	29	21.2
330° ~ 360°	6	54	60	43.8
Total	37	100	137	100

Table 4 The buccolingual distribution of the IAN in relation to the lower third molar, as reported in previous studies

	This study	Ueda et al. [27]	Ghaeminia et al. [16]	Tantanapornk-ul et al. [26]	De Melo Albert et al. [28]	Ohman et al. [17]	Monoco et al. [9]	Maegawa et al. [15]
Buccal	8.9 %	45.5 %	17 %	25 %	45 %	31 %	25 %	51 %
Lingual	11.8 %	32.4 %	49 %	26 %	48 %	33 %	19 %	26 %
Between roots	0.7 %	0.7 %	15 %	4 %		10 %	5 %	4 %
Inferior	78.6 %	21.4 %	19 %	45 %	7 %	26 %	51 %	19 %
Number	136	145	53	142	31	90	73	47

setting the IAN requiring protection as the origin and then observing the relative position of the nearby molar. Therefore, in the present study, we used a cylindrical co-ordinate system to categorize the relationship between the IAN and lower third molar. The advantage of using the cylindrical coordinate system is that it simplifies classifying the relationship between the third molars and IAN. The two parameters identified by this system—namely, the relative angle and shortest distance between the mandible canal and third molars—provide quantitative data and a detailed understanding for further investigation. The angle data not only reveal the distribution between the IAN and lower third molar, but may also prevent misunderstanding among clinical practitioners and researchers. Furthermore, the shortest distance between the lower third molar and mandible canal provides additional information regarding the distance between the mandible canal and third molar root, which is not available when using the Cartesian coordinate system. The shorter the distance is between these two structures, the greater the possibility for IAN injury during extraction of the lower third molar. Therefore, determining this distance is crucial. As shown in Table 3, an increment of 1 mm was adopted as the scale. Our observations indicated that for 75 % of all cases (75 cases), the distance between the IAN and lower third molar exceeded 3 mm, and for 3 % of cases (3 cases) the distance was shorter than 1 mm. In two of these three cases, removing the impacted third molars presented greater difficulty (the IAN was located on the lingual side relative to the lower third molar); thus, removal of impacted lower third molars necessitates additional caution.

To prevent situations where whether the IAN is located in the buccal or inferior region (or in the lingual or inferior region) cannot be determined, the position (r, θ) of the IAN relative to the lower third molar can be determined using the cylindrical coordinate system. Although Miller et al. [30] proposed inferior–lingual and inferior–buccal classifications regarding the relationship between the IAN and lower third molars, communication (particularly verbal) between clinical practitioners remain vague; by comparison, the cylindrical coordinate system (r, θ) provides superior clarity.

This study was subject to several limitations. First, all human samples were of Asian ethnicity, and whether the differences would occur in other ethnic groups was not explored. Second, the effects of gender and age were not investigated because of the small sample. Third, given the current status of the cylindrical coordinate system, the segmentation of impacted lower third molars was based on a manual approach. In future, an automated approach should be developed to enhance the clinical application of this system. Finally, unlike the prevalent use of the Cartesian coordinate system, the cylindrical coordinate system remains a new method for analyzing the relationship between the IAN and lower third molar. Comprehensive investigations are necessary to further verify the academic results and clinical applicability of this approach.

Conclusion

This study proposes a cylindrical coordinate system as a new analysis system for clarifying the anatomical relationship between the lower third molars and IAN. The Cartesian coordinate system revealed that the highest distribution is on the inferior side (78.6 %), followed by the lingual side (11.8 %), buccal side (8.9 %), and then between the roots (0.7 %). Based on the results of the study, using the cylindrical coordinate system to present the relationship between the IAN and lower third molar as (r, θ) might provide clinical practitioners with a more explicit and objective description of the relative position of both sites. However, comprehensive research on and cautious application of this system in the future remain necessary.

Abbreviations
IAN: Inferior alveolar nerve; CT: Computed tomography.

Competing interests
The authors declare that they have no competing interests.

Authors' contributions
MC, HH, and JH participated in the design of the study. WW, LF, and MT performed the measurement. MT and HH conducted the statistical analysis. WW and JH conceived the study, participated in its design and coordination, and drafted the manuscript. All authors read and approved the final manuscript.

Acknowledgment

This research was supported by the National Science Council of Taiwan (NSC 100-2815-C-039-048-B) and Ministry of Science and Technology (MOST 103-2221-E-039 -002).

Author details

[1]School of Dentistry, College of Medicine, China Medical University, 91 Hsueh-Shih Road, Taichung 40402, Taiwan. [2]Department of Dentistry, China Medical University and Hospital, Taichung 404, Taiwan. [3]Department of Bioinformatics and Medical Engineering, Asia University, Taichung 413, Taiwan. [4]Department of Biomedical Engineering, Hungkuang University, Taichung 433, Taiwan.

References

1. Au AH, Choi SW, Cheung CW, Leung YY. The efficacy and clinical safety of various analgesiccombinations for post-operative pain after third molar surgery: A systematic review and meta-analysis. PLoS One. 2015;10(6): e0127611.
2. Bouloux GF, Steed MB, Perciaccante VJ. Complications of third molar surgery. Oral Maxillofac Surg Clin North Am. 2007;19(1):117.
3. Tymofiyeva O, Rottner K, Jakob P, Richter EJ, Proff P. Three-dimensional localization of impacted teeth using magnetic resonance imaging. Clin Oral Investig. 2010;14(2):169–76.
4. Gaddipati R, Ramisetty S, Vura N, Kanduri RR, Gunda VK. Impacted mandibular third molars and their influence on mandibular angle and condyle fractures–A retrospective study. J Craniomaxillofac Surg. 2014;42(7):1102–5.
5. Engelke W, Beltrán V, Cantín M, Choi E-J, Navarro P, Fuentes R. Removal of impacted mandibular third molars using an inward fragmentation technique (IFT)–Method and first results. J Craniomaxillofac Surg. 2014;42(3):213–9.
6. Susarla SM, Blaeser BF, Magalnick D. Third molar surgery and associated complications. Oral Maxillofac Surg Clin North Am. 2003;15(2):177–86.
7. Robert RC, Bacchetti P, Pogrel MA. Frequency of trigeminal nerve injuries following third molar removal. J Oral Maxillofac Surg. 2005;63(6):732–5.
8. Tay A, Zuniga J. Clinical characteristics of trigeminal nerve injury referrals to a university centre. Int J Oral Maxillofac Surg. 2007;36(10):922–7.
9. Monaco G, Montevecchi M, Bonetti GA, Gatto MR, Checchi L. Reliability of panoramic radiography in evaluating the topographic relationship between the mandibular canal and impacted third molars. J Am Dent Assoc. 2004;135(3):312–8.
10. Kipp DP, Goldstein BH, Weiss Jr W. Dysesthesia after mandibular third molar surgery: a retrospective study and analysis of 1,377 surgical procedures. J Am Dent Assoc. 1980;100(2):185–92.
11. Rud J. Third molar surgery: relationship of root to mandibular canal and injuries to the inferior dental nerve. Tandlaegebladet. 1983;87(18):619.
12. Chiapasco M, De Cicco L, Marrone G. Side effects and complications associated with third molar surgery. Oral Surg Oral Med Oral Pathol. 1993;76(4):412–20.
13. Sameshima GT, Asgarifar KO. Assessment of root resorption and root shape: periapical vs panoramic films. Angle Orthod. 2001;71(3):185–9.
14. Nakagawa Y, Ishii H, Nomura Y, Watanabe NY, Hoshiba D, Kobayashi K, et al. Third molar position: reliability of panoramic radiography. J Oral Maxillofac Surg. 2007;65(7):1303–8.
15. Maegawa H, Sano K, Kitagawa Y, Ogasawara T, Miyauchi S, Sekine J, et al. Preoperative assessment of the relationship between the mandibular third molar and the mandibular canal by axial computed tomography with coronal and sagittal reconstruction. Oral Surg, Oral Med, Oral Pathol, Oral Radiol Endodontol. 2003;96(5):639–46.
16. Ghaeminia H, Meijer GJ, Soehardi A, Borstlap WA, Mulder J, Berge SJ. Position of the impacted third molar in relation to the mandibular canal. Diagnostic accuracy of cone beam computed tomography compared with panoramic radiography. Int J Oral Maxillofac Surg. 2009;38(9):964–71.
17. Ohman A, Kivijarvi K, Blomback U, Flygare L. Pre-operative radiographic evaluation of lower third molars with computed tomography. Dentomaxillofac Radiol. 2006;35(1):30–5.
18. Nakayama K, Nonoyama M, Takaki Y, Kagawa T, Yuasa K, Izumi K, et al. Assessment of the relationship between impacted mandibular third molars and inferior alveolar nerve with dental 3-dimensional computed tomography. J Oral Maxillofac Surg. 2009;67(12):2587–91.
19. Byun B-R, Kim Y-I, Yamaguchi T, Maki K, Ko C-C, Hwang D-S, et al. Quantitative skeletal maturation estimation using cone-beam computed tomography-generated cervical vertebral images: a pilot study in 5-to 18-year-old Japanese children. Clin Oral Investig. 2015;19(8):2133–40.
20. Zhao D, Chen X, Yue L, Liu W, Mo A, Yu H, et al. Assessment of residual alveolar bone volume in hemodialysis patients using CBCT. Clin Oral Investig. 2015;9(7):1619–24.
21. Jaju PP, Jaju SP. Clinical utility of dental cone-beam computed tomography: current perspectives. Clin Cosmet Investig Dent. 2014;6:29-43.
22. Chang H-W, Huang H-L, Yu J-H, Hsu J-T, Li Y-F, Wu Y-F. Effects of orthodontic tooth movement on alveolar bone density. Clin Oral Investig. 2012;16(3):679–88.
23. Hsu J-T, Chang H-W, Huang H-L, Yu J-H, Li Y-F, Tu M-G. Bone density changes around teeth during orthodontic treatment. Clin Oral Investig. 2011;15(4):511–9.
24. Hsu J-T, Chen Y-J, Ho J-T, Huang H-L, Wang S-P, Cheng F-C, et al. A comparison of micro-CT and dental CT in assessing cortical bone morphology and trabecular bone microarchitecture. 2014;9(9):e107545.
25. Hsu J-T, Wang S-P, Huang H-L, Chen Y-J, Wu J, Tsai M-T. The assessment of trabecular bone parameters and cortical bone strength: A comparison of micro-CT and dental cone-beam CT. J Biomech. 2013;46(15):2611–8.
26. Tantanapornkul W, Okouchi K, Fujiwara Y, Yamashiro M, Maruoka Y, Ohbayashi N, et al. A comparative study of cone-beam computed tomography and conventional panoramic radiography in assessing the topographic relationship between the mandibular canal and impacted third molars. Oral Surg Oral Med Oral Pathol Oral Radiol Endod. 2007;103(2):253–9.
27. Ueda M, Nakamori K, Shiratori K, Igarashi T, Sasaki T, Anbo N, et al. Clinical significance of computed tomographic assessment and anatomic features of the inferior alveolar canal as risk factors for injury of the inferior alveolar nerve at third molar surgery. J Oral Maxillofac Surg. 2012;70(3):514–20.
28. de Melo Albert DG, Gomes AC, do Egito Vasconcelos BC, de Oliveirae Silva ED, Holanda GZ. Comparison of orthopantomographs and conventional tomography images for assessing the relationship between impacted lower third molars and the mandibular canal. J Oral Maxillofac Surg. 2006;64(7):1030–7.
29. Sato H, Kawamura A, Yamaguchi M, Kasai K. Relationship between masticatory function and internal structure of the mandible based on computed tomography findings. Am J Orthod Dentofacial Orthop. 2005;128(6):766–73.
30. Miller CS, Nummikoski PV, Barnett DA, Langlais RP. Cross-sectional tomography. A diagnostic technique for determining the buccolingual relationship of impacted mandibular third molars and the inferior alveolar neurovascular bundle. Oral Surg Oral Med Oral Pathol. 1990;70(6):791–7.

Permissions

All chapters in this book were first published in MI, by BioMed Central; hereby published with permission under the Creative Commons Attribution License or equivalent. Every chapter published in this book has been scrutinized by our experts. Their significance has been extensively debated. The topics covered herein carry significant findings which will fuel the growth of the discipline. They may even be implemented as practical applications or may be referred to as a beginning point for another development.

The contributors of this book come from diverse backgrounds, making this book a truly international effort. This book will bring forth new frontiers with its revolutionizing research information and detailed analysis of the nascent developments around the world.

We would like to thank all the contributing authors for lending their expertise to make the book truly unique. They have played a crucial role in the development of this book. Without their invaluable contributions this book wouldn't have been possible. They have made vital efforts to compile up to date information on the varied aspects of this subject to make this book a valuable addition to the collection of many professionals and students.

This book was conceptualized with the vision of imparting up-to-date information and advanced data in this field. To ensure the same, a matchless editorial board was set up. Every individual on the board went through rigorous rounds of assessment to prove their worth. After which they invested a large part of their time researching and compiling the most relevant data for our readers.

The editorial board has been involved in producing this book since its inception. They have spent rigorous hours researching and exploring the diverse topics which have resulted in the successful publishing of this book. They have passed on their knowledge of decades through this book. To expedite this challenging task, the publisher supported the team at every step. A small team of assistant editors was also appointed to further simplify the editing procedure and attain best results for the readers.

Apart from the editorial board, the designing team has also invested a significant amount of their time in understanding the subject and creating the most relevant covers. They scrutinized every image to scout for the most suitable representation of the subject and create an appropriate cover for the book.

The publishing team has been an ardent support to the editorial, designing and production team. Their endless efforts to recruit the best for this project, has resulted in the accomplishment of this book. They are a veteran in the field of academics and their pool of knowledge is as vast as their experience in printing. Their expertise and guidance has proved useful at every step. Their uncompromising quality standards have made this book an exceptional effort. Their encouragement from time to time has been an inspiration for everyone.

The publisher and the editorial board hope that this book will prove to be a valuable piece of knowledge for researchers, students, practitioners and scholars across the globe.

List of Contributors

Pernilla Sahlstrand-Johnson and Magnus Jannert
Department of Oto-Rhino-Laryngology, Faculty of Medicine, Lund University, Skåne University Hospital, Malmö, Sweden

Anita Strömbeck and Kasim Abul-Kasim
Division of Neuroradiology, Diagnostic Centre for Imaging and Functional Medicine, Faculty of Medicine, Lund University, Skåne University Hospital, Malmö, Sweden

Jon Holm
Division of Medical Physics, Karolinska University Hospital, Huddinge, Stockholm 14186, Sweden

Louiza Loizou, Nils Albiin, Nikolaos Kartalis and Bertil Leidner
Department of Clinical Science, Intervention and Technology (CLINTEC), Karolinska Institutet, 17177 Stockholm, Sweden

Louiza Loizou, Nils Albiin, Nikolaos Kartalis and Bertil Leidner
Department of Radiology, Karolinska University Hospital, Huddinge, 14186 Stockholm, Sweden

Anders Sundin
Department of Radiology, Karolinska University Hospital, Solna, 17176 Stockholm, Sweden

Anders Sundin
Department of Molecular Medicine and Surgery, Karolinska Institutet, Stockholm 17176 Sweden

Huijuan Xiao, Hongna Tan, Pan Liang, Bo Wang, Lei Su, Suya Wang and Jianbo Gao
The Department of Radiology, The First Affiliated Hospital of Zhengzhou University, No.1, East Jianshe Road, Zhengzhou, Henan Province 450052, China

Yihe Liu
The No.7 People's Hospital of Zhengzhou, 17 Jingnan 5th Road, Zhengzhou Economic and Technological Development Zone, Zhengzhou, Henan Province 450000, China

Yasutaka Ichikawa, Kakuya Kitagawa, Naoki Nagasawa, Shuichi Murashima and Hajime Sakuma
Department of Radiology, Mie University Hospital, 2-174 Edobashi, Tsu, Mie 514-8507, Japan

Thorsten Jentzsch, James Geiger, Samy Bouaicha, Ksenija Slankamenac and Clément ML Werner
Division of Trauma Surgery, Department of Surgery, University Hospital Zuerich, Zuerich, Switzerland

Thi Dan Linh Nguyen-Kim
Institute of Diagnostic and Interventional Radiology, University Hospital Zuerich, Zuerich, Switzerland

John Fleming, Joy Conway and Michael Bennett
National Institute of Health Research Biomedical Research Unit in Respiratory Disease, University Hospital Southampton NHS Foundation Trust, Southampton, UK

John Fleming
Department of Medical Physics and Bioengineering, University Hospital Southampton NHS Foundation Trust, Southampton, UK

Joy Conway
Faculty of Health Sciences, University of Southampton, Southampton, UK

Georges Caillibotte, Spyridon Montesantos, Caroline Majoral, Ira Katz and John Fleming
Medical R&D, Air Liquide Santé International, Centre de Recherche Claude-Delorme, Les Loges-en-Josas, France

Ira Katz
Department of Mechanical Engineering, Lafayette College, Easton, PA, USA

John Fleming
Department of Nuclear Medicine, Southampton General Hospital, Mail Point 26, Southampton SO166YD, UK

David S Wack
The University at Buffalo, State University of New York, Buffalo, NY, USA

Kenneth V Snyder and Adnan H Siddiqui
Dept. of Neurosurgery and Toshiba Stroke and Vascular Research Center, The University at Buffalo, State University of New York, Buffalo, NY, USA

Kevin F Seals
School of Medicine, The University at Buffalo, State University of New York, Buffalo, NY, USA

Tobias Penzkofer, Eva Donandt, Peter Isfort, Christiane K Kuhl, Andreas H Mahnken and Philipp Bruners
Department of Diagnostic and Interventional Radiology, Aachen University Hospital, RWTH Aachen University, Pauwelsstr. 30, 52074 Aachen, Germany

Tobias Penzkofer
Surgical Planning Laboratory, Department of Radiology, Brigham and Women's Hospital, 75 Francis Street, 02115 Boston, USA

Philipp Bruners Andreas H Mahnken, Peter Isfort and Tobias Penzkofer
Applied Medical Engineering, Helmholtz-Institute Aachen, RWTH Aachen University, Pauwelsstr. 20, 52074 Aachen, Germany

Thomas Allmendinger
Siemens Healthcare, CT Division, Forchheim, Germany

Andreas H Mahnken
Department of Diagnostic and Interventional Radiology, University Hospital Marburg, Philipps University of Marburg, Marburg, Germany

Shoaleh Shahidi
Biomaterial Research Center, Department of Oral and Maxillofacial Radiology, School of Dentistry, Shiraz University of Medical Sciences, Shiraz, Iran

Ehsan Bahrampour
Department of Oral and Maxillofacial Radiology, School of Dentistry, Shiraz University of Medical Sciences, Shiraz, Iran

Elham Soltanimehr
Department of Pediatric Dentistry, School of Dentistry, Shiraz University of Medical Sciences, Shiraz, Iran

Alireza Mehdizadeh and Ali Zamani
Medical Physics and Medical Engineering Department, School of Medicine, Shiraz University of Medical Sciences, Shiraz, Iran

Morteza Oshagh
Private Practice,Tehran, Iran

Marzieh Moattari
Faculty of Nursing and Midwifery, Shiraz University of Medical Sciences, Shiraz, Iran

Michael Behnes, Ibrahim Akin, Benjamin Sartorius, Christian Fastner, Ibrahim El-Battrawy and Martin Borggrefe
First Department of Medicine, University Medical Center Mannheim, Faculty of Medicine Mannheim, University of Heidelberg, Theodor-Kutzer-Ufer 1-3, 68167 Mannheim, Germany

Holger Haubenreisser, Stefan O. Schoenberg, Thomas Henzler and Mathias Meyer
Institute of Clinical Radiology and Nuclear Medicine, University Medical Center Mannheim, Faculty of Medicine Mannheim, University of Heidelberg, Theodor-Kutzer-Ufer 1-3, 68167 Mannheim, Germany

Joost J. A. de Jong and Joop P. W. van den Bergh
NUTRIM School for Nutrition and Translational Research in Metabolism, Maastricht University, Maastricht, The Netherlands

Piet P. Geusens, Joop P. W. van den Bergh and Joost J. A. de Jong
Department of Rheumatology, Maastricht University Medical Center, Maastricht, The Netherlands

Arno Lataster
Department of Anatomy and Embryology, Maastricht University, Maastricht, The Netherlands

Bert van Rietbergen and Jacobus J. Arts
Faculty of Biomedical Engineering, Eindhoven University of Technology, Eindhoven, The Netherlands

Paul C. Willems and Jacobus J. Arts
Department of Orthopedic Surgery, Maastricht University Medical Center, Maastricht, The Netherlands

Paul C. Willems, Piet P. Geusens and Jacobus J. Arts
CAPHRI School for Public Health and Primary Care, Maastricht University, Maastricht, The Netherlands

Piet P. Geusens and Joop P. W. van den Bergh
Faculty of Medicine and Life Sciences, Hasselt University, Hasselt, Belgium

Joop P. W. van den Bergh
Department of Internal Medicine, VieCuri Medical Center, Venlo, The Netherlands

Taro Yanagawa, Sachiko Takamizawa and Makoto Taniguchi
Department of Neurosurgery, Tokyo Metropolitan Neurological Hospital, 2-6-1 Musashidai, Fuchu 1830042, Japan

Hirokazu Iwamuro
Department of Research and Therapeutics for Movement Disorders, Juntendo University Graduate School of Medicine, 2-1-1 Hongo, Bunkyo-ku, Tokyo 1138421, Japan

Petr Martynov, Nikolai Mitropolskii, Katri Kukkola, and Anssi Mäkynen
Optoelectronics and Measurement Techniques Unit, University of Oulu, Finland

Ilkka Lindgren and Monika Gretsch
Department of Radiology, Oulu University Hospital, 90029 Oulu, Finland

Vesa-Matti Koivisto
Department of Radiology, Lapland Hospital District, 96101 Rovaniemi, Finland

Jani Saunavaara
Medical Imaging Centre of Southwest Finland, Turku University Hospital, 20521 Turku, Finland

Jarmo Reponen
Finntelemedicum, Research Unit of Medical Imaging, Physics and Technology, University of Oulu; Department of Radiology, Hospital of Raahe, PL 25, 92101 Raahe, Finland

Chang-Mo Nam, Kyong Joon Lee, Yousun Ko, Kil Joong Kim and Kyoung Ho Lee
Department of Radiology, Seoul National University Bundang Hospital, Seoul National University College of Medicine, 82 Gumi-ro 173 Beon-gil, Bundang-gu, Seongnam-si, Gyeonggi-do 13620, Korea

Bohyoung Kim
Division of Biomedical Engineering, Hankuk University of Foreign Studies, Oedae-ro 81, Mohyeon-myeon, Cheoin-gu, Yongin-si, Gyeonggi-do 17035, Korea

Giasemi Koutouzi, Monika Danielak-Nowak, Henrik Leonhardt and Mårten Falkenberg
Department of Radiology, Institute of Clinical Sciences, Sahlgrenska Academy, Gothenburg, Sweden

Behrooz Nasihatkton
K. N. Toosi University of Technology, Tehran, Iran

Fredrik Kahl
Department of Electrical Engineering, Chalmers University of Technology, Gothenburg, Sweden

Fredrik Kahl
Center for Mathematical Sciences, Lund University, Lund, Sweden

Tingting Liu, Hetao Cao and Dongmei Hou
Department of Medical Imaging, Affiliated Hospital of Nantong University, Shi, Jiangsu Sheng, Nantong 226001, China

Jianpeng Ma
Department of Magnetic Resonance Imaging, Dingbian County People's Hospital, Dingbian, Yulin 718600, Shaanxi, China

Lin Xu
Department of Radiology, PLA general hospital, No.28 Fuxing Road, Haidian District, Beijing 100000, China

Sören Strandberg, Marie-Louise Wretling and Adel Shalabi
Department of Radiology, Karolinska University Hospital, Karolinska Institutet, Stockholm, Sweden

Torsten Wredmark
Department of Orthopaedic Surgery, Karolinska University Hospital, Karolinska Institutet, Stockholm, Sweden

Abbas Aroua, Eleni-Theano Samara, François O Bochud and Francis R Verdun
Institute of Radiation Physics, Lausanne University Hospital, Lausanne, Switzerland

Reto Meuli
Department of Diagnostic and Interventional Radiology, Lausanne University Hospital, Lausanne, Switzerland

Kristina Imeen Ringe, Christian von Falck, Hoen-oh Shin and Frank Wacker
Department of Diagnostic and Interventional Radiology, Hannover Medical School, Carl-Neuberg Str. 1, 30625, Hannover, Germany

Bastian Paul Ringe
Department of General, Visceral and Transplantation Surgery, Hannover Medical School, Carl-Neuberg Str.1, 30625, Hannover, Germany

Thomas Becker
Department of General and Thoracic Surgery, University Hospital Schleswig-Holstein, Arnold-Heller Str.1, 24105, Kiel, Germany

Eva-Doreen Pfister
Department of Pediatric Gastroenterology and Hepatology, Hannover Medical School, Carl-Neuberg Str. 1, 30625, Hannover, Germany

Burckhardt Ringe
Drexel University, College of Medicine, 216 N Broad Street, Philadelphia, PA 19102, USA

Joshua Tambe and Boniface Moifo
Department of Radiology and Radiation Oncology, University of Yaounde 1, Yaounde, Cameroon

Emmanuel Fongang, Emilienne Guegang and Alain Georges Juimo
Yaounde General Hospital, Yaounde, Cameroon

Robert D Prins, Raymond H Thornton, C Ross Schmidtlein, Brian Quinn, Hung Ching and Lawrence T Dauer
Department of Medical Physics, Memorial Sloan-Kettering Cancer Center, 1275 York Ave. New York, NY 10021, USA

Robert D Prins
Department of Environmental Health Sciences, Mailman School of Public Health, Columbia University, 722 West 168th Street, New York, NY 10032, USA

Ke-Zeng Li, Ru Zhang, Yuan-Yuan Tian and Tao Hu DDS
State Key Laboratory of Oral Diseases, Departments of Operative Dentistry and Endodontics, West China School of Stomatology, Sichuan University, Chengdu, P.R. China

Bin Guo
Institute of Stomatology of Chinese PLA General Hospital, Beijing, P.R. China

Wei-Quan Wang
School of Dentistry, College of Medicine, China Medical University, 91 Hsueh-Shih Road, Taichung 40402, Taiwan

Hu Wang
Department of Radiology, West China School of Stomatology, Sichuan University, Chengdu, China

Xuan Yu
Department of Stomatology, Yinzhou People's Hospital, Ningbo, Zhejiang, P.R.China

Lih-Jyh Fuh and Michael Y. C. Chen
Department of Dentistry, China Medical University and Hospital, Taichung 404, Taiwan
School of Dentistry, College of Medicine, China Medical University, 91 Hsueh-Shih Road, Taichung 40402, Taiwan

Jui-Ting Hsu and Heng-Li Huang
Department of Bioinformatics and Medical Engineering, Asia University, Taichung 413, Taiwan
School of Dentistry, College of Medicine, China Medical University, 91 Hsueh-Shih Road, Taichung 40402, Taiwan

Ming-Tzu Tsai
Department of Biomedical Engineering, Hungkuang University, Taichung 433, Taiwan

Index

www.ingramcontent.com/pod-product-compliance
Lightning Source LLC
Chambersburg PA
CBHW082017190326
41458CB00010B/3215